G000167758

RECENT ADVANCES IN HEMATOLOGY RESEARCH

QUALITY MANAGEMENT IN TRANSFUSION MEDICINE

Recent Advances in Hematology Research

Additional books in this series can be found on Nova's website under the Series tab.

Additional e-books in this series can be found on Nova's website under the e-book tab.

Public Health in the 21ST Century

Additional books in this series can be found on Nova's website under the Series tab.

Additional e-books in this series can be found on Nova's website under the e-book tab.

RECENT ADVANCES IN HEMATOLOGY RESEARCH

QUALITY MANAGEMENT IN TRANSFUSION MEDICINE

CEES TH. SMIT SIBINGA
EDITOR

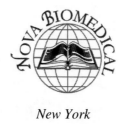

New York

Copyright © 2013 by Nova Science Publishers, Inc.

All rights reserved. No part of this book may be reproduced, stored in a retrieval system or transmitted in any form or by any means: electronic, electrostatic, magnetic, tape, mechanical photocopying, recording or otherwise without the written permission of the Publisher.

For permission to use material from this book please contact us:
Telephone 631-231-7269; Fax 631-231-8175
Web Site: http://www.novapublishers.com

NOTICE TO THE READER

The Publisher has taken reasonable care in the preparation of this book, but makes no expressed or implied warranty of any kind and assumes no responsibility for any errors or omissions. No liability is assumed for incidental or consequential damages in connection with or arising out of information contained in this book. The Publisher shall not be liable for any special, consequential, or exemplary damages resulting, in whole or in part, from the readers' use of, or reliance upon, this material. Any parts of this book based on government reports are so indicated and copyright is claimed for those parts to the extent applicable to compilations of such works.

Independent verification should be sought for any data, advice or recommendations contained in this book. In addition, no responsibility is assumed by the publisher for any injury and/or damage to persons or property arising from any methods, products, instructions, ideas or otherwise contained in this publication.

This publication is designed to provide accurate and authoritative information with regard to the subject matter covered herein. It is sold with the clear understanding that the Publisher is not engaged in rendering legal or any other professional services. If legal or any other expert assistance is required, the services of a competent person should be sought. FROM A DECLARATION OF PARTICIPANTS JOINTLY ADOPTED BY A COMMITTEE OF THE AMERICAN BAR ASSOCIATION AND A COMMITTEE OF PUBLISHERS.

Additional color graphics may be available in the e-book version of this book.

Library of Congress Cataloging-in-Publication Data

ISBN: 978-1-62618-665-1

Library of Congress Control Number: 2013936633

Published by Nova Science Publishers, Inc. † *New York*

Contents

Preface

Quality has so many terms, from quality assurance, quality systems, quality control and a multitude of others, especially in the many various dialects and languages.

However, there are commonalities as quality relates intimately to life – personal or private, social or environment and professional. Quality is essential in all aspects of daily life, 24 hours a day, every day of the year, without exception.

Standards must be set and the effects monitored and evaluated if the desired and expected behaviour changes and benefits in the quality of life are to be attained. Humans are prone to err, but are often reluctant to recognise or accept error and the deviations from set norms and standards. Keeping an open mind is the first step to learning what has erred or deviated. This step is important in leading to corrective actions and above all prevention of reoccurrence. To master these situations the collection of evidence through documentation is paramount, a *conditio sine qua non.*

Over time the environment and conditions of life, whether personal, social or professional will inevitably change. As a consequence these changes should be recognised, standards adjusted and novel technologies and methodologies developed, which will allow quality to grow with the changes. That requires an attitude or culture that reaches beyond the narrow boundaries of regular routine life and environment. Change is often experienced as endangering and full of risk – the threat of the unknown, the darkness outside lighted houses and shelters. To overcome and continue the journey of improvement, leadership is needed at all levels in life.

Quality is not for sale, it has to be created and carefully maintained. That can be achieved individually, but also group or team wise – family and friends, peers and colleagues, in sports and culture, as well as in a vocation and professional environment. Quality is mutual and is best experienced in an intimate relationship – giving or provision and reception or acceptance as suppliers and customers of whatever is used and needed in life from cradle to grave.

Transfusion Medicine is one of the younger disciplines in the medical sciences and practices, but has come a long way to being developed recognized and appreciated for its beneficiary contribution to life – moral and ethical, in society as part of human solidarity and in medicine through its important supportive role in treatment and prevention of morbidity and mortality. However, like in many other aspects of human life, there are also 'hidden devils' that may strike and cause serious harm, even take life if not observed and attended.

To secure the prevention of the often unexpected striking of these devils, quality as a well managed structure and system in life is needed – personal attitude and a continuous alertness, the commitment to observe, communicate and report what went well but more importantly what deviated and went wrong are paramount to guarantee quality of life. When these unexpected deviations occur, they can be identified and corrective actions taken.

Quality is often seen as something expensive to create and maintain. The opposite is true, as quality improves life, prevents unnecessary costs and allows efficacy, consistency and safety.

This publication provides a broad array of almost all of these aspects and principles as applicable to Transfusion Medicine, the bridging science between the healthy community and those who, unfortunately by birth or during life, experience an imbalance of the physical quality of life with a dependence on the support with some of the 'elixer of life', human blood.

The 14 chapters have been written by experts in the field from all over the world and from disciplines and sciences that all are of importance for the development and continuation of quality as a culture, an on-going journey of which the destination is infinity.

Cees Th. Smit Sibinga
Professor of International Development of Transfusion Medicine (IDTM),
University of Groningen, NL

November 2012.

Foreword

Transfusion Medicine has evolved rapidly from an intervention mainly perceived as a laboratory prepared product to save life, usually in dramatic circumstances due to trauma and excessive blood loss, as in complications resulting from conflict, pregnancy and surgery, to the recognition that blood and blood products for clinical use must meet the highest standards of safety and efficacy.

The word quality began its journey as the understanding of a laboratory quality control measurement. However, as the clinical practice of blood transfusion evolved through the discovery that transfusion can transmit infectious agents and can also the cause harm to the recipient. Clinicians, scientists and regulators recognised the importance to fully understand, define and implement quality in all facets of transfusion medicine.

In the latter part of the 20th Century quality in clinical transfusion assumed the recognition and importance, which had been long overdue. International and regional organisations responsible for health policies, regulations and recommendations prioritised quality as the key to safety in transfusion medicine. The World Health Organisation (WHO) joined with other leading authorities by prioritising quality in transfusion medicine and in 2000 Blood Transfusion Safety was decreed one of WHO's seven priorities of work.

Quality of blood services was defined by WHO, in 1993, as: *"The consistent and reliable performance of services or products in conformity with specified standards"*.

This definition means that the "products" are blood and blood components and plasma derived products, which are both safe and effective for clinical transfusion, or other specified uses and that a quality based approach in all procedures ensures maximum safety for recipients, donors and staff, and results in maximum clinical effectiveness.

This publication benefits from the collective and invaluable experience of authors, many of whom have had extensive knowledge and involvement in all aspects of transfusion medicine. They have taken part in defining, developing and implementing quality management systems in developed and developing countries. This experience results from decades of work as leaders in national transfusion services, regulatory authorities. Many have participated as members of committees and in an advisory capacity to WHO and other recognised international authorities on the subject.

This publication is unique in many aspects as it provides an insight into quality management by bringing together the expertise and collective experience of internationally recognised experts from a range of related professions and backgrounds, including those from medical, scientific, quality management, organisational management, pharmaco-economics, medical sociology, international funding management and regulatory authority experts.

Each chapter provides an insight into different aspects and experiences in quality management and contains practical and current issues in quality management. There are many instances where the information provided is of a practical and instructive nature, from which the reader will be able to harness examples, ideas and advice.

The editor and authors have endeavoured to provide chapters, which are interesting and practical. Readers, particularly in economically restricted environments, both in developed and developing environments will find the information provided both helpful and useful.

Dr Jean C Emmanuel MD; MCPCP

In: Quality Management in Transfusion Medicine
Editor: Cees Th. Smit Sibinga

ISBN: 978-1-62618-665-1
© 2013 Nova Science Publishers, Inc.

Chapter I

History of Quality Management in Transfusion Medicine

John R. Hess[1,], Cees Th. Smit Sibinga[2,†] and Paul D. Mintz[3,‡]*

[1] U. of Maryland School of Medicine,
Baltimore, MD, US
[2] ID Consulting for International Development of
Transfusion Medicine (IDTM), University of Groningen,
AE Zuidhorn, NL
[3] Division of Hematology,
Office of Blood Research and Review,
CBER, FDA, Rockville, MD, US

Abstract

The development of Transfusion Medicine has come with many advances. It has not been until the second half of the 20th century, that Quality Management has received more focused attention together with the development of vein-to-vein responsibility. Outbreaks of diseases transmissible through blood triggered this development from a purely product and procedure orientation into a process and system orientation with the recognition of quality system essentials and haemovigilance.

This first chapter depicts the key moments in the developments, describes how the developments took place and illustrates how in different parts of the world initiatives to contain quality and safety were born and developed.

Keywords: Blood safety, process improvement, national blood program development, standards, statistical control, haemovigilance

* Tel: +1-301-706-6865. E-mail: JHESS@umm.edu.
† Tel: +31-6-2223.4325. E-mail: c.sibinga@planet.nl.
‡ Tel: +1-240.447.2308. E-mail: pdmintz@gmail.com.

1. The Early Days

Quality management of blood transfusion is as old as transfusion itself. On June 15, 1667, Jean-Baptiste Denis, a physician, (with the assistance of Paul Emmerez, a surgeon), performed the first recorded transfusion of blood to a human. Denis chose a lamb as the donor reasoning that animal blood had fewer impurities than human blood, as animals were not subject to "*all the passions that trouble the life of man and corrupt the whole substance of the blood*". [1a] In this procedure, a sixteen year-old boy with recurrent fevers was transfused an unspecified amount of blood. He had a strong sensation of heat in the arm receiving the blood but had no other ill effects. Shortly thereafter, Denis performed a second transfusion from a lamb to a healthy male who also noted a feeling of heat at the infusion site, but who had no other adverse reactions.

Blood had long been associated with vitality in human cultures. The Egyptians rubbed heads with oil containing blood to treat graying hair and baldness. [1a] They also employed blood baths for resuscitation and recuperation. The Greeks believed blood the most important of the four humours. The Romans are reported to have entered the gladiatorial arena to drink the blood of the dying as a method of generating courage.

The physiologic basis for the pioneering work of Denis was described in 1628 when William Harvey, an English physician, published that blood circulates and is pumped by the heart. The ability of vascular infusion to modify behavior was demonstrated in 1656 when Christopher Wren injected wine and ale into the veins of a dog inducing noticeable drunkenness. In 1665, Richard Lower performed dog-to-dog transfusions in England creating a model for Denis. At this time, Lower and other English investigators were contemplating animal to human transfusion and saw themselves in competition with Denis. Several distinguished members of the English Royal Society approached the physician-director of the Bedlam asylum and asked him to procure a patient to be transfused with animal blood. He refused to do so, thus setting an early example of prospective transfusion review. Subsequently, in November 1667, the same investigators persuaded a man to receive a transfusion from a lamb in return for monetary payment. An estimated ten ounces of blood was transfused.

Several hours after the transfusion, the subject developed a fever and profuse sweating lasting through the night, but he was well thereafter. The following month the experiment was repeated on the same subject with the same transient reaction. The subject declined a third transfusion, unless he should be transformed entirely into a sheep "*without as well as within*". [1b] Subject autonomy prevailed and no further transfusion was performed.

In December 1667, Denis transfused his third human subject with lamb's blood on two occasions a few days apart. During the second transfusion, the subject felt heat in the arm receiving the transfusion and shortly thereafter developed what we now know was a hemolytic transfusion reaction manifested by fever, nausea, diarrhea, a nosebleed, and "*black urine*". He apparently made a full recovery from the transfusion reaction but died suddenly and, at first inexplicably, fewer than two months later. Denis stated that his widow approached him and tried to extort money so that she wouldn't report that the transfusions had led to her husband's death. A judicial inquiry in April 1668 resulted in his widow being convicted of poisoning her husband with arsenic. Denis was exonerated of any wrongdoing. However, the judge's verdict included the stipulation that "*no transfusion should be made upon any human body but by the approbation of the physicians of the Parisian Faculty (of Medicine).*" This conservative faculty at the Sorbonne had long opposed Denis' experiments, and this court order directing prospective utilization review of all transfusions had the immediate effect of stopping all human transfusion activity. In December, 1669 the French parliament upheld the court's edict. This action was followed by a proclamation from the Roman Catholic Pope who suggested transfusion was satanic and cannibalistic. No further human transfusions are known to have been performed for the next 150 years.

James Blundell revived the study of transfusion in animals and performed the first human to human transfusion in 1818 (Figure 1).

He published a description of the unsuccessful attempt the following year. [2] Ten years later, he had performed 10 transfusions, five successful, and wrote a description of his technique and a discussion of considerations to improve the safety and effectiveness of transfusion. [3] His efforts to improve transfusion quality centred on the observation that blood exposed to the air clotted quickly, and his solutions were to work "expediently" and use a device of his invention, the Gravitator, which reduced the exposure of blood to air. The majority of his second paper is a step by step description of his procedure for using the device and explanations of why he though the steps in the procedure were important. His injunction to work expediently persists in the modern rule that a unit of whole blood should be collected in 6-10 minutes to limit clotting in the collection line as does the use of a gravity-fed fluid column to prevent air embolism. Blundell's injunction to watch the patient and stop the transfusion if any of a number of signs occurs is especially important. His clearly described step-by-step procedure and discussion of the consequences of changing the procedure have a decidedly modern feel.

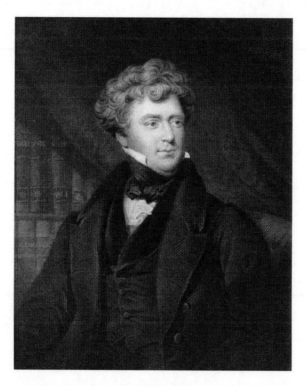

Figure 1. The Scottish Obstetrician Dr. James Blundell (1791 – 1878).

Fifty years later, Chadwick reviewed the scientific and technical status of transfusion for the Massachusetts Medical Society. [4] Despite a thoughtful discussion of the indications for and methods of transfusion, his belief that animal to human transfusion was safe and his cavalier approach to patient symptoms during transfusion and to basic cleanliness in blood handling clearly date his work. As safe forms of intravenous fluids such as Ringer's and Locke's solutions became available at the end of the 19th century, the reputation of transfusion and transfusionists sank very low.

2. The 20th Century Onset – Impact of WWI and WWII

At the beginning of the 20th century, transfusion was limited scientifically by a lack of understanding of transfusion reactions and infections and technically by the lack of reliable equipment and methods to anticoagulate blood. Scientific and technical progress over the next two decades, led by Karl Landsteiner's discovery of the ABO blood group system reversed most of this decline (Figure 2).

Once the ABO system had been identified, Ottenberg and Kaliski showed that ABO cross matching could prevent major acute transfusion reactions, Roger Lee showed that group 'O' was universal donor, and Peyton Rous showed that haemaglutination matching was as good as haemolysin matching, less cumbersome, and faster. [5-7] Roger Lee (Figure 3a) also demonstrated that citrate was an excellent anticoagulant for human blood, Richard Lewisohn experimentally determined the safe dose of citrate, and Rous and Turner used citrate and glucose to store rabbit red cells for 4 weeks.

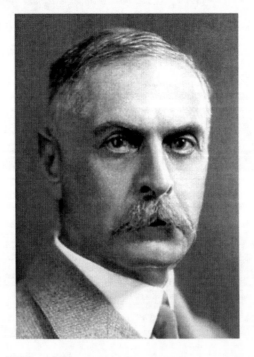

Figure 2. Karl Landsteiner (1868 – 1943).

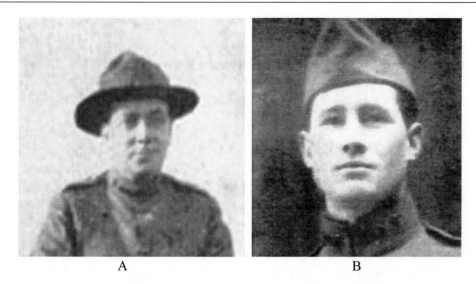

Figure 3. A and B – Harvard professor A) Roger I. Lee oversaw the development of the world's first blood bank by B) Oswald H Robertson while serving on the Western Front in World War I. Lee insured appropriate attention to blood typing, infectious disease testing, and bacteriologic safety. Robertson designed blood collection bottles and demonstrated the safety and efficacy of 26 day red cell storage.

Learning from all of these advances, Oswald Robertson, who had worked with Roger Lee as a medical student at Harvard (Figure 3b) and with Peyton Rous as a post-doctoral researcher at the Rockefeller Institute in 1916, went back to Harvard in 1917 and joined Lee when the Harvard Medical Unit went to France in World War I. [11] In France, Robertson built the world's first blood bank, storing Lee's universal donor whole blood in citrate in transfusion bottles of his own design, resuscitating wounded soldiers triaged as too deeply in shock to benefit from surgery and saving their lives. Robertson also stored red cells for longer periods in Rous-Turner solution, but a committee of his fellow medical officers voted that this was dangerous because of the risk of bacterial contamination. [12] As a result the standard became 5-day storage in citrate only.

Approximately 30,000 transfusions were performed in 1918, the final year of World War I, but with the end of the war, the 24-hour-a-day surgical care associated with the forward Casualty Clearing Stations and the farther back Base Station Hospitals disappeared and so did routine transfusion. Nevertheless, the British Army declared transfusion to be the most important medical advance of the War [13].

Advances in quality control had made the initial development and rapid proliferation of blood banking possible. To a remarkable degree, they were driven by the organization in which Robertson served, the United States Army. The U.S. Army had contracted the first manufacture of rifles or any form of machinery with interchangeable parts. Interchangeable parts required standards and tracking with 'serial' numbers to see which ones worked and which ones did not. By the time of the U.S. Civil War, Major Jonathan Letterman had extended interchangeability to standards for the training and practice of surgeons, operating field ambulances, and hospital sanitation generally. [14, 15] As medical knowledge grew, Major John Shaw Billings assembled the Army Medical Library and wrote the Index Medicus of all scientific medical publications, the forerunners of the U.S. National Library of Medicine and PubMed, and he built the Army Medical Museum and designed the Johns

Hopkins Hospital. [16] Major George Sternberg discovered the *Pneumococcus*, confirmed the microscopic blood parasite that caused malaria, and wrote his Manual of Bacteriology, the first textbook of the new science. [17] As Surgeon General Sternberg, he sent Major Walter Reed to discover the routes of transmission of typhoid and yellow fever. Major William Gorgas used Reed's findings to control yellow fever in Panama, allowing the building of the Panama Canal. [18]

When Gorgas became Surgeon General of the Army in early 1914 he worked out the arrangement with Harvey Cushing at Harvard and the American Red Cross to recruit the Harvard Medical Unit in which Robertson served. After Robertson had demonstrated successful transfusion, he was transferred to the Army's central medical laboratory in France where he ran a school for transfusionists and conducted transfusion research until the end of the war [19].

Over the same period of time, mathematicians developed an interest in the role of numeric standards to inform decisions. In the 1880s, Francis Galton, the English polymath, described the 'central tendency' of biologic data and its standard deviation and popularized correlation and regression analysis. [20] In his will Galton established the first chair of mathematical statistics at Cambridge where Carl Pearson, the first professor of statistics, invented the Chi-squared test. [21] In industry, Guinness brewery supported the work of William Gosset who developed the 'student's' t-test. In government, the English agricultural research station at Rothamsted supported Robert Fisher and his development of randomized block testing and the analysis of variance. [22, 23] Industrial quality control, based on a full understanding of the meaning of the degrees of freedom in the analysis of variance as described by W. Edwards Deming, blossomed. [24] These developments meant that by the time of World War II, the basis for statistical quality control had been established (Figure 4).

As World War II approached, mathematical statistics informed the work Elmer DeGowin as he demonstrated that whole blood could be shipped on ice for long distances by plane and train without undue haemolysis. [25] Even more important, work was carried out by the New York Chapter of the American Red Cross in its 'Blood for Britain' programme, where it became clear that despite the best efforts at open sterile methods using Robertson bottles, 9.4% of units of whole blood-derived plasma collections became bacterially contaminated. Only the use of autoclaved needle sets and vacuum bottles containing 3% citrate solution prevented the high rates of contamination.

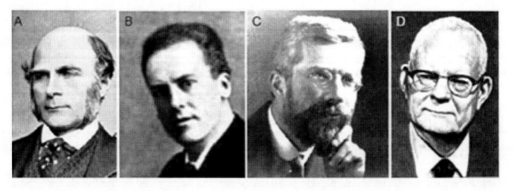

Figure 4. Individuals important in the development of statistical quality control included A) Sir Francis Galton, B) Karl Pearson, C) Sir Ronald Fisher, D) W. Edwards Deming. All contributed to our mathematical understanding of biological variability and quality control.

These findings set the stage for the most important practical advance in blood logistics of the war, the development of acid citrate dextrose (ACD) the first autoclavable whole blood storage solution and its deployment in sterile 600 mL vacuum bottles, the second standard container in blood banking. That development in turn set in motion a massive validation of the whole U.S. blood banking system, from its 25 American Red Cross regional donor centres and their 13 million collections to the ability to ship 600,000 bottles of whole blood on the floors of DC-3s across the North Atlantic to Paris and the Central Pacific to the Philippines. [26] Standards for manufactured products, arm cleaning, syphilis testing, refrigerator temperatures, and storage duration were developed and validated with bacterial testing, haemoglobinometry, and Ashby counts. By the time the war was over, DeGowin, Alsever, and Hardin could write a book on Blood Transfusion containing technical advice that was evidence-based [27].

3. The Blood Safety Crises

Appropriate indications for transfusion were recognized early as a critical safety issue as transfusion became commonplace in the developed world. In 1936, Bock emphasized that clear indications for transfusion practices should be created. [28] The following year Fantus concluded that too many transfusions were being given at Cook County Hospital in Chicago and described the development of a multidisciplinary committee to review blood transfusion practices at this hospital. [29] In 1951, the Ministry of Health in England requested reviews of blood transfusion practices, [30] and an editorial in the New England Journal of Medicine the same year called attention to inappropriate transfusion practices. [31] In 1953, the Medical Staff of Providence Hospital in Washington DC adopted in its bylaws indications for blood transfusion. [32] Also in 1953, Strauss and Torres asserted that 49 of 290 transfusions were not indicated and recommended educational programmes to improve transfusion practices. [33] Other reports in the 1950s supported these findings and underscored potential liability of physicians for adverse events from unnecessary transfusions. [34-38] In 1960, Graham-Stewart said, *"all routine dogma concerning transfusion should be abandoned and each case should be dealt with on its merits"*. [39] As noted below, in 1961 in the United States, the Joint Commission incorporated the review of transfusion practices into its accreditation process. [40] In 1962, the Joint Blood Council called for a review of transfusion practices by medical staff committee. [41] That same year, Crosby called on hospitals to create a 'transfusion board' to review transfusion practices and to educate clinicians. [42] In 1964, Walz demonstrated that a hospital transfusion committee could effectively decrease unnecessary transfusions. [43] In 1984, JAMA published an article addressing the utilization review of transfusion practices providing national prominence to this activity. [44] More recently, the development of transfusion medicine as a distinct clinical specialty and the presence of transfusion safety officers in some hospitals have contributed significantly to quality management efforts. Appropriate blood use remains one of the four fundamental objectives of the World Health Organization's Blood Safety Policy, and has proven the most difficult objective to achieve. General medical oversight of blood use turned out not to be sufficient to protect the public in a series of blood-related public health crises of the second half of the twentieth century. These crises are best remembered by the names of the underlying infectious diseases that drove them: syphilis, hepatitis-B, HIV/AIDS, hepatitis-C, and mad cow. The transmission of syphilis in fresh whole blood transfusions was a problem in the 1950s, but has largely disappeared in the developed world with the advent of testing. In part this was because testing identified contaminated units, but also because holding blood at room or refrigerator temperatures long enough for routine testing led to the death of the organism. Hepatitis B transmission occurred in at least 1 in 6 blood transfusions at the U.S. National Institutes of Health (NIH) in the 1960s, ultimately leading to the identification of the organism. [45] The elimination of paid blood donors, the testing of individual units, and a vaccine have all contributed to the reduction of this transfusion transmitted disease. HIV-AIDS was first recognized in 1981 and has spread rapidly through a number of high-risk populations to now infect some forty million people world-wide. Transmission through blood transfusion was recognized in the second year of the epidemic and led to the death of two-thirds of the world's haemophilia patients. The social consequences of the HIV-AIDS epidemic led to the restructuring of the national blood systems of Europe e.g. France, the Netherlands, the UK, and in Canada. Hepatitis-C, which was occurring in 8% of all transfused patients at the NIH during the 1970s, is being reduced by testing. But a large reservoir of infected people in the population and the lack of a vaccine means that risk will continue into the forseeable future. Mad cow disease, spread by the contamination of the ruminant food chain with animal tissue was recognized as having spread to humans in Britain in 1996 as variant Creutzfeld Jacob Disease (vCJD) and as a transfusion transmitted disease a decade later. Obtaining blood from the safest portion of the population and testing it rigorously for significant blood-borne pathogens are two more of the pillars of WHO's Safe Blood Policy. Different organizations and nations have approached these goals in different ways.

4. International Initiatives

4.1. World Health Organization

Since 1975, the World Health Organization (WHO) has been a leader in the movement to improve blood safety. Successive World Health Assembly resolutions have addressed this goal since 1975. [46] The objective of the WHO Blood Transfusion Safety (WHO/BTS) program has been to ensure universal access to safe, high-quality and efficacious blood products for transfusion, their appropriate use, and also to ensure donor safety.

In recognition of the importance of the provision of safe blood products, the Director-General established a blood safety programme in the late 1980s. In 2000, safe blood was declared an Organization-wide priority and blood safety was designated the theme of World Health Day 2000. The need for safe blood products (whole blood and plasma derived) has been stressed in several resolutions adopted by regional committees, the Executive Board and the Health Assembly. These have contributed to making the matter a high priority on national and global health agendas. WHO has been involved in setting evidence-based norms and standards for the quality and safety of blood products and in supporting their appropriate application. The WHO Secretariat initiated a major program to support the development of high-quality systems for all aspects of blood transfusion through a global quality management program. WHO has also provided guidance, support and capacity building in strengthening blood transfusion services in selected countries. This support has been through policy advice and technical guidance and support, advocacy, mentoring, technology transfer, networking, and working to assure funding.

WHO/BTS has committed to –

- supporting the development of national blood systems
- preventing the transmission of infectious agents
- building collaboration and partnerships for global blood safety and working with countries, international partners, collaborating centres, local institutions and communities
- advocating for political support and consistent resources for sustainable, nationally-led blood transfusion services
- developing scientific and evidence-based guidance on the safety, quality, availability and use of blood products
- strengthening the capacity and quality of national blood systems
- improving clinical transfusion practices

The Quality Management Project (QMP) was launched in 2000 under the auspices of World Health Day. The project addresses the need to adopt the principles of quality management in all areas of blood transfusion services and has been developed as an innovative initiative designed to build regional and national capacity in quality management for blood transfusion services throughout the world and to promote the establishment of effective quality systems in blood transfusion at all levels of the health system in member states. The QMP is coordinated at a global level by the Blood Transfusion Safety Team in the Department of Essential Health Technologies, at WHO Headquarters. At the regional level, the QMP is coordinated by WHO Regional Offices, in partnership with Regional Quality Training Centres, WHO Collaborating Centres, national blood transfusion services, international nongovernmental organizations and experts in quality and transfusion medicine. The first full Quality Management Training course was conducted through WHO EURO at the WHO Collaborating Centre in Groningen and hosted the Middle European countries from the Baltics to the Balkan. The QMP is intended to be a long-term project. The QMP aims to assist blood transfusion services and national authorities in all WHO Member States to implement effective quality systems through:

- Development of regional and national capacity in quality management
- Identification and strengthening of regional quality training centers
- Development of advocacy and training materials on quality management
- Training of facilitators
- Establishment of external quality assessment schemes
- Development of a monitoring and evaluation system for the provision of post-training support and follow-up
- Creation of effective quality networks
- Development of the Quality Management Training: facilitator's toolkit as a comprehensive set of teaching materials to support a training course for quality managers in blood transfusion services.

WHO has been an international leader for more than 35 years in bringing sustained quality management programs to transfusion services throughout the world [47].

4.2. The Council of Europe

The Council of Europe (CoE) was founded in 1949 as a non-political socio-economic organization with currently over 40 Member States. One of the founding principles is increasing cooperation between Member States to improve the quality of life. Within the context of this cooperation the CoE has consistently selected ethical problems for study, of which one of the most important so far has been the non-commercialisation of human blood, organs and tissues. The CoE is based in Strasbourg, France and has a Directorate for the Quality of Medicines and HealthCare (EDQM) that covers also the blood quality and safety issues. In the 1950 cooperation between Member States started on blood transfusion, inspired by a number of guiding principles e.g. promotion of voluntary and non-remunerated donation of blood, mutual assistance in promotion of the rights of donors and recipients, and a rational use of blood and blood components. As a first result in 1958 the European Agreements on the Exchange of Therapeutic Substances of Human Origin, the Exchange of Blood Grouping Reagents and the Exchange of Tissue-typing Reagents were adopted. Based on these three agreements, the CoE established a blood transfusion programme with the objective to ensure good quality of blood and blood components. Since then the CoE has adopted a series of Recommendations to the Member States, covering ethical, social, scientific and education aspects of blood transfusion. These Recommendations are policy statements to governments proposing a common course of action to be implemented and followed. In the field of blood transfusion the two major Recommendations are Recommendation R (88) 4 on the responsibilities of Member State Health Authorities and the Recommendation R (95) 15, which contains a technical appendix – Guidelines on the Preparation, Use and Quality Assurance of Blood Components. Work on this R (95) 15 started in 1986 with a Select Committee of Experts in Quality Assurance in Blood Transfusion Services which published the First proposals on quality assurance on blood transfusion. Based on these proposals a more comprehensive guide on blood components was published in 1995. The immediate and successful response among the Member States lead to adoption of this guide as an appendix to Recommendation No R (95) 15. [48] It was agreed that the appendix 'Guide to the Preparation, Use and Quality Assurance of Blood Components' would be regularly updated, which actually happens annually. The Guide has become an international reference to facilitate ongoing improvements on the preparation, use and quality assurance of blood components through education (courses) and recommendations.

4.3. European Union (EU)

After World War II, moves towards European integration were seen by many as an escape from the extreme forms of nationalism that had devastated the continent. One such attempt to unite Europeans was the European Coal and Steel Community, which was declared to be "*a first step in the federation of Europe*", starting with the aim of eliminating the possibility of further wars between its member states by means of pooling the national heavy industries. The founding members of the Community were Belgium, France, Italy, Luxembourg, the Netherlands, and West Germany. The originators and supporters of the Community include Jean Monet, Robert Schuman, Paul-Henri Spaak, and Alcide De Gasperi.

The European Union (EU) is an economic and political entity and confederation of 27 Member States which are located primarily in Europe. The EU traces its origins from the European Coal and Steel Community (ECSC) formed by six countries in 1951 (Belgium, France, Germany, Italy, Luxemburg and the Netherlands). In 1957, these six countries signed the Treaty of Rome, which extended the earlier cooperation within the European Coal and Steel Community (ECSC) and created the European Economic Community, (EEC) establishing a customs union. They also signed another treaty on the same day creating the European Atomic Energy Community (Euratom) for cooperation in developing nuclear energy. Both treaties came into force in 1958. In the intervening years the EU has grown in size by the accession of new Member States (1973, 1981, 1986, 1995, 2004 and 2005) and in power by the addition of policy areas to its remit. The Maastricht Treaty established the European Union under its current name in 1993. The latest amendment to the constitutional basis of the EU, the Treaty of Lisbon, came into force in 2009.

The EU operates through a system of supranational independent institutions and intergovernmental negotiated decisions by the member states. Important institutions of the EU include the European Commission (EC), the Council of the European Union, the European Council, the Court of Justice of the European Union, and the European Central Bank. The European Parliament is elected every five years by EU citizens. The European Commission is the politically independent institution which represents and upholds the interests of the EU as a whole. It is actually the driving force within the EU institutional system. It proposes legislations and their regulations (Directives), policies and programmes of action and is responsible for the implementation of the decisions of the EU Parliament and Council (Competent Authority).

The EU has developed a single market through a standardised system of laws (Directives) which apply in all member states. Within the Schengen Area (which includes 22 EU and 4 non-EU states) passport controls have been abolished. EU policies aim to ensure the free movement of people, goods, services, and capital, enact legislation in justice and home affairs, and maintain common policies on trade, agriculture, fisheries and regional development. A monetary union, the eurozone, was established in 1999 and is composed of 17 member states. Although the EU has no major competences in the field of health care, Article 35 of the Charter of Fundamental Rights of the European Union affirms that "*A high level of human health protection shall be ensured in the definition and implementation of all Union policies and activities*". All the member states have either publicly sponsored and regulated universal health care or publicly provided universal health care. The European Commission's Directorate-General for Health and Consumers seeks to align national laws on the protection of people's health, on the consumers' rights, on the safety of food and other products. This also applies to the procurement and clinical use of human blood and blood components. The EC Communication of 21 December 1994 on blood safety and self-sufficiency in the European Community identified the need for a blood strategy in order to reinforce confidence in the safety of blood transfusion chain and promote Community self-sufficiency. In its Resolution of 2 June 1995, on blood safety and self-sufficiency in the Community the Council invited the commission to submit appropriate proposals in the framework of the development of a blood strategy. In its resolution of 12 November 1996 on a strategy towards blood safety and self-sufficiency in the European Community, the Council invited the Commission to submit proposals as a matter of urgency with a view to encouraging the development of a coordinated approach to the safety of blood and blood products. In its resolutions of 14 September 1993, and 17 April 1996 on blood safety and self-sufficiency through voluntary unpaid donations in the European Community, the European Parliament stressed the importance of ensuring the highest level of blood quality and safety and has reiterated its continued support for the objective of Community self-sufficiency. In its resolutions of 14 September 1993, and 17 April 1996 on blood safety and self-sufficiency through voluntary unpaid donations in the European Community, the European Parliament stressed the importance of ensuring the highest level of blood safety and has reiterated its continued support for the objective of Community self-sufficiency.

As a result the European Parliament and the Council adopted on 27 January 2003 the Directive 2002/98/EC setting standards of quality and safety for the collection, testing, processing, storage and distribution of human blood and blood components and amending Directive 2001/83/EC that sets standards for plasma for the production of medicinal products such as albumin and immunoglobulins. [49] A key element of this EU directive is in the establishing of a uniform quality management through a quality system and haemovigilance. In the preamble of the directive it is mentioned that –

(16) Blood establishments should establish and maintain quality systems involving all activities that determine the quality policy objectives and responsibilities and implement them by such means as quality planning, quality control, quality assurance, and quality improvement within the quality system, taking into account the principles of good manufacturing practice as well as the EC conformity assessment system.

(17) An adequate system to ensure traceability of whole blood and blood components should be established. Traceability should be enforced through accurate donor, patient, and laboratory identification procedures, through record maintenance, and through an appropriate identification and labeling system. It is desirable that a system is developed in order to enable the unique and unmistakable identification of donations of blood and blood components in the Community. In the case of blood and blood components imported from third countries, it is important that an equivalent level of traceability be ensured by the blood establishment in the stages preceding importation to the Community. The same requirements of traceability which apply to blood and blood components collected in the Community should be ensured in the stages following importation.

(18) It is important to introduce a set of organized surveillance procedures to collect and evaluate information on the adverse or unexpected events or reactions resulting from the collection of blood or blood components in order to prevent similar or equivalent events or reactions from occurring thereby improving the security of transfusion by adequate measures. To this end a common system of notification of serious adverse events and reactions linked to the collection, processing, testing, storage, and distribution of blood and blood components should be established in Member States.

Attached to this mother Directive 2002/98/EC are a number of regulatory Commission Directives set to implement technical requirements for blood and blood components (Commission Directive 2004/33/EC), traceability requirements and notification of serious adverse reactions and events (Commission Directive 2005/61/EC) and standards and specifications relating to a quality system for blood establishments (Commission Directive 2005/62/EC) [50-52].

Since the objectives of the set of Directives, namely

1) to contribute to general confidence both in the quality of donated blood and blood components and in the health protection of donors;
2) to attain self-sufficiency at a Community level;
3) to enhance confidence in the quality and safety of the transfusion chain among the Member States, cannot be sufficiently achieved by the Member States alone, these – by reason of its scale and effects – be better achieved at Community level.

For this reason the EU through its EC has instituted a regulatory body, the competent authority, to which Member States report regularly and which holds frequent meetings with the appropriate delegations of the Member States. As it is necessary that the best possible scientific advice is available to the Community in relation to the quality and safety of blood and blood components, in particular as regards adapting the provisions of the Directive to scientific and technical progress, the EC is advised by the Scientific Committee for Medicinal Products and Medicinal Devices as well as international experience in this field.

4.4. The International Federation of Red Cross and Red Crescent Societies

The Red Cross idea was born in 1859, when Henry Dunant, a young Swiss man (Figure 5), came upon the scene of a bloody battle in Solferino, Italy, between the armies of imperial Austria and the Franco-Sardinian alliance.

Some 40,000 men lay dead or dying on the battlefield and the wounded were lacking medical attention. Dunant organized local people to bind the soldiers' wounds and to feed and comfort them. On his return, he called for the creation of national relief societies to assist those wounded in war, and pointed the way to the future Geneva Conventions.

"Would there not be some means, during a period of peace and calm, of forming relief societies whose object would be to have the wounded cared for in time of war by enthusiastic, devoted volunteers, fully qualified for the task?" he wrote.

The Red Cross was established in 1863 in Geneva, Switserland, when five Swiss men, including Dunant, set up the International Committee for Relief to the Wounded, later to become the International Committee of the Red Cross. Its emblem was a red cross on a white background, the inverse of the Swiss flag. The following year, 12 governments adopted the first Geneva Convention; a milestone in the history of humanity, offering care for the wounded, and defining medical services as 'neutral' on the battlefield.

The International Federation of Red Cross and Red Crescent Societies (IFRC) was founded in 1919 in Paris in the aftermath of World War I. The war had shown a need for close cooperation between Red Cross Societies, which, through their humanitarian activities on behalf of prisoners of war and combatants, had attracted millions of volunteers and built a large body of expertise.

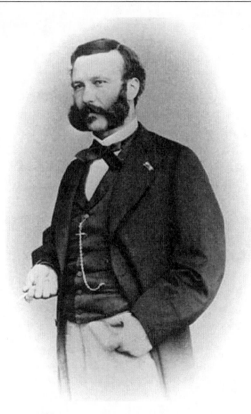

Figure 5. Henri Dunant (1828 – 1910) at the time of the battle of Solferino.

A devastated Europe could not afford to lose such a resource. It was Henry Davison, president of the American Red Cross War Committee, who proposed forming a federation of these National Societies. An international medical conference initiated by Davison resulted in the birth of the League of Red Cross Societies (LRCS), which was renamed in October 1983 to the League of Red Cross and Red Crescent Societies LRCRCS), and then in November 1991 to become the International Federation of Red Cross and Red Crescent Societies (IFRCRCS).

The first objective of the IFRCRCS was to improve the health of people in countries that had suffered greatly during the four years of war. Its goals were "*to strengthen and unite, for health activities, already-existing Red Cross Societies and to promote the creation of new Societies*" There were five founding member Societies: Britain, France, Italy, Japan and the United States. This number has grown over the years and there are now 187 recognized National Societies - one in almost every country in the world.

4.4.1. Quality Provision in Blood Services of the IFRCRCS

In many spheres of health care around the world, the concept of the provision of quality services has been actively pursued. It is clear that quality programmes need to be extended to blood services in order to ensure the quality and safety of blood and blood products supplied to all communities and to enhance the confidence of the public in blood services. The International Federation of Red Cross and Red Crescent Societies either provides, or assists in the provision of, at least one third of the world's blood supply, and thus has the responsibility to ensure that blood and blood products provided by Red Cross and Red Crescent are as safe as can be in the particular circumstances of the country concerned. The policy addresses specific responsibilities within blood programmes, and provides principles and guidelines for the implementation of quality procedures in blood programmes associated with Red Cross and Red Crescent. The global emphasis is on the promotion of voluntary and non-remunerated blood donation.

Since the outbreak of the HIV/AIDS epidemic and its global spread, a number of National Red Cross Blood Transfusion Service got involved in dramatic stories of patients infected through contaminated blood. This generated a more vigilant approach of the IFRCRCS and the adoption of a strict policy for those National Blood Services that continued their operations. National Red Cross or Red Crescent Societies must therefore ensure that all blood programmes with which they are associated are in compliance with this policy; that all staff and volunteers participating in blood programmes are aware of the rationale and details of the policy and act accordingly; and that all relevant governmental and non-governmental partners are adequately informed of this policy. This policy was adopted by the 12th Session of the General Assembly of the International Federation of Red Cross and Red Crescent Societies, October 1999 and replaces all previously established policies on Quality Provision in Blood Services.

In 1997 the 11th Session of the General Assembly in Seville, Spain was to develop a Blood Quality Programme. There were two instructive manuals produced in 1998 to support the development of quality management in blood transfusion:

- Blood Programme Quality Manual; [53].
- Blood Programme Development Manual. [54]

5. The Developments in the United States

After the Second World War, U.S. Army support for the American Red Cross's national blood service was withdrawn, so only a few large hospitals retained their own local blood banks. However, following the Texas City disaster in 1947 (an industrial explosion and fire), President Truman recommended that every city should have a blood bank, and in response, the American Association of Blood Banks was formed. One of its first acts was to begin developing and publishing technical recommendations. The recommendations eventually grew into the AABB's Technical Manual and Standards. Responsibility for regulating the new blood banks passed from the National Research Council to the National Institutes of Health's Laboratory of Biological Standards. The Laboratory oversaw the use of newly available radioisotopes, first iron and then chromium, as red cell labels and the development of accurate measures of red cell recovery and survival after storage. These isotope studies informed the debate about the addition of phosphate and adenine to red cell storage solutions. In 1972, authority for the regulation of blood banks was transferred to the Food and Drug Administration. The activities of these and other organizations are discussed in more detail below.

Quality management of blood banking and transfusion practice has been a critical element of regulatory and accreditation processes in the United States. The activity has been directed at both the products transfused (e.g. by the United States Food and Drug

Administration) and patient care (e.g. by the Joint Commission). The Food and Drug Administration (FDA), the AABB (formerly the American Association of Blood Banks), the Joint Commission (TJC, formerly the Joint Commission for the Accreditation of Healthcare Organizations), and the College of American Pathologists (CAP) have all addressed quality management in this field. Recently, a Biovigilance Network (a component of the National Healthcare Safety Network) was established in 2006 as a unique public-private collaboration between the U.S. Department of Health and Human Services, including the Centers for Disease Control and Prevention, and organizations involved in blood collection, transfusion, tissue and organ transplantation, and cellular therapies. The goal of the network is to enhance patient safety and protect donor health while also reducing overall health care-related costs. The AABB and CDC have developed the Hemovigilance Module of the Network which will allow the aggregation and analysis of nationwide data relating to adverse events and near-misses in order to develop recommendations for practice improvements.

5.1. United States Federal Government

5.1.1. The US Food and Drug Administration

The US Food and Drug Administration (FDA) considers blood and blood components to be both drugs and biologics and has a long history of regulating the quality of these products. Biologics were initially regulated in the US under the Biologics Control Act of 1902, but the regulation of blood components was not addressed at that time. In 1944, the Biologics Control Act was incorporated into the Public Health Service (PHS) Act, and in 1970, the definition of a biological product within the PHS Act was expanded to explicitly encompass both whole blood and blood components. [55] The PHS Act requires blood components to be proven safe, pure, potent and effective before they can be shipped in interstate commerce. As a drug, blood components are also regulated under the Federal Food Drug and Cosmetic (FDandC) Act of 1938. [56] The FDandC Act requires blood establishments to be registered with FDA, licensed by FDA before engaging in interstate commerce and inspected periodically by FDA investigators. Under the FDandC Act, a drug is considered adulterated if the facilities, methods and controls used for manufacturing are not in conformance with current good manufacturing practice. Subsequently, FDA promulgated Current Good Manufacturing Practices (CGMP) regulations to assure blood components are made according to the highest attainable standards using properly controlled processing procedures to produce blood components of uniform high quality. [57] The CGMP regulations for blood and blood components became effective in December 1975 and were codified in Title 21 of the Code of Federal Regulations in April 1976 [58].

FDA noted the release of unsuitable blood components during FDA inspections and also while reviewing error and accident (now called biological product deviations) reports submitted to FDA. In a FDA memorandum to blood establishments dated April 6, 1988, FDA's Center for Biologics Evaluation and Research (CBER) requested that blood establishments review their procedures and employee training programs to determine if adequate safeguards are in place to prevent the release of unsuitable blood components [59].

In 1995, the FDA issued a document, 'Guideline for Quality Assurance in Blood Establishments', the stated purpose of which was "*to assist manufacturers of blood and blood components, including blood banks, transfusion services, and plasmapheresis centers, in developing a quality assurance program in their effort to be consistent with recognized principles of quality assurance and current good manufacturing practice.*" [60] Blood establishments were advised they may follow the guideline or may choose to use alternative procedures.

The document asserts that to ensure the continued safety of the nation's blood supply, it is essential that establishments implement effective control over manufacturing processes and systems through the development of a written and managed quality assurance program which is designed to recognize and prevent the causes of recurrent deficiencies in performance. It states, "*A quality control unit having the responsibility and authority to ensure product quality is required by 21 CFR 211.22(a).....Parts 210 and 211 and Parts 600 through 680 clearly require a program of activities to control the manufacturing process to prevent the release of unsuitable products.*" The document notes that a quality assurance function should be established to control the manufacturing process to prevent the release of unsuitable products. It recommends that the quality control unit report to management personnel who would have the authority to implement corrective actions when necessary. This document defines the elements of a quality program to include having standard operating procedures, training and education, competency evaluation, proficiency testing, validation, equipment, error/accident reports, complaints, adverse reactions, records management, lot release, and quality assurance audits.

In 2004, FDA stated it would begin using a quality systems approach of its own to improve the predictability, consistency, integration, and overall effectiveness of its entire regulatory operation. In 2006, FDA released a guidance recommending implementation of a comprehensive quality systems model for human and veterinary pharmaceutical products, including biological products, to facilitate compliance with 21 CFR parts 210 and 211. [61] FDA acknowledged that the CGMP regulations were somewhat different in organization and in certain elements from other quality management systems; however, FDA noted they share underlying principles. The guidance states, "*More recently developed quality systems stress quality management, quality assurance, and the use of risk management tools, in addition to quality control.*" FDA decided that it would be useful to examine how the CGMP regulations and the elements of a modern, comprehensive quality system fit together in contemporary manufacturing practice. In the conclusion, FDA states, "*The central goal of a quality system is the consistent production of safe and effective products and ensuring that these activities are sustainable. Quality professionals are aware that good intentions alone will not ensure good products. A robust quality system will promote process consistency by integrating effective knowledge-building mechanisms into daily operational decisions.*"

In the U.S., a formal quality assurance program is required by the Centers for Medicare and Medicaid Services (CMS) which regulates all laboratory testing (except research) performed on humans in the U.S. through the Clinical Laboratory Improvement Amendments (CLIA). In 1988, CLIA established quality standards for clinical laboratories to ensure the accuracy, reliability, and timeliness of patient test results regardless of where the test is performed. CMS data indicates that CLIA has helped to improve the quality of testing in the United States [62].

In 1983, the FDA entered into an agreement with the Health Care Financing Administration (HCFA), now called CMS. A Memorandum of Understanding between the FDA and CMS was developed that consolidated within CMS responsibility for the inspection and surveying of unregistered transfusion services in order to minimize the duplication of effort and also to reduce the burden on the affected institutions. [63] Transfusion services which engage in compatibility testing and transfusion of blood components, but which do not routinely collect or process blood components, are now inspected by CMS. CMS, state survey agencies, including those in CLIA-exempt states, and accreditating organizations (such as CAP and AABB) conduct routine biennial surveys of transfusion services on behalf of FDA. FDA does not routinely survey unregistered transfusion services, although the FDA may inspect any transfusion service at any time.

5.2. The Joint Commission (TJC)

The Joint Commission (TJC), formerly the Joint Commission for the Accreditation of Healthcare Organizations (JCAHO) was the first agency in the United States to require utilization review of transfusion practices. This activity became a part of the TJC's accreditation process in 1961 [64].

In 1978, the TJC introduced a Medical Staff standard on Blood Utilization Review which required hospitals to collect data on blood use. [65] Between 1985 and 1991, the JC required utilization review of every blood transfusion with the caveat that when blood usage review consistently supported the justification and appropriateness of blood use, the review of an adequate sample of cases was acceptable. Although only a few hospitals were ever reported as complying with this standard, this element of JC accreditation was the most influential force driving enhanced blood utilization review in the U.S. Since 1991, the JC has made a series of changes to this requirement and developed several others relating to blood transfusion.

In 1996, the JC added Medical Staff standard MS.8.1.3 requiring medical staff to be involved in performance improvement activities for blood and blood use. [66] In 2002, the JC established its National Patient Safety Goals (NPSGs) program; the first set of NPSGs was effective January 1, 2003. [67] NPSGs were developed to help accredited organizations address specific areas of concern relating to patient safety and are assessed on each survey. The first set included NPSG (National Patient Safety Goal 1a). stipulating that two identifiers be used to identify a patient for blood transfusion as well as when other treatments are provided or when procedures are performed. NPSG.01.03.01 requiring the organization to "*eliminate transfusion errors related to patient misidentification*" became a goal in 2010. [68] In 2009, to be effective January 1, 2010, the JC introduced standard UP (Universal Protocol).01.01.01 requiring a standardized pre-operative list including blood product availability. [69] (This is a NPSG and, as such, is surveyed each time as well). In 2010, the JC added standard PC (Patient Care).02.01.01, Element of Performance 15 requiring that transfusions be administered per law (Federal and state) and medical staff policy [70].

All of the above numbered standards are still in force today. In addition, at present, the JC also requires hospitals to collect data on all reported and confirmed transfusion reactions (PI.01.01.01 Element of Performance 8). [71] This requirement, along with the requirement noted above requiring hospitals collect data on blood use (PI.01.01.01 Element of Performance 7), refers to a standard that directs leaders to give priority to high-volume, high-risk or problem-prone processes for performance improvement activities [LD (Leadership)], (04.04.01, Element of Performance 2). The requirement relating to transfusion reactions links to a standard that mandates the hospital to "*provide and encourage the use of systems for blame-free internal reporting of a system or process failure, or the results of a proactive risk assessment*" (LD.04.04.05, Element of Performance 6).

The JC standards do not define further the specific details of the utilization review of blood transfusions, in order to allow organizations flexibility in applying measures according to their specific practices.

5.3. College of American Pathologists (CAP)

The College of American Pathologists (CAP) has played an active role in quality management in transfusion medicine. Through its Proficiency Testing (PT) Surveys, Laboratory Accreditation, and Quality Management Tools programs, CAP members and collaborating partners have developed and participated in a variety of activities. The cornerstone of CAP's external quality assurance offerings is the CAP Surveys program which was initiated in 1949. Today, the CAP's Transfusion Medicine Resource Committee oversees more than 25 surveys related to blood banking and transfusion medicine. The Resource Committee also supports the use of the RhIG Dose Calculator, located on the Transfusion Medicine Topic Center of the CAP Web site, which allows laboratories to calculate the recommended dose of Rh immune globulin for Rh immunoprophylaxis by a standard and reliable method.

Along with PT, the CAP's Laboratory Accreditation Program founded in 1961 specifically addresses laboratory practices in Transfusion Medicine with an extensive checklist used as part of the inspection and accreditation of a laboratory offering transfusion medicine services. Additionally, CAP's Quality Practices Committee has developed numerous 'Q-PROBES' specific to Transfusion Medicine. Q-PROBES are an external peer-comparison program that addresses process-, outcome-, and structure-oriented quality assurance issues. This allows laboratories to establish benchmarks through external database comparisons and compare their performance to establish laboratory goals and improve performance. Since 1989, the CAP has introduced more than 15 Transfusion Medicine-specific Q-PROBES that include:

- Appropriateness of Plasma Transfusions
- Quality of Transfusion Documentation
- Utilization of RBC Transfusions
- Blood Bank Safety Practices
- T and S Completion for Scheduled Surgical Procedures
- Transfusion Errors
- Blood Component Preparation Turnaround Time
- Operating Room Blood Delivery Turnaround Time
- Small Hospital: Blood Bank Control of Usage and Wastage
- Autologous Blood Transfusion Practices
- Transfusion Errors
- Transfusion Appropriateness
- Autologous Blood Utilization
- Blood Utilization

Specifically, there were Q-PROBE studies comparing blood utilization statistics between institutions in 1989, 1990, and 1991, and there was a Q-PROBE study in 1993 on transfusion appropriateness.

5.4. AABB (Formerly American Association of Blood Banks)

The AABB was founded in 1947. Article III of the AABB's constitution states that one of its purposes is *"to keep currently aware of and encourage high standards of service"*. In 1953, to help fulfill its mission, the AABB published the first edition of a manual titled 'Technical Methods and Procedures' (subsequently renamed the Technical Manual). The introduction to this first edition noted that AABB *"has prepared this Manual in the interest of improving the quality of service rendered by blood banks"* [72].

In 1958, the AABB began issuing standards for its institutional members, an activity that has continued to the present. The first sentence of the Preface of the first edition of the AABB's 'Standards for Blood Banks and Transfusion Services' (BBTS) (then titled as 'Standards for a Blood Transfusion Service') stated : *"These Standards have been prepared ....for the purpose of improving the quality and safety of human blood transfusions."* [73] The term quality management first appeared in the fifteenth edition as the title of Standard A2.000 under which A2.100 stated: *"Each blood bank and transfusion service shall establish a program of quality assessment and improvement, under the supervision of a designated person, to ensure that policies and procedures are properly maintained and executed."* [74] The twentieth edition included credit for the first time to a Quality Management Subcommittee of the Standards Program Committee. [75] This Subcommittee has been credited in each subsequent edition. In 1958, the AABB also established a committee on inspection and accreditation and an international assessment and accreditation programme was born. In 1985, the AABB's Transfusion Practices Committee published a prominent report in JAMA outlining a method for the utilization review of blood transfusions. This prescient work coincided with the JC's attention to this practice as outlined above and called attention to the AABB's interest in transfusion utilization review. [76] In this regard, the 14th edition of the BBTS Standards was the first to address peer-review of transfusion practices. Standard A4.000 stated: *"All transfusing facilities shall use a peer-review program that documents monitoring of transfusion practices including ordering, use and waste of blood components. This program shall include criteria for evaluating transfusion practice."* [77] This requirement has been retained in revised form through all subsequent editions.

In 1991, the AABB board of directors created two committees, 1) the Technical Quality Assurance Committee and 2) the Transfusion Service Quality Assurance Committee, and charged them to develop a quality assurance programme appropriate for the activities performed within member institutions. [78] The AABB also incorporated the requirement for a program of quality assurance into its Standards for Blood Banks and Transfusion Services. [79] Subsequently, the Board selected January 1, 1998, as the deadline for implementation of a quality programme for institutional members of the AABB. In 1994, the AABB's Technical Quality Assurance Committee provided members with a quality plan manual and a self-assessment manual in a single binder to help them develop, implement, evaluate and sustain a quality programme. [80] In 1997, the AABB defined the minimum elements that must be addressed in a quality management system. [81, 82] These 'Quality System Essentials'

(QSEs) were developed to be compatible with ISO 9001 standards, the aforementioned FDA Guideline for Quality Assurance in Blood establishments and other FDA quality documents. The purposes of the quality system essentials were to (1) define the generic elements that must exist in a quality programme if that programme was to meet AABB Standards for Blood Banks and Transfusion Services and (2) identify the minimum quality programme requirements that must be in place to meet the January 1, 1998 deadline for institutional members who wished to be accredited by the AABB. [83, 84] The intent of the QSEs is to ensure that quality principles are applied consistently throughout an entire organization, not just within individual operational areas. [85] They have been updated with each edition of standards. The implementation of a quality programme such as that embodied in AABB's Standards, which includes the establishment of a quality system while also involving all operational systems, affords the means of changing the institution's approach to quality, if necessary, from one of detection to one of prevention [84].

6. Development and Initiatives in Selected Other Countries

As blood transfusion is largely a local activity, and transfusion system development is a regional and national activity, the pathways that different nations have chosen in transfusion system safety development are all different and filled with important useful lessons. This book is too short to list them all. However, several are mentioned here briefly as examples.

6.1. France

France emerged from World War I with many skilled transfusionists. The most notable was Arnault Tzanck (Figure 6) who organized transfusion donor services, developed transfusion devices and systems of blood storage, collected transfusion statistics, built organizations for transfusionists, and ultimately founded the scientific journal Revue d'Hématologie and in 1949 the Centre National de Transfusion Sanguine (National Blood Transfusion Center) of which he became the first director [86].

All blood collection in France was subsequently consolidated into a national blood collection system, the French Blood Establishment, with regional centres for component processing and research. This government agency's close ties with the prison system and use of prisoner blood donors led to significant transmission of hepatitis and HIV and a major re-evaluation of its safety systems in the late 1980s. The result was the development of a unique vein to vein quality management programme called haemovigilance. The haemovigilance programme seeks to identify systematically the risks of transfusion so that interventions can be developed to protect the patients. This practice was introduced in France in the early 1990s and has been developed in several European countries as a mix of governmental and non-governmental programs [87].

The French Institute Pasteur has been highly active in helping to build transfusion systems in Francophone Africa. [88] There was particular success in Tunisia and considerable achievement in Morocco and the Ivory Coast.

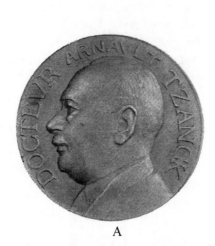
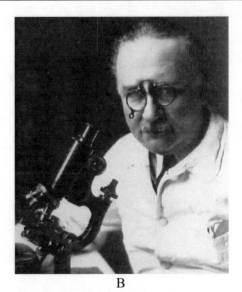

A   B

Figure 6. Arnault Tzanck (1886 – 1954).

6.2. Netherlands

Since the beginning of the 20st Century the Netherlands Red Cross Society has been involved in the recruitment of volunteers to donate blood in the hospitals. The donations were performed in the direct method (see picture Chapter 4) using a Jubé syringe and a stop cock. The tubing connecting the stop cock with donor and recipient were of a rubber and anticoagulation was not done. In 1926 Dr. H.C.J.M. van Dijk launched the idea to organize a blood bank with a stock of blood to cope with emergencies, instead of having to rush in donors. He approached the Board of the Netherlands Red Cross with the request to take responsibility for a neutral national organization coordinating the various blood transfusion services in the country. In 1930 his ideas and efforts were substantiated with the creation of the first Red Cross Blood Transfusion Service in the Saint Fransiscus Hospital in Rotterdam, followed by Amsterdam and Groningen. The Netherlands Red Cross decided to establish a Central Laboratory for the Blood Transfusion Service (CLB) in Amsterdam to initiate research and coordinate the Red Cross Blood Transfusion Services in the country. A next step was the creation of a Central Medical Blood Transfusion Committee (CMBC) as a scientific and practical advisory body.

Key scientists were among others Prof. A. Pondman, Prof Jochem.G.G. Borst who developed a citrate containing glass receptaculum that allowed an aseptic collection and preservation of the blood, Dr. Joep Spaander and Prof. Dr. Jochem J. van Loghem who developed with his charisma the CLB into an internationally well reputed spearhead research institute largely focused on immunohaematology with a formalized relation to the University of Amsterdam (Figure 7). In 1940 an initiative developed in Groningen by Dr. Leendert .J. Zielstra and medical technically supported by Prof. Tekke. Huizinga (hospital pharmacist) and Prof. Willem J. Kolff (internist and the inventor and creator of the first renal dialysis machine), lead to the set up of a ⌐regional⌐blood bank to accommodate the three Groningen City hospitals – Foundation Blood Bank Groningen..

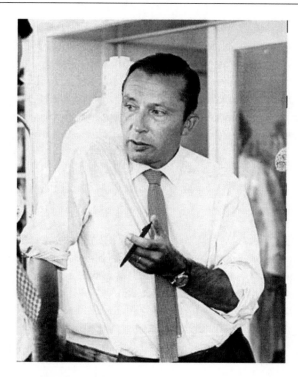

Figure 7. Jochem van Loghem (1914 – 2005).

Following the French legislative model blood transfusion and in particular the collection of blood became regulated in 1961. This 'Law on Human Blood' was replaced in 1982 by a more stringent 'Law on Blood Transfusion' to address the diversity of the practices of the 22 Regional Red Cross Blood Banks that had been created since 1973, regionalize the operations, and to harmonize the practices. However, the principles of quality remained restricted to products rather than to processes or the management of the processes in a structured way. In 1984 a group of blood bank directors adjusted the AABB Standards to the Dutch situation, but unfortunately that initiative did not reach a sufficiently broad consensus platform to be implemented. In the mid 1980s the Netherlands Red Cross Blood Banks united in a Federation to be able to respond appropriately to the new 1982 Law. This Federation of Netherlands Red Cross Blood Banks developed the idea to set up an accreditation system based on a peer inspection structure to inspect for compliance with these standards. In 1990 the Dutch Inspection and Certification Policy committee was created under the leadership of Dr. Cees Th. Smit Sibinga from the Northern Blood Bank in Groningen. This Blood Bank became the first non-American civilian blood centre accredited in 1981 by AABB and as a consequence he had become an AABB I and A programme inspector. The quality and quality management concepts were developed and spread over the country as well as internationally through a series of annual International Symposia on Blood Transfusion. [89] Dr. Smit Sibinga's experience was used to create a major change in the Netherlands - the development of a quality culture among the Dutch institutes and a good start of harmonizing GMP practices [90] in anticipation of the EU developments for safe and quality blood transfusions. [91] In 1997 the Federation decided to initiate a national haemovigilance programme that over the years had matured in an independent National Haemovigilance Bureau TRIP (Transfusion Reactions In Patients). Established in 2001 and based in The Hague [92] Trip is a Foundation in which all professional medical associations involved in prescription and transfusion of blood are united. The first report was published in 2003.

The blood supply in the Netherlands changed in 1998 into one national structure, based on the third Law on Blood Supply that came in force December 1997. The Foundation Sanquin Blood Supply accommodates both the former research and plasma fractionation institute CLB, which operate market conform, and the non-for-profit blood supply. Sanquin Blood Bank. [93] Sanquin is based in Amsterdam with branches in Rotterdam, Nijmegen and Groningen.

6.3. Australia

The Australian Red Cross Blood Service (ARCBS) is a branch of the Australian Red Cross (ARC). It is the body primarily responsible for blood donation and related services in Australia. Australian Red Cross Blood Service employs around 4000 employees across scientific, medical and support services, processing over half a million non-remunerated blood donations each year. The Blood Service is funded by the governments of Australia There are five strategic operational units in Queensland, New South Wales and the Australian Capital Territory, Victoria and Tasmania, South Australia, Western Australia and Northern Territory.

The Australian Red Cross blood services were initially managed by state-level organisations. Victoria's Blood Transfusion Service was founded in 1929, and by 1941 each state had its own Organ Transfusion Service. Also in 1941, the National Emergency Blood Transfusion Service (later the National Blood Transfusion Committee) was formed to coordinate the state groups. In 1945, the Red Cross took over blood and serum preparation units established by the Australian Army. In 1995, a government report recommended the foundation of a separate national structure, and the ARCBS was formed in 1996, encompassing the old state and territory blood donation and transfusion services. In 1999, the then Ministry for Health and Aged Care, established the Review of the Australian Blood Banking and Plasma Product Sector (The Stephen Review), chaired by Sir Ninian Stephen. The Stephen Review was conducted primarily in response to rapidly increasing costs, administrative inefficiencies and the lack of a national focus in the blood sector. The goal was to ensure that patients in Australia continued to have ongoing access to a safe and secure supply of blood and blood components. At that time there were over 30 agreements in existence between the various stakeholders, including governments, the Australian Red Cross Blood Service and Commonwealth Serum Laboratory Ltd (CSL). In addition, supply costs had tripled between 1991 and 1999. This made Australia's blood supply system fragmented with little leverage over escalating costs and containment of quality. The Stephen Review was released in 2001 and recommended the strengthening of the arrangements for the coordination and oversight of Australia's blood supply, including the establishment of a National Blood Authority (NBA) to manage Australia's blood supply at a national level [94].

Under the *National Blood Agreement*, the NBA is responsible for "in consultation with each Party, and for the approval of the Ministerial Council or the Jurisdictional Blood Committee, to undertake annual supply and production and budgeting …" The national blood supply is a national scheme for the subsidised supply of blood and blood products into the Australian health sector. It is analogous to other national health subsidy schemes such as e.g.

Medicare, the Pharmaceutical Benefits Scheme, the Aged Care Scheme, and the National Diabetes Services Scheme.

Key aspects which distinguish the national blood supply (Figure 1) from other national subsidy Schemes are the particular:

- policy aims and objectives agreed by all governments under the *National Blood Agreement*
- shared funding framework established under the *National Blood Agreement*, in which costs are essentially shared on a 63%:37% basis between the Australian Government and State/Territory governments
- method for the delivery of the subsidy, through centralised supply contracts agreed and administered by the NBA, operating within the Australian Government procurement and financial accountability framework.

The national blood supply is wholly government funded (no co-payment mechanisms apply) for the management and purchase of blood and blood components and plasma derived products. Under the scheme, blood and blood products are ultimately provided free of charge to patients in Australia. Blood donated in Australia has been tested for Hepatitis B since 1972, HIV-1 since 1985, Hepatitis C since 1990, HIV-2 since 1992/3, and HTLV-1 since 1993. As with other blood transfusion services, the ARCBS has to strike a balance between protecting blood recipients against infection, and accepting enough donors to maintain an adequate supply of blood. In the development of quality and quality management, ARCBS adopted in an early stage the CoE Guide [48] as their set of national (technical) standards. There is a major attention on the clinical use of blood as well as on education.

To manage the quality, the Australian Committee on Standards of Quality in Health Care (ACSQHC) developed the National Safety and Quality Health Service (NSQHS) Standards to drive the implementation and use of safety and quality systems and improve the quality of health service provision in Australia. [95] The Standards also provide a nationally consistent statement of the level of care consumers should be able to expect from health services. Standard 7 is the Blood and Blood Products standard and the NBA provided detailed input into the development of the standard. The NBA continues to work with the Commission to ensure the standard is implemented and imbedded.

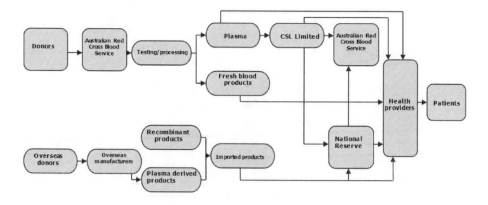

Figure 8. The Australian blood supply chain.

As a consequence haemovigilance is a key focus area for the Australian Red Cross Blood Service. The National Blood Authority has overall responsibility for haemovigilance in Australia under the governance of the Haemovigilance Advisory Committee. The Blood Service, however, plays a significant role in haemovigilance through its links with the jurisdictional programs (such as STIR, BloodSafe, Blood Watch and QiiT), and as an intrinsic part of the 'vein-to-vein' transfusion process through its collection, manufacture and supply of blood components and as provider of transfusion expertise. Following discussions with the National Blood Authority (NBA) in 2006, jurisdictional stakeholders identified the collection and reporting of haemovigilance data as a clear priority. During 2007, a minimum dataset of transfusion-related adverse events was developed, defined and recommended by the NBA Haemovigilance Project Working Group (HPWG) and endorsed by the Jurisdictional Blood Committee.

However, Australian states and territories are at different points of development in their capacity to report against the agreed minimum dataset, and investment will be required to enable all to report to the same level. The HPWG noted the requirement for a quality analysis of the costs associated with transfusion-related adverse events to assist with formulating an understanding of the benefit of public investment in haemovigilance at the local, state and national levels. An enduring national haemovigilance programme has been established under the governance of a Haemovigilance Advisory Committee constituted under the National Blood Authority Act that builds on the successful outcomes of the National Haemovigilance Project. The programme has as its overarching rationale improvement in transfusion safety and quality to bring about better patient outcomes. Improvements in quality of data will be achieved by states and territories continuing to work towards reporting of data that align with the agreed minimum dataset [96].

Australian governments work collaboratively with clinical colleges and the ARCBS to scope, assess and, where appropriate, promote a stronger awareness and wider adoption of comprehensive patient blood management strategies through the development of an advanced e-learning programme as an integral part of quality management. Reducing exposure to allogeneic blood and blood products will reduce exposure to transfusion risks. Special consideration is given to strategies used internationally, such as active management of pre-operative anaemia, intra-operative cell salvage, reduction of unnecessary blood tests, further understanding of anaemia tolerance to assist the adoption of conservative transfusion triggers, and use of alternative pharmacological therapies where appropriate.

6.4. United Kingdom

Blood transfusion started in the United Kingdom under the responsibility of the British Red Cross Society. The first more organized actions took place during World War I. In 1926 the British Red Cross instituted the first human blood transfusion service in the world. Over the recession years several hospital based blood banks were created based on voluntary and non-remunerated blood donors. Also during WWII the British Red Cross was the coordinating organization for the blood supply for the wounded of the German V2 air raids and the patients in the hospitals. With the end of the war, it was realised that the structure, which had proved so successful for blood collection, should be preserved and the National Blood Transfusion Service was founded in England and Wales.

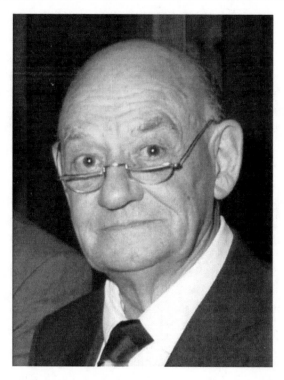

Figure 9. Fred Stratton (1913 - 2001).

Over the decades following the war the hospital based blood transfusion services were merged into Regional Blood Transfusion Services with a better economy of scale to handle costs and quality of the blood supply. A system of mobile team sessions was created to reach out into the community and stimulate the spirit of voluntary and non-remunerated blood donation. A basic departmental structure of the regional services was established following the flow of the primary process of collection, processing, testing/QC, storage and distribution. Quality culture and management developed gradually over the years and was further stimulated by the creation in May 1983 of the British Blood Transfusion Society (BBTS) which had its inaugural first meeting in December 1983 in Cambridge under de leadership of the first president Professor Fred Stratton (Figure 9).

With the global outbreak of HIV-AIDS the need for more stringent quality rules in the procurement of blood became obvious. Unfortunately the country was hit by transmissions of HCV and in the 1990s the outbreak of Mad Cow disease and the likelihood of transmission of the causative prions through blood. This was the start of a major re-organization of the blood services in England under the responsibility of the National Health Service (NHS). [97] The National Blood Authority (NBA) was established in April 1993, and took over responsibility in England for what was previously known as the National Blood Transfusion Service (NBTS) in April 1994. This development sought to change a regionally-based service into a national one. In September 1994, the NBA published its proposals for the future of the Regional Blood Transfusion Services, now to be called the National Blood Service (NBS). The proposals included the establishment of three administrative Zones to replace the previous regional structure. In 1995 the Department of Health approved the establishment of the National Blood Service (NBS) with 3 administrative Zones to replace the previous structure of Regional Transfusion Centres. Independent National and Zonal Blood User Groups (NBUG and ZBUGs) were established to oversee the new arrangements on behalf of the users of the services. In 1996 a haemovigilance system based on voluntary participation of the hospitals was created – Serious Hazards of Transfusion or SHOT, which published its first report in 1998 drawing attention to the large number of avoidable transfusion errors. The message was clear and the UK Chief Medical Officer (CMO) organized a Seminar on 'Evidence-based Blood Transfusion' in London attended by a multidisciplinary audience including blood users, representatives of Blood Services, NHS managers and patients. The factors leading to this initiative included –

- concerns about the blood supply in the face of increases in the demand for blood and intermittent blood shortages,
- increases in the cost of blood associated with universal leucocyte-depletion of blood components and nucleic acid testing,
- data from the Serious Hazards of Transfusion (SHOT) scheme showing that the safety of transfusion should be improved, and
- concerns about the transmission of variant Creutzfeldt-Jakob (vCJD) disease by blood transfusion.

Based on recommendations from the Seminar the Health Services Circular 'Better Blood Transfusion' (HSC 1998/224) was issued in December 1998. It detailed actions required of NHS Trusts and clinicians to improve transfusion practice, including –

- Establishment of a Hospital Transfusion Committee to oversee all aspects of transfusion
- Participation in the SHOT scheme
- Development of agreed and disseminated local protocols for transfusion practice, based on national guidelines and supported by in-house training
- Consideration of the use of autologous transfusion, particularly peri-operative cell salvage

In 1999 the 3 NBS Zones were integrated into a new national management structure and the ZBUGs were disbanded. The focus had definitely shifted from the quality aspects of the procurement processes to patient oriented quality handling and practice – the chain approach with the consumer being the leading factor for quality management and improvement. The strategy was a complete integration of blood transfusion in the health care. In 2001 a second UK CMO Seminar on 'Better Blood Transfusion' was held in London, focusing on –

- Providing better information to patients;
- Avoiding unnecessary transfusion;
- Making transfusion safer;
- Ensuring 'Better Blood Transfusion' is an integral part of NHS care

In 2005 the NHS Blood and Transplant (NHSBT) was established to replace NBS, and to encompass organ donation across the UK [98].

In 2006 two further quality management measures were introduced –

1) National Patient Safety Agency (NPSA) issued the Safer Practice Notice setting out measures to improve the safety of blood transfusions, including training and competency testing of staff, photo-identification cards for regularly transfused patients and electronic tracking systems for patients and blood.
2) Oxford group produced a specification for electronic transfusion management systems on behalf of the NPSA and NHS Connecting for Health.

In 2011 a national Seminar on Modernisation of Transfusion Services was held in London, which triggered a change in focus of the *Better Blood Transfusion* initiative to *Patient Blood Management* (PBM) [99].

Conclusion

That human to human transfusion has been subject to various kinds of review and quality management from concerned individuals, medical and scientific bodies, regulatory agencies of governments and accrediting organizations throughout its history is understandable. This has contributed greatly to public health and patient safety especially since the dramatic effects of blood borne disease over the last quarter of the 20st century. Where the focus in the beginning was on immunohaematology to achieve proper compatibility, it shifted over the second half of the 20st century to processing of blood and machine collections of specific blood collections.

Only over the last quarter quality and its structured management started to grow, ultimately changing the emphasis from the narrow product orientation to the broad chain and customer orientation – the integration of blood transfusion in the national health care. After all, history has shown that from very early onset on it has never been the test tube that was to be transfused, but the patient at the bedside.

Acknowledgment

The findings and conclusions in this chapter related to the U.S. Food and Drug Administration have not been formally disseminated by the Food and Drug Administration and should not be construed to represent any Agency determination or policy.

References

[1]   a. Tucker, Holly. *Blood Work: A tale of medicine and murder in the scientific revolution.* 1st Edition. New York: W.W. Norton and Company, Inc., 2011. Pg.133. b. Tucker, Holly. *Blood Work: A tale of medicine and murder in the scientific revolution.* 1st Edition. New York: W.W. Norton and Company, Inc., 2011. Pg.169.

[2]   Blundell J. Some account of a case of obstinate vomiting in which an attempt was made to prolong the life by injection of blood into the veins. *Med. Chir. Trans.* 1819; 10:296-311.

[3]   Blundell J. Observations on transfusion of blood. *Lancet* 1828; 2:321-324.

[4]   Chadwick JR. Transfusion. *Boston Med. Surg. J.* 1874; 41:25-32.

[5]   Ottenberg R, Kaliski DJ. Accidents in transfusion: their prevention by preliminary blood examination: based on an experience with one hundred twenty-eight transfusions. *J. Amer. Med. Assoc.* 1913. 61:2138.

[6]   Lee RI. A simple and rapid method for the selection of donors for transfusion by the determination of blood groups. *Brit. Med. J.* 1917; 2:684-685.

[7]   Rous P. A rapid and simple method of testing donors for transfusion. *J. Amer Med. Assoc.* 1915; 64:1980-1982.

[8]   Lee RI, Vincent B. The coagulation of normal human blood: an experimental study. *Arch. Intern. Med.* 1914; 13:398-425.

[9]   Lewisohn R. A new and greatly simplified method of blood transfusion. *Med. Rec.* 1915; 87:141-142.

[10] Rous P, Turner JW. The preservation of living red blood cells in vitro. *J. Exp. Med.* 1916 Feb. 23:219-237.

[11] Stansbury LG, Hess JR. Blood transfusion in World War I: The roles of Lawrence Bruce Robertson and Oswald Hope Robertson in the most important   medical advance of the war. *Transfus. Med. Rev.* 2009; 23:232-236.

[12] Transfusion of blood for the recently injured in the United States Army. Paris: Medical Division of the American Red Cross Society in France, 1918.

[13] McPherson WG, Boeley AA, Wallace C: Blood transfusion, Chap 5, pp 108-132, in *History of the Great War, Medical Services, Surgery of the War.* London, His Majesty's Stationery Office, 1922.

[14] Oblensky FE, Jonathan Letterman, Dec. 1824 –15 Mar. 1872. *Mil. Med.* 1968; 133:312-315.

[15] Blair JS. Major Jonathan Letterman, Director of Medical Services, Union Army. J. R. Army Med. Corps. 2004; 150:61-62.

[16] Hurd HM. Dr. John S. Billings, bibliographer and librarian. *Bull. Med. Libr. Assoc.* 1990; 78: 172.

[17] Malkin HM. The trials and tribulations of George Miller Sternberg (1838-1915)--America's first bacteriologist. *Perspect. Biol. Med.* 1993; 36:666-678.

[18] Craddock WL. The achievements of William Crawford Gorgas. *Mil. Med.* 1997; 162: 325-327.

[19] Hess JR, Schmidt PJ. The first blood banker: Oswald Hope Robertson. *Transfusion* 2000; 40:110-113.

[20] Galton F. Regression toward mediocrity in hereditary stature. *J. Anthropol. Institute* 1886: 15: 246-263.

[21] Pearson K. On the criterion that a given system of deviations from the probable in the case of a correlated system of variables is such that it can be reasonably supposed to have arisen from random sampling. *Philosophical Magazine*, Series 5. 1900: 50:157–175.

[22] Student (Gossett WS). The probable error of a mean. *Biometrica* 1908; 6:1-25.

[23] Fisher RA. The correlation between relatives on the supposition of Mendelian inheritance. *Philosophical Transactions of the Royal Society of Edinburgh* 1918; 52: 399–433.

[24] Deming WE. The Chi-test and curve-fitting. *J. Amer. Statist. Assoc.* 1934; 29:372-382.

[25] DeGowin EL, Harris JE, Plass ED. Studies on preserved human blood . I. Various factors influencing hemolysis. *J. Amer. Med. Assoc.* 1940; 114:850-855.

[26] Kendrik DB. *Blood program in World War II.* Washington, Office of the Surgeon General, 1964.

[27] DeGowin EL, Hardin RC, Alsever JB. *Blood Transfusion.* London, WB Saunders; 1949.

[28] Bock AV. Use and abuse of blood transfusions. *N. Engl. J. Med.* 1936; 215:412-5.

[29] Fantus B. The therapy of Cook County Hospital. *J. Amer. Med. Assoc.* 1937; 109: 128-31.

[30] Use of blood transfusion. *Lancet* 1951 ;ii:1044.

[31] Garland J, Smith RM, Lanman TH, et al. Abuse of transfusion therapy (editorial). *N. Engl. J. Med.* 1951;245:745-6.

[32] McCoy KL. The Providence Hospital blood conservation program. *Transfusion* 1962; 2:3-6.

[33] Straus B, Torres JM. Use and abuse of blood transfusion. *J. Amer. Med. Assoc.* 1953; 151: 699-701.

[34] Crisp WE. One pint of blood. *Obstet. Gynecol.* 1956;7:216-17.

[35] Cantor D. *A legal look at blood transfusions.* GP 1957;16:82-4.

[36] Crosby WH. Misuse of blood transfusions. *Blood* 1958;13:1198-200.

[37] Crosby WH. Misuse of blood transfusions. *Med. Bull. U S Army,* Europe 1958;15:7.

[38] Friesen R. The use and abuse of blood in abortions. *Can. Med. Assoc. J.* 1959;80:802-5.

[39] Graham-Stewart CW. A clinical survey of blood transfusions. *Lancet* 1960;ii:421-24.

[40] *Bulletin of Joint Commission on Accreditation of Hospitals, publications* 26, March 1961. Oakbrook Terrace, IL: Joint Commission on Accreditation of Hospitals, 1961.

[41] Joint Blood Council. Transfusion review program. *J. Amer. Med. Assoc.* 1962; 180: 230-1.

[42] Crosby WH. The hospital transfusion board. *Transfusion* 1962; 2:1-2.

[43] Walz DV. An effective hospital transfusion committee. *J. Amer. Med. Assoc.* 1964; 189:660-2.

[44] Grindon, Al; Tomasulo PS; Bergin JJ. et al. "The hospital transfusion committee." *J. Amer. Med. Assoc.,* Vol 253.No. 4 (Jan 25, 1985): 540-43.

[45] Alter HJ, Klein HG. The hazards of blood transfusion in historical perspective. *Blood.* 2008; 112:2617-2626.

[46] WHA28.72 Utilization and supply of human blood and blood products. 1975 *Handb. Res.,* Vol. I, 1.5.2.2; 8.2.4 Thirteenth plenary meeting, 29 May 1975.

[47] The World Health Organization, *Blood Safety Program* (accessed 21 Jun 2012) http://www.who.int/bloodsafety/en.

[48] Guide to the Preparation, Use and Quality Assurance of Blood Components. *Annex to Recommendation No. R(95)15,* Committee of Ministers of the Council of Europe. Council of Europe Publishing, Strasbourg, F, 1995.

[49] Directive 2002/98/EC of the European Parliament and of the Council of 27 January 2003 setting standards of quality and safety for the collection, testing, processing,

storage and distribution of human blood and blood components and amending Directive 2001/83/EC. *Official Journal of the European Union,* L33, 8/02/2003.

[50] Commission Directive 2004/33/EC of 22 March 2004 implementing Directive 2002/98/EC of the European Parliament and of the Council as regards certain technical requirements for blood and blood components. *Official Journal of the European Union,* L91, 30/03/2004.

[51] Commission Directive 2005/61/EC of 30 September 2005 implementing Directive 2002/98/ EC of the European Parliament and of the Council as regards traceability requirements and notification of serious adverse reactions and events. *Official Journal of the European Union,* L256, 1/10/2005.

[52] Commission Directive 2005/62/EC of 30 September 2005 implementing Directive 2002/98/ EC of the European Parliament and of the Council as regards Community standards and specifications relating to a quality system for blood establishments. *Official Journal of the European Union.* L256, 1/10/2005.

[53] *Blood Programme Quality Manual.* 1998, IFRCRCS, Geneva, CH.

[54] *Blood Programme Development Manual,* 1998, IFRCRCS, Geneva, CH.

[55] *Public Health Service Act.* Regulation of Biological Products. Title 42 United States Code, Chapter 6A, Part F, Section 262 (42USC262). (accessed 12 Jun 2012). www.fda.gov/RegulatoryInformation/ Legislation/ucm148717.htm.

[56] *Federal Food, Drug and Cosmetic Act.* Drugs and Devices. Chapter V, Subchapter A. (accessed on 12 Jun 2012) www.fda.gov/RegulatoryInformation/Legislation/Federal FoodDrugandCosmeticActFDCAct/FDCActChapterVDrugsandDevices/default.htm.

[57] *FDA, Code of Federal Regulations,* Title 21, parts 210, 211, and 606 US Government Printing Office, Washington, DC, April 1, 2010. (accessed on 12 Jun 2012). http://www.accessdata.fda.gov/scripts/cdrh/cfdocs/ cfcfr/cfrsearch.cfm.

[58] Human blood and blood products: collection, processing and storage. Federal Register. 40 FR 53531, November 18, 1975.

[59] *FDA Memorandum to All Registered Blood Establishments: Control of Unsuitable Blood and Blood Components,* April 6, 1988. (accessed 12 Jun 2012). http://www.fda. gov/BiologicsBloodVaccines/GuidanceComplianceRegulatoryInformation/Other RecommendationsforManufacturers/MemorandumtoBloodEstablishments/default.htm.

[60] *FDA Guideline for Quality Assurance in Blood Establishments,* July 11, 1995. (accessed on 12 Jun 2013). www.fda.gov/BiologicsBloodVaccines/Guidance ComplianceRegulatoryInformation/Guidances/Blood/default.htm.

[61] *FDA Guidance for Industry: Quality Systems Approach to Pharmaceutical CGMP Regulations,* September 2006. (accessed on 12 Jun 2012). http://www.fda.gov/Biologics BloodVaccines/GuidanceComplianceRegulatoryInformation/Guidances/General/ucm21 7665.htm.

[62] *Clinical Laboratory Improvement Amendments (CLIA).* (accessed 12 Jun 2012). http://www.cms.gov/Regulations-and-Guidance/Legislation/CLIA/index.html?redirect=/ CLIA/.

[63] *Memorandum of Understanding between the Health Care Financing Administration and the Food and Drug Administration.* FDA 225-80-4000, June 6, 1983. (accessed on 12 Jun 2012) http://www.fda.gov/ AboutFDA/PartnershipsCollaborations/Memoranda ofUnderstandingMOUs/DomesticMOUs/ucm116313.htm.

[64] *Bulletin of Joint Commission on Accreditation of Hospitals, publications* 26, March 1961. Oakbrook Terrace, IL: Joint Commission on Accreditation of Hospitals, 1961.

[65] *Accreditation Manual for Hospitals,* Chicago, IL: Joint Commission on Accreditation of Hospitals, 1978, p.87, MS IV.

[66] *Accreditation Manual for Hospitals,* volume I, Oakbrook Terrace, IL: Joint Commission on Accreditation of Healthcare Organizations, 1996, p.245.

[67] "JCAHO Approves National Patient Safety Goals for 2003", *Joint Commission Perspectives,* 2002;22:1-3.

[68] "Approved: 2010 National Patient Safety Goals", *Joint Commission Perspectives,* 2009; 29: 1,20-31.

[69] "Approved: 2010 National Patient Safety Goals", *Joint Commission Perspectives,* 2009; 29: 30-31].

[70] Hospital Accreditation Standards, 2010, Oakbrook Terrace, IL: *Joint Commission Resources,* 2010, p.PC-16.

[71] Hospital Accreditation Standards 2012, Oakbrook Terrace, IL: *Joint Commission Resources,* 2012.

[72] *Technical methods and procedures.* Dallas, TX: American Association of Blood Banks, 1953.

[73] Strumia MM, Jennings ER, eds. *Standards for a blood transfusion service.* 1st ed. Washington, DC; Chicago, IL: AABB, 1958.

[74] Widmann FK, ed. *Standards for blood banks and transfusion services.* 15th ed. Bethesda, MD: AABB, 1993.

[75] Gorlin JB, ed. *Standards for blood banks and transfusion services.* 20th ed. Bethesda, MD: AABB, 2002.

[76] Grindon, Al; Tomasulo PS; Bergin JJ. et al. "The hospital transfusion committee." *J. Amer. Med. Assoc.;* 1985;253:540-43.

[77] Widmann FK, ed. *Standards for blood banks and transfusion services.* 14th ed. Arlington, VA: AABB, 1991.

[78] Otter, J; Cooper, E.S. "What do the Accreditation Organizations Expect?." *Arch. Pathol. Lab. Med.* 1999;123: 468-71.

[79] Widmann FK, ed. *Standards for blood banks and transfusion services.* 14th ed. Arlington, VA: AABB, 1991.

[80] *Quality Program.* Vols 1 and 2. Bethesda, MD: American Association of Blood Banks; 1994.

[81] Quality program implementation. *Association bulletin #97-4.* Bethesda, MD: AABB, 1997.

[82] Smith , Dennis M., Otter, Jean. "Performace improvement in a hospital transfusion service." *Arch. Pathol. Lab. Med.* 1999;123:585-591.

[83] Smith DM. *Quality Program Implementation.* Bethesda, Md: American Association of Blood Banks; August 1, 1997.

[84] Otter J, Cooper, Shannon E. "What do the Accreditation Organizations Expect?" *Arch. Pathol. Lab. Med.* Vol 123 June (1999): 468-71.

[85] Smith , Dennis M.,Otter, J. "Performace improvement in a hospital transfusion service." *Arch. Pathol. Lab. Med.* 1999;123: 585-91.

[86] Schneider WL. Arnault Tzanck, MD (1886-1954). *Transfus. Med. Rev.* 2010; 24:147-150.

[87] Smit Sibinga CTh, Murphy MF. "Hemovigilance: An Approach to Risk Management in Transfusion Medicine." Chap 28. *Transfusion Therapy: Clinical Principles and Practice*. Ed. Paul D. Mintz. 3rd ed. Bethesda, MD: AABB Press, 2011. 797-811.

[88] Schneider WH, Drucker E, Blood transfusion in the early years of AIDS in Sub-Saharan Africa. *Amer. J. Public Health* 2006;96:984–994.

[89] Smit Sibinga CTh, Das PC, Taswell HF eds. *Quality Assurance in Blood Banking and its Clinical Impact Proceedings of the seventh annual Symposium on Blood Transfusion,* Groningen 1982. Dordrecht NL, Martinus Nijhoff Publs, 1984.

[90] Smit Sibinga CTh, Das PC, Heiniger HJ, eds Good Manufacturing Practice in Transfusion Medicine. *Proceedings of the eighteenth International Symposium on Blood Transfusion*, 1993. Dordrecht NL, Kluwer Academic Publs. 1994.

[91] TRIP National Hemovigilance Office (Netherlands), *Transfusion and Transplantation Reactions in Patients* (accessed on 3 Sep 2012). http://www.tripnet.nl/pages/en/.

[92] Council Recommendation 98/463/EC on the suitability of blood and plasma donors and the screening of donated blood in the European Community, *Official Journal of the European Union* 1998; L203:14-26.

[93] Foundation Sanquin Blood Supply URL: http://www.sanquin.nl/ , accessed 03 September 2012.

[94] *Review of the Australian Blood Banking and Plasma Product Sector*. A report to the Commonwealth Minister for Health and Aged Care by a committee chaired by the Rt Hon Sir Ninian Stephen. 2001. (accessed on 12 Jun 2012). www.nba.gov.au/policy/pdf/report.pdf.

[95] Australian Commission on Safety and Quality in Health Care (ACSQHC) *National Safety and Quality Health Service Standards.* (accessed 12 Jun 2012) www.transfusion.com.au/sites/default/files/ NSQHS%20Standards%20(2).pdf.

[96] National Blood Authority Haemovigilance Project Working Group . *Initial Australian Haemovigilance Report* 2008. (accessed 12 Jun 2012). www.nba.gov.au/haemovigilance/nba_hemreport08.pdf.

[97] Murphy MF, Robinson EAE, Gordon-Smith EC. The Chief Medical Officer's National Blood Transfusion Committee. 2003 In: *SHOT Annual Report* 2001/02. Manchester, UK: p43-46. (accessed 12 Jun 2012) www.shotuk.org/shot-reports/reports-and-summaries-2001-2002/.

[98] *UK National Health Service, Blood and Transplant*, (accessed 3 Aug 2012). http://www.nhsbt.nhs.uk/about/.

[99] *UK National Health Service, Blood and Transplant, Transfusion Guidelines* (accessed on 3 Aug 2012) http://www.transfusionguidelines. org.uk/index.aspx?Publication= BBT.

In: Quality Management in Transfusion Medicine
Editor: Cees Th. Smit Sibinga

ISBN: 978-1-62618-665-1
© 2013 Nova Science Publishers, Inc.

Chapter II

Need for Quality Management in Transfusion Medicine

Jerry A. Holmberg[1], and Neil Rosin[2],†*

[1] Novartis Vaccines and Diagnostics, Inc. Former Senior Advisor
for Blood Policy, Department of Health and Human Services, US
[2] Position Managing Director - Quality Management and
Improvement Consultancy (Ltd), Remuera,
Auckland, New Zealand

Abstract

The focus of this chapter is how quality and quality management evolved in the manufacturing industry leading to the same concepts being applied in blood transfusion medicine. Although Transfusion Medicine is a relatively young subspecialty of medicine, it involves both the clinical practice and laboratory controlled practices. It includes not only service but a manufactured product. The manufacturing of biological products is produced in compliance to national, international and professional standards to credibility of safety, potency, and efficacy. All of the steps from recruitment to transfusion of the final product must be maintained in controlled processes. Historical aspects of the Quality System in Transfusion Medicine have evolved much from those found in other industries. Total Quality Management, Continuous Process Improvement, Haemovigilance and national governance models are discussed with the emphasis on understanding risk and mitigating those risks in a controlled process. The need for a Quality System has been largely demanded by the consumer (patient and clinician) as well as the government. Expectation of a safe and reliable blood supply in light of past experience of transfusion transmitted infections and adverse events have been identified.

* Jerry A. Holmberg, PhD, MT(ASCP)SBB: Novartis Vaccines and Diagnostics, Inc. Former Senior Advisor for Blood Policy, Department of Health and Human Services, US. 34845 Apple Pride Court, Round Hill, VA, US 20141. Tel: +1(510)289-2927; E-mail: Jerry. Holmberg@novartis.com.
† Neil Rosin, MBA, NHD MED TECH, NHD TQM: Position Managing Director - Quality Management and Improvement Consultancy (Ltd). Address: 4/633 Remuera Road, Remuera, Auckland, New Zealand. Tel: +6421676237; E-mail: neilrosin@gmail.com.

Keywords: Quality, Transfusion, Medicine, Blood, Haemovigilance, Safety

1. Introduction

Quality defined as lack of variation, is evident in all aspects of life and can even be traced back to the B.C. era. Structures in India and Egypt show evidence of measurement and inspection. Look at the precisely cut stones used for the pyramids and forts. Such precision in engineering could only be achieved through consistent methods of shaping and cutting using precise measurement devices for that era. Such consistency has led to 'quality' structures.

The need for quality stems back to the first documented evidence in 1832 of a quality concern. A merchant named John Welburgham of Canterbury was fined a six pence for selling rotten and unwholesome fish. [1]

Before the industrial revolution skilled craftsman served as both manufacturers and inspectors (quality control), of their own work through building quality into their pride of workmanship. The first two steps towards the provision of a quality product was inspection and quality control. This led to an independent quality control department which focused on testing of product allowing management to concentrate on production quantity and efficiency. Quality control is defined as *"the operational techniques and activities that are used to fulfil requirements for quality"*.(BS.4778, Part 1. 1987 ISO 8402, 1986). Under such a system of quality control one can expect raw material testing, some self-inspection of operators of product during the process and final product testing. Organizations whose approach is based on inspection and quality control are operating in a detection mode (finding and fixing mistakes). [2]

The Industrial revolution changed the concept from holistic manufacturing to production efficiency concepts, smaller job tasks and reliance on others through a manufacturing value chain, was introduced by the likes of Jefferson and Taylor.

This concept was not without problems, products were produced and prior to release for sale products were inspected and rejects removed after inspection.

In the 1920s statistical theory began to be applied effectively to quality control, and in 1924 Shewhart made the first sketch of a modern control chart. [3] His work was later developed by Deming and the early work of Shewhart, Deming, Dodge and Romig constitutes much of what today comprises the theory of statistical process control (SPC).

2. Quality Assurance/Quality Management

Quality Assurance/Quality Management principles were initiated post World War I which focused on systems to manufacture 'Right First Time'. Elements including documented procedures, personnel training, continuous improvement programmes and internal audit programmes were developed to ensure that products of consistency and quality were produced with less focus on final inspection. Quality Assurance is defined as *"All those planned and systematic actions necessary to provide adequate confidence that a product or service will satisfy given requirements for quality."* (BS.4778, Part 1. 1987 ISO 8402, 1986). Examples of additional features acquired when progressing from quality control to quality assurance include comprehensive standard operating procedures to increase uniformity and conformity, training of staff, assessment tools such as internal quality audits, external quality assessment schemes, continuous improvement through corrective and preventative action. This creates a shift from detection towards prevention of non-conformances. More emphasis is placed on quality planning, improving the design of the product, improving the control over processes and involving and motivating staff.

To aid the adaptation of quality control and quality assurance (termed quality management), procedures and systems have been continuously codified over the years resulting in all embracing general purpose international standards. International Standardisation Organisation (ISO) 9000 has become the internationally recognised standard for quality management systems which may comprise a number of standards that specify the requirements for the development and maintenance of a quality system. Examples of such include, but not limited to ISO9000 (Manufacturing and Service Industries), ISO 13485 (Medical Devices), ISO 17025 (Calibration and test laboratories), ISO 15189 Medical Laboratories.

Quality System (QS) requirements for medicinal products have been internationally recognized as a way to assure product safety and efficacy and customer satisfaction since at least 1983, and were instituted as requirements in a final rule published on October 7, 1996. The US Food and Drug Administration (FDA) had documented design defects in medical devices that contributed to recalls from 1983 to 1989 that would have been prevented if QS had been in place. The rule is promulgated at 21 CFR 820. According to current Good Manufacturing Practice (GMP), medical device manufacturers have the responsibility to use good judgment when developing their quality system and apply those sections of the FDA QS Regulation that are applicable to their specific products and operations, in Part 820 of the QS regulation. As with GMP, operating within this flexibility, it is the responsibility of each manufacturer to establish requirements for each type or family of devices that will result in devices that are safe and effective, and to establish methods and procedures to design, produce, and distribute devices that meet the quality system requirements. [4] The FDA has identified in the QS regulation the essential elements that a quality system shall embody for design, production and distribution, without prescribing specific ways to establish these elements.

Country specific standards have also been developed. For example The British Standard (BS) 5750 for quality systems had been published in 1979.

3. The TQM Concept of Excellence

As we move into the 21st century, Total Quality Management (TQM) has developed in many countries into holistic frameworks, aimed at helping organisations achieve excellent performance, particularly in customer and business results. Definition of Total Quality Management is *"A management philosophy embracing all activities through which the needs and expectations of the customer and the community, and the objectives of the organization are satisfied in the most efficient and cost effective way by maximising the potential of all employees in a continuing drive for improvement."*

In Europe, a widely adopted framework is the so-called 'Business Excellence' or 'Excellence' Model, promoted by the European Foundation for Quality Management (EFQM), in the UK by the British Quality Foundation (BQF) and in US the Malcolm Baldridge Award institutionalised in 1987 by US government. In Canada, the National Quality Institute presents the 'Canada Awards for Excellence' on an annual basis to organisations that have displayed outstanding performance in the areas of Quality and Workplace Wellness, and have met the Institute's criteria with documented overall achievements and results. The Criteria address critical aspects of management that contribute to performance excellence: leadership; strategic planning; customers; measurement, analysis, and knowledge management; the workforce; operations; and results.

The structure of Standards has led to independent external assessments to verify that quality standards have been implemented and to ensure formal recognition thereof:

1   Companies or consultants can be hired into any business to 'accredit' that the QA system in place and its operation complies with a national or international code. Such accreditation offers 'assurance' within a supply chain that the product has been reliably and safely produced;

2   Regulators in the form of Government to assess compliance to regulations and manufacturing codes e.g., Good Manufacturing Practice (GMP), FDA regulations. [5]

Harmonization of quality standards has become a prerequisite to ensure industries operate according to standards. Pharmaceutical Inspection Convention and Pharmaceutical Inspection Co-operation Scheme (PIC/S) is leading the international development, implementation and maintenance of harmonised GMP standards and quality systems of inspectorates in the field of medicinal products. This is to be achieved by developing and promoting harmonised GMP standards and guidance documents; training competent authorities in inspection, in particular inspectors; assessing (and reassessing) inspectorates; and facilitating the co-operation and networking of competent authorities and international organisations.

Integration of various standards is also an opportunity to improve quality outcomes. The pharmaceutical industry has traditionally focused upon the application of GMP, it has been slow to consider the potential benefits to be gained by implementing an EN ISO 9001 Quality Management System (QMS). Conseil Européen des Féderations de l'Industries Chimique (CEFIC) commissioned a working group of experts drawn from several major industrial Active Pharmaceutical Ingredients (API) producers to prepare a practical, user-friendly guidance document integrating current GMP requirements into the EN-ISO 9001 QMS framework. To achieve this the working group have taken relevant features from the August 1996 CEFIC/EFPIA publication *"Good Manufacturing Practice for Active Ingredients Manufacturers"* and combined these with the relevant complementary requirements of EN-ISO 9001 *"Quality Systems: Model for quality assurance in design, development, production, installation and servicing"*. In the blood transfusion sector such integration has also taken place in South Africa. A comparison was made of ISO 9001, ISO Guide 25 Blood Transfusion Standards and current GMP (cGMP) Model of a Quality Management System within the Blood Transfusion Sector of South Africa. 1997.

Quality management was pioneered in industrial manufacturing but has found its way into healthcare sectors, blood transfusion services, medical pathology laboratories, hospitals and more recently finding its way in the service industry e.g., FedEx, and hotel chains.

Quality systems and quality management in transfusion medicine have gained considerable attention since the outbreak of the Human Immunodeficiency Virus (HIV) and the resultant Acquired Immunodeficiency Disease Syndrome (AIDS) epidemic. Risks of transmitting HIV, hepatitis C virus (HCV) and hepatitis B virus (HBV) are real threats to safety of transfusion lending itself to governments imposing higher standards in Blood Transfusion Practice (BTP). This has continued in the 21st century with the observed transmission through blood of prions (variant Creutzfeldt-Jakob disease), West Nile virus and Dengue virus. [6]

Much of the developed world has invested heavily in ensuring that blood and blood components are of exceptional quality. Extraordinary measures have been embraced to minimize the risk of transfusion-transmitted infection. These measures have included the introduction of Regulatory frameworks for blood and blood components and enhancing the applied science and technologies that support improved blood donor selection and screening and blood component manufacture.

4. What Constitutes a Quality Management System

Although quality management systems are documented international standards, the concepts for implementation is varied in different countries dependant on the human and financial resources, and social and economic infrastructure of a country.

The Human Development Index (HDI) is a composite statistic of life expectancy, education, and income indices to rank countries into four tiers of human development (Very High, High Medium and Low) published by the United Nations Development Programme[1]. [7] Countries with Low HDI would possibly lack the capacity for implementation of a quality system as quality gurus would define it. Quality system in these countries would be trying to maintain functional equipment, with associated reagent to perform testing possibly with documented procedures and a rudimentary system for staff training on the bench. On the other side of the continuum in a country classified as Very High HDI is the implemented quality system that is regulated by an inspection body to international standards with a system of process and product continuous improvement.

To ensure the provision of safe blood and blood components governments are developing strategies to ensure blood transfusion services operate within a regulatory environment.

Governments are dedicated to ensuring blood and blood components are manufactured in line with international Quality Standards. This may be national blood transfusion standards created by country work groups, national blood transfusion standards adopted from another country with appropriate similarities in standards, or government standards used for the manufacture of therapeutic products and pharmaceutical products i.e., cGMP guidelines (UK, Australia) or FDA guidelines or regulations (US). Harmonization of standards is more

---

[1] See also Chapter 15, Annex 4: HDI ranking.

common place. European Directorate for the Quality of Medicines and Healthcare (EDQM) has initiated a steering committee to define and promote the implementation of quality and safety standards in blood and blood components collection, storage, distribution and usage. (Guide to the Preparation, Use and Quality Assurance of Blood Components - current edition). [8]

To achieve such standards there are a number of organizations with specific blood transfusion expertise that support the development, implementation and maintenance of a quality system.

The World Health Organisation (WHO) supports the development of quality systems through technical advice, training and development of guidelines for quality system in blood transfusion. AABB operates in a consultancy capacity to train and support Blood Transfusion Services (BTS) in quality system implementation and is an accreditation body to assess the quality system operations of BTS according to AABB accreditation requirements. Blood Transfusion Societies are playing a pivotal role in the support of quality system implementation in developing countries with ISBT utilizing a quality management workgroup to develop quality indicators.

The African Society of Blood Transfusion (AfSBT) is hard at work in the development of a step-wise accreditation programme which will support Blood Transfusion Services in Africa to work towards implementation of a structured quality system and ultimately accreditation.

With harmonization of standards and assessment of Blood Transfusion Practices will create a more standardized approach to the implementation and maintenance of quality systems for the provision of safe blood to patients.

Like the rest of the developed world we now know that residual risks to the safety of transfused patients is predominantly in the hospital environment. Transfusing the wrong blood component to the wrong patient is the dominant risk of transfusion. The literal confusion of blood sample, blood component and patient identities results in the unintended transfusion of a blood component into the wrong patient at an unacceptable frequency.

Despite the relative tolerance of the blood group antigen systems to such mishaps, these 'wrong blood' episodes occasionally produce major morbidity and even fatalities.

It is recognized that as a community we have particular responsibilities and accountabilities with respect to transfusion safety and appropriateness. These reflect the need to meet the reasonable expectations of blood donors who entrust their precious gift to a collective of professionals. Blood donors anticipate that their gift will be optimally used by these professionals to improve the health of those in our community who depend on transfusion support. Additionally we face the very high expectations of those requiring transfusion, with expectations regarding safety for this supportive therapy being significantly greater than our community's typical expectations regarding safety of healthcare interventions. These expectations can only be achieved by applying the blood transfusion process (donor mobilization, blood collection, processing, testing and issuing of blood) to a suitable quality management system.

Lack of a unified body to take an overview of all aspects of blood safety sometimes making it difficult aligning effort with risks. Technological advances such as viral genomic detection may be mandated by regulatory authorities but prevention of transfusion errors requires local managerial and leadership commitment.

Much is known about best practice models of transfusion that offer optimum transfusion safety. These models have often been developed and predominantly discussed in environments 'outside' the environments where most blood often transfusion of blood and blood components actually occurs (hospital environments).

Much of contemporary Transfusion Medicine expertise lies in the areas of acute medical and surgical care. It is often the case that much of the knowledge regarding optimal transfusion practice has resided within the hospital Blood Bank, rather than being grounded within the clinical units and healthcare professional groups who commonly transfuse blood components to their patients. [9]

Transfusion Medicine expertise has largely resided within Blood Transfusion Societies, rather than being strong interests of those medical and nursing special interest groups who use transfusion as a common supportive therapy. Internationally it is the WHO, ISBT, AABB and other bodies that have enthusiastically embraced transfusion safety programmes rather than the international clinical societies whose members actively transfuse blood and blood components. WHO advocates that a well-organised, nationally co-ordinated blood transfusion service with an effective national quality system to achieve that blood components are safe, clinically effective and of appropriate and consistent quality.

The QS should cover all aspects of its activities and ensure traceability, from the motivation, mobilization and selection of blood donors to the transfusion of blood and blood components to patients. It should also reflect the structure, needs and capabilities of the BTS, as well as the needs of the hospitals and patients that it serves.

Blood Transfusion Services are moving towards a national governance model. However, this model has focused on the legislative and regulatory framework and setting up a National Blood Transfusion Service (NBTS) with a central national management structure to manage the motivation and mobilization of donors, blood collection, processing, testing and issuing of blood and blood components. While it has not significantly progressed into the arena of clinical transfusion practice, this arena offers the greatest potential to see changes in transfusion practice translate into enhanced patient safety.

4.1. National Governance Model for Blood

At present the impact of this transition has largely been apparent in the supply-side of the vein-to-vein transfusion 'safety chain'. There is support for the translation of a national governance model to include clinical transfusion practice.

Hospital Transfusion Committees and Hospital Transfusion Teams must be supported to allow meaningful monitoring and transfusion practice improvement and a national system of Haemovigilance.

Even more importantly there needs to be postgraduate workplace training in the pragmatics of safe and appropriate transfusion, including approaches to informing patients of the risks and benefits of transfusion.

There is a growing national and international experience of the use of a specially trained person within hospitals to support transfusion safety and appropriateness agendas. Indeed the experience of the pilot of the introduction of Transfusion Practitioners in Scotland has been followed by the national roll-out of Transfusion Nurses as a key platform within their national *"Better Blood Transfusion Programme"*.

Transfusion Nurses (Scotland) or Transfusion Safety Officers (North America) act as educators, trainers, coordinators of data collection, project managers and change agents. They are a critical component of hospital 'transfusion teams' and provide invaluable support for the efforts of the Hospital Transfusion Committee

These key individuals have various titles (Transfusion Nurse, Transfusion Nurse Specialist or Consultant, Transfusion Safety Officer, Haemovigilance Officer, Specialist Practitioner of Transfusion). They are usually recruited from nursing backgrounds. They act a vital 'bridge' between the different provider groups engaged in the transfusion 'safety chain', in particular those beyond the hospital laboratory

5. The Need and the Benefit of Quality

There is a continual need for introducing quality and the management thereof into organizations. Quality systems are designed implemented and maintained in organizations to ensure [10-13]:

Product Quality – Some primary aspects of product quality include: performance, reliability and durability. Through the use of a quality management programme, the organization can produce a product that performs according to international specifications and its stated promises. Quality management programmes help to improve the quality of a product, ensure that the product will endure normal everyday use and to design new products. Example of product quality in the blood transfusion sector may relate to final product meeting standards e.g., platelet concentration at a dosage level and within appropriate pH and volume.

Increased revenues – A quality management programme also removes inefficient processes within the system. By removing unnecessary processes, employee productivity usually increases since the employee is spending less time on activities that do not contribute to the product's quality. As a result, the employee is producing more work in less time while the company has not increased the salary. Quality management programmes help recapture lost monies due to inefficiencies. Many BTS are parastatal and funded by government. Hense there are restrictions on their operations and restricts acquisition of new equipment; but Quality Management System will enable process efficiencies which in turn will allow for funds to be used more effectively. Quality Management Systems are also beneficial in BTS which operate with a cost recovery system as a surplus of revenue can be used for process improvements, staff salaries, or acquisition of new equipment.

Customer Satisfaction – A Quality Management System ensures customer satisfaction:

a   Regular customer satisfaction surveys (donor and users) should be conducted to understand the qualities of the product important to the customer. Customer surveys can be used to target those features of a product or service that need improvement;

b   Customer satisfaction programmes should include systems for reporting and acting on product and service complaints to improve the organizations commitment to customer satisfaction;

c   A Haemovigilance programme provides for a surveillance system relating to serious adverse or unexpected events or reactions in donors or recipients, and the epidemiological follow-up of donors.

Reduce Waste – Quality management means that there is a systematic approach to keeping inventories at acceptable levels without incurring waste. Blood components have a shortened shelf life and as blood is a scarce commodity it is crucial to minimize wastage. Accurate data of blood usage as well as quality efficient testing and processing regimes are critical to reduce wastage. Procurement strategies for commodities to ensure First in First Out (FIFO) and economic order quantities (EOQ) are maintained will reduce the amount of inventory held that costs the organization money and occupies valuable space.

Teamwork – Quality Management Systems force organizational departments to work as a team. Different areas of the organization become reliant upon one another to produce a quality product that meets and exceeds the customers' expectations. A QS incorporates measures linking the various operations departments (donor motivation and mobilization , blood collection , processing, testing and issuing) with each other and with support services such as Information Technology (IT), Finance, Human Resource (HR) and Quality.

Quality systems will minimize clerical and process errors which if undetected may cause harm to patient. Any error, regardless of its severity and whenever it occurs in the chain of events leading to a transfusion , can have a detrimental effect on the outcome. All quality activities will help to ensure safe blood supply

Volunteer, non-remunerated blood donors create a unique social contract between themselves, BTS and those charged with ensuring optimal patient outcomes (the clinicians). Blood donors have a vested interest in knowing that the blood donated is handled and tested to strict quality standards ensuring that their donated blood will benefit not harm the patient.

Governments and industry in the developing and least developed countries make serious efforts to increase exports and reach new international markets. To attain success in global markets, it is essential that customers are satisfied with both non-price and price factors. Quality of the product and its conformance to customer requirements is very often the single most important consideration in securing export growth. In the blood transfusion environment there is less emphasis on export of products as blood is procured within a country to National or even International (EU) Blood Transfusion Standards and blood is generally issued within that country. However, excess frozen plasma is often exported to unique and specialised fractionation plants for further processing into derivatives such as albumin, Factor VII:C and immunoglobulins. As part of the manufacturers quality system the plasma (raw material) would need to comply to stringent internationally acceptable blood transfusion standards for collection and testing of blood donations. Final product manufactured by the fractionation plants according to cGMP (Pharmaceutical manufacturing codes) are then exported to other countries.

Standards/Guidelines for Blood Transfusion ensure that blood is collected tested and issued according to National/International standards and if the BTS or Blood Establishment is certified/accredited to international certification/

accreditation standards or manufactured according to cGMP there is good assurance that all precautions have been taken to provide safe , quality blood and blood components.

Quality and its management relating to blood donation testing is paramount in ensuring blood donations are free from Transfusion Transmissible Infections (TTI). Validation of methods for sensitivity and specificity for transfusion transmissible infection testing will improve safety of the blood supply.

Lower HIV prevalence in donors achieved through stringent selection and screening based on appropriate monitoring and evaluation activities.

Reduced seroprevalence rates in regular donors achieved by the application of quality principles to donor retention activities.

Good quality and good clinical outcomes promote voluntary blood donations as customers provide positive feedback to public which promotes voluntary blood donations.

Documentation and record keeping is a requirement in the quality system enabling process optimization with clear instructions for performing the work. Work records are maintained which provide traceability of all activities and an audit trail from donation to administration of blood to patient. In the event of look-back or recall of product the Quality Management System will support the action to trace the units and identify the status thereof.

6. Community Expectations

In a perfect world one would think that mankind would evolve to a higher order of perfection and with the evolution of cells, tissues, organs, systems would become more efficient over time. In a perfect world there would be order and predicted outcomes that would continuously improve processes to deliver optimal results for a better quality of life. In a perfect world there would be no loss of control, no change, no resource constraints, no external influencing factors, no human factors, and no physical factors to jeopardize the outcome. To achieve process control would require a vacuum from external influences, but the product will be influenced by the external environment once removed from the controlled setting.

As we try to understand the need for quality in Transfusion Medicine products and services, it may be helpful to explore the laws of entropy and the laws of physics. The law of entropy or the second law of thermodynamics is commonly used to explain order and disorder. Complementing this is the law of Maximum Entropy Production that considering the constraints, a system will select a path or paths to minimize the potential at the fastest rate. In other words, if dynamics that minimize the potential at the fastest rate considering the constraints, and if order is more efficient than disorder, then it is logical that order would and should be selected whenever possible. Ordered processes produce entropy faster than disorder. [14] Ensuring order out of disorder or minimizing disorder is the goal of quality in transfusion medicine.

Continuing the comparison to the world of physics, it is generally accepted that the laws of physics are universal and they serve as the basis for more modern physics. There is no doubt that humanity and quality of live have been enhanced by the both classic and modern physics. Although Sir Isaac Newton's understanding of physics may be attributed to a headache from the failing apple, the laws of physics which include mass and motion may help us understand the need for quality in products and services. The three laws of motion expressed in classical physics simply stated include:

- First law of motion or inertia states that an object continues at rest or uniform motion unless a force is applied;
- Second law states that if a net force is applied to an object the object will accelerate;
- The third law states that for every action there is an equal and opposite reaction.

The first law should be looked at as two parts. The first part of this law may appear intuitive; that is an object will continue at rest. But the second part of the law may be more difficult to understand since it states that the object will continue at a uniform velocity unless acted upon by an external force. If one looks at resistance, the friction of resistance can inhibit the velocity of the object. However if an external net positive force is applied to an object, as stated in the second law, the object will accelerate. The second law is based on mass and acceleration of the net force. The third law explains that if one force exerts force on another, it can either remain unaffected or have an equal and opposite effect on the first object.

In the biological world of Transfusion Medicine, products and services are also influenced by other objects, pathways or variables. Understanding the desired outcome and the controls that are required to deliver consistent products and services are influenced by many factors let alone the initial product or service attributes or requirements. Therefore comparison to the laws of physics in the desire to maintain properties of transfusion products and services may be helpful to understanding the need for quality.

Quality drives every aspect of designing the right product or service for the right reason or purpose, at the right time, at the desired and expected level of performance for the desired outcome. In other words, the goal of quality on product or service is to ensure the effectiveness, efficacy, and potency to deliver consistently upon expectations! So it could be safe to say that quality is determined by expectations. As the great US automotive industrialist Henry Ford said: "*Quality means doing it right when no one is looking.*"

The need for quality of Transfusion Medicine products and services starts with identification of consumers' needs and desired outcomes. Product, including service requirements must address who, what, when, why, where and all factors that influence the outcome. In other words identification of intended and unintended product requirements must be a robust process that includes the consumer. In Transfusion Medicine, the consumer includes the patient, the physician, and the society.

Unfortunately what has been missing for many decades, if not in the last century in medicine has been the focus on the patient as the consumer. Patient centric paradigm has been missing and hopefully should be the driver for quality in transfusion medicine. Continuing with the thoughts of order and disorder, it is helpful to look at the Rubik's cube to understand the paradigm shift needed to see new patterns in quality of patient care in transfusion medicine. For too long transfusion medicine has been industry focused and not patient focused. [15] Only when transfusion medicine focuses on patient requirements and patient blood management through the quality system will the new pattern of transfusion medicine emerge.

In 2011, Hofmann reported on five drivers that should be considered in shifting the paradigm from an industry view to the patient. [16] Hofmann points out that the modern health care system needs to shift from product focus, even if viewed from 'appropriate use', to patient blood management (PBM). The first driver is the aging population and the inherent increase in blood utilization in the elderly versus the decreasing donor population in developed countries. The complexity of Transfusion Medicine and the many different cost centers drives the product cost. The third driver is prevention of known, new and re-emerging pathogen while facing uncertainty over potential long silent carrier states. Fourth is the independent risk factor of adverse events associated with transfusion of blood products and finally the lack of evidence of benefit associated with transfusions. [16]

Over the years as transfusion medicine has evolved, it has become clear that the quality system must and should be the foundation of everything that is done in providing blood products and services to the patients and their physicians.

Just as the patient should be at the centre of our actions, the health care professionals and those within blood services should embrace the quality system. Since many variables can affect the quality of products and services, every person from the board of directors to the facility's maintenance staff must embrace the QS. Embracing includes not only awareness but participation in establish the need and monitoring processes.

In a perfect world Transfusion Medicine professionals and industry would perform and produce blood products based on the quality system to provide the right product based on patient requirements at the right time to ensure safety, efficacy and potency of the product. In a perfect world, the quality system would be embraced at all levels and processes would be controlled and monitored. In a perfect world, policies, processes, and procedures to ensure that expected quality of safety, efficacy and potency would be maintained. In a perfect world, training of the quality system and training to policies, processes, and procedures would be a normal expectation from the blood industry to the clinician to the patient.

7. Legal Aspects and Responsibilities/Accountability/Liabilities

In a perfect world we would also not need government policies and regulations to enforce quality of blood products used in transfusion medicine. Unfortunately we don't live in a perfect world and breaches in quality have lead government policies and regulations to step in in order to protect the patient. Many times these interventions were at the cost of life and via political intervention.

All one has to do is to go back three decades to view the evolution of quality in transfusion medicine and the blood/plasma production industry.

As with many improvements, risk to the patient, regulatory consequences, financial loss, and liability have been the primary drivers in establishment of the quality system within transfusion medicine.

Root cause analysis and risk analysis of forces or variables that could influence the safety, effectiveness and potency of blood products have been influential tools in improving quality outcomes to patients. The power of a risk analysis that leads to effective risk management and communication has created change in Transfusion Medicine.

In doing a risk analysis in a transparent environment facilitates public and patient trust. As risks are identified, whether infectious or non-infectious safety issues, risk management needs to contribute to the Quality System in a controlled process called risk communication (Figure 1). Although many risks have been associated with infectious diseases, the inherent risk of a blood donation and ultimate transfusion is a reality. When risks are identified the management needs to include a mechanism to engineer out the risk. The engineering process can be donor questions for potential deferral, testing strategies, pathogen reduction technologies, or physical engineering of equipment.

Within governments the need to ensure the quality of blood products to protect the patient and the donor requires a coordinated system which not only includes policy and regulations but also surveillance and research. Figure 2 represents a model that used in the United States to advance public health and protect patients and donors of blood components. The intersection of the Venn diagram is theoretically where all aspects of public health intersect for the protection of donor health and patient health.

There are several agencies within the US Department of Health and Human Services that have regulatory control, although the immediate impression is the FDA, agencies such as the Health Resources and Services Administration (HRSA) and the financial arm of health care, that is the Centers for Medicare and Medicaid Services (CMS) empower regulatory control which drive the needs in quality control.

Research that affects quality through the advancement of science and medicine is not only influenced by the National Institutes of Health (NIH) but also the Centers for Disease Control and Prevention (CDC) and the FDA. Surveillance of public health is also performed by the CDC, HRSA through contracts managed under contracts with the organ community, and the FDA for the monitoring of adverse reactions of licensed products and fatal outcomes.

As mentioned previously, the quality systems in many biological products were introduced into in the 1980s. Unfortunately the momentum for this was driven by the emerging infectious disease that was eventually known as HIV and the clinical manifestation of AIDS.

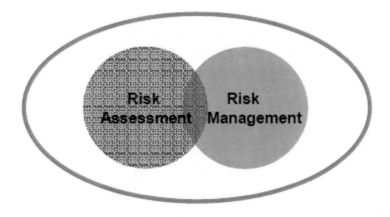

Risk Communication

Figure 1. The communication between risk assessment and risk management.

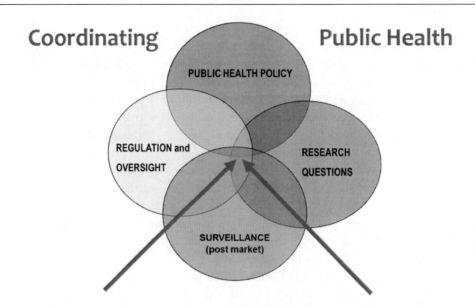

Figure 2. Interaction of various public health agencies in the US model to monitor patient and product safety within the quality system.

The introduction of HIV into the blood and plasma supply forced public health to ensure that look back from recipient to donor and also from donor to recipient was instituted.

Quality was gradually introduced to ensure the safety of the blood supply although some blood collections refused conform. In the late 1980's the American Red Cross (ARC) was put on warning for its quality breaches and out of control processes; eventually in 1993 the FDA lowered the boom. [17] The FDA has procedures to resolve disagreements in findings with the licensed facility. [18] A consent decree is the final attempt to court mediate compliance to GMPs. By the late 1990s the ARC and others such as the New York Blood Center and the Blood Systems Inc. were all under court ordered consent decrees; collectively this represented the majority of the US blood supply. Fortunately the New York Blood Center and Blood Systems, Inc. have been able to satisfy the court. Both organizations emerged from this compliance order as new organizations embracing the quality system. [19]

The ARC remains under its second consent decree and continues to be under the quality magnifying glass of the FDA as well as the Federal Courts. [20] In April 2012, the ARC paid over $9.5M in fines for its latest failures to comply. [21] Under the 2003 Consent Decree fines can be assessed against the ARC as follows:

- $10,000 per event (and $10,000 per day) for any violation of an ARC standard operating procedure (SOP), the law, or consent decree requirement and timeline. SOPs are written procedures that are designed to help ensure product quality;
- $50,000 for the preventable release of each unit of blood for which FDA determines that there is a reasonable probability that the product may cause serious adverse health consequences or death, as well as $5,000 for the release of each unit that may cause temporary problems, up to a maximum of $500,000 per event;

- $50,000 for the improper re-release of each unsuitable blood unit that was returned to ARC inventory;
- $10,000 for each donor inappropriately omitted from the National Donor Deferral Registry, a list of all unsuitable donors.

North of the US border, Canada also faced turbulent judicial review of their blood supply system. Under Judge Krever's investigation, the quality and effectiveness of the Canadian blood supply was questions and recommendations resulted in a total revamping of the Canadian system. [22] The Canadian Red Cross was reorganized to form Canadian Blood Service. Patients infected with hepatitis were compensated for transfusion transmission through the blood and plasma supply.

In the early 1990s questions started to percolated through the political channels to question the lack of action that lead to the spread of HIV through the blood and plasma supply. The HIV crisis and the lack of the quality system especially in the decision making process had an enormous impact of the lives of over 16,000 haemophiliacs. The lack of decisions to protect the blood supply continues to be felt by the brotherhood of haemophiliacs that have endured the trauma of the lack of the quality decision making processes to protect them from HIV and hepatitis, both hepatitis B and C.

In 1993, US Senators Kennedy and Graham requested former Secretary of Health and Human Services, Donna Shalala to have the Institute of Medicine (IOM) to review the events of the 1980 and the introduction of HIV into the blood supply. Although there was a general understanding that the US blood supply was the safest in the world, there was general consensus that results of such a study would be beneficial in strengthen the quality systems of the blood and plasma supply. The IOM convened its study and called expert witness to discuss the tragic events and the decision making processes. The IOM reviewed the events of the past decision making process and the public health organization that supported those decision. The report, *HIV and the Blood Supply: An Analysis of Crisis Decision Making, made 14 recommendations in 1995.* [23]

Based on this report, former Secretary Donna Shalala established a task force headed by the Assistant Secretary of Health. During 1996, this task force reviewed the IOM report and investigated the blood safety decision making process. Based on the internal HHS task force, former Secretary Shalala testified before Congress about changes in HHS she would make to enhance blood safety and availability.

Former Secretary Shalala testified before the House Committee on Government Reform and Oversight that she designated the Assistant Secretary for Health (ASH) as the HHS Blood Safety Director who would respond to blood safety issues with broad public health and societal implications that cannot be resolved through analysis of scientific data alone. Although this role has not been codified in written legislation since Secretary Shalala's testimony, the ASH has acted on behalf of the Secretary in the role of Blood Safety Director. Thus, the ASH coordinates blood safety and availability issues across the Government. This coordination relies on experts within the government as well as external to the government. Advisory committees from the private and public sector supports the President's Executive Branch to make recommendations to ensure blood safety, quality, surveillance, and availability of blood components and plasma derivatives.

Another major event that created the need for data elements of the quality system was the establishment of the Patient Safety and Quality Improvement Act of 2005 also known as the

Patient Safety Act provided for establishment of Patient Safety Organizations (PSOs). Through non-government funded organizations, confidential data could be collected, aggregated, and analyzed regarding the quality and safety of healthcare delivery. As authorized by the Secretary of HHS, its Agency for Health and Research Quality was charged to coordinate the development of a set of common definitions and reporting formats that allowed healthcare providers to voluntarily collect and submit standardized information regarding patient safety events. This introduction of voluntary collection and analysis was a boost to haemovigilance, a significant element of the quality system. In 2008 the AABB was recognized as a PSO with the requirement to report back to its participants every 24 months. This system complements the a system established within the CDC's National Healthcare Surveillance Network. Both the PSO and the CDC's haemovigilance are protected under law. This is significant in voluntary reporting errors and adverse outcomes for continuous process improvement and standards for quality. As a result of both of these programmes, transfusion safety officers have started to be employed within healthcare systems.

As mentioned in the preceding paragraphs, professional standards establish the need for quality and the data to monitor process control. Not only is the AABB influential in establishing standards of practice not only for blood products, but cellular therapies. The Plasma Protein Therapeutic Association (PPTA) accredits plasma centres against its quality standards. Although these two organizations are specific for blood, plasma, and cellular products within transfusion, the College of American Pathologist also establishes quality standards for the general laboratory.

An effort toward patient blood management was first approached by the Society for Advancement of Blood Management (SABM). The Joint Commission (TJC) for healthcare facilities recognized the importance of the patient quality measures that were being fostered by organizations such as SABM and AABB. This recognition by TJC resulted in the establishment of a technical advisory panel to develop a matrix for performance measures. The performance measure framework was a proposed systematic approach to the establishment of criteria that potentially could influence quality and ultimately patient care. The panel systematically approached transfusion management from the patient. Peer reviewed data was sought for support of the transfusion parameters, unfortunately the parameters often lacked significant controlled data to support performance measures. This was unfortunate since the data collection by itself would have built a body of knowledge needed in transfusion medicine. As a result the National Quality Forum turned down the elements in 2011. [24] The parameters remain in TJC library and can be used as quality measures by any facility.

Most recently quality issues continue to come to the attention of both the medical professional and politicians. The FDA's Blood Product Advisory Committee received a statement by the AABB on the organizations position on bacterial contamination and their standard to address the issue. Bacterial contamination of platelet concentrates is a problem that plagues the quality system and platelet manufacturing. [25, 26] Progress has been made with initial blood diversion pouches from the collection site. Yet, both technical and engineering solutions need to be focused on this health hazard.

In October 2012, the National Association for Healthcare Quality offered five recommendations to improve institutional quality, safety reporting and staff protection.

These recommendations include accountability on safety and quality, ensuring accurate, comprehensive and transparent data collection, promoting teamwork and enhanced communication. These recommendations should not come as a surprise since they embrace fundamentals of the quality system, rather they emphasis the need for continuous process improvement in the quality journey.

Conclusion and Take Home Message

Transfusion Medicine and the blood, plasma and cellular therapies' have focused on the quality system. This sense of quality has strengthened the blood supply and is now viewed as its foundation. As a result the world's blood supply continues to improve towards a safety system. Although residual risk of transfusion of blood, plasma or cellular therapies remain, the supply is viewed today as safe. The journey to this destination was encountered by challenges such as the AIDS crisis but the outcome was quality standards established by professional organizations and regulations. The many victims of the AIDS crisis and the consequences of poor quality standards of the past, is a constant reminder to the Transfusion Medicine specialist and the blood bank professional that the journey to excellence is not a final destination but a continuous pathway for improvement.

Quality principles have migrated from inspection to quality control which focuses on testing of product to ensure that product complies. The paradigm shift is the change from quality assurance to management of quality (Quality Management and then Total Quality Management). Current quality improvement cultures are measured through business excellence models such as the European Foundation for Quality Management (EFQM), in the UK the British Quality Foundation (BQF), in US Malcolm Baldrige Award and in Canada 'Canada Awards for Excellence'. Overarching International Quality Management standards such as ISO have been developed by committees to set global requirements for managing quality in a range of industries (manufacturing, service, laboratories). Industry specific standards, for example Blood Transfusion Standards/Guidelines have been developed nationally and internationally (e.g., EC implementation Directives 2004/33 and 2006/62) for the provision of safe blood to patients, and National *e.g., AABB and BBTS) and International Societies (e.g., ISBT) are providing quality support through the extension of a quality management body of knowledge to blood transfusion practices. In many countries the Blood Transfusion Practices are incorporated into the pharmaceutical cGMP regulatory system. There are extensive lists of various quality management standards and guidelines across different industries and countries. Harmonization of standards is at present an opportunity to minimize variations in standards and is ongoing (e.g., EU, CoU, AABB, AfSBT). The need for quality and its management is paramount to achieving a quality product that meets the needs of the customers. Quality Management has become a science in all industries across the globe and this is evident when researching current trends in quality management and the large number of Quality Managers employed in organizations to manage quality. Blood Transfusion Sectors are dependent on the adequate design, implementation and maintenance of quality systems to ensure the provision of adequate, safe, quality blood and blood components to patients and aim to achieve recognition of the fully implemented Quality Management System through accreditation/certification.

References

[1]   http://www.slideshare.net/krishnakant1/02historyquality

[2]   Dale, B. G. *Managing Quality.* 2nd edition. 1994. UK. Prentice Hall International.

[3]   http://www.businessballs.com/dtiresources/quality_management_ history.pdf

[4]   http://en.wikipedia.org/wiki/Quality_management_system#Concept_of_quality_-historical_ background

[5]   http://www.qualityregister.co.uk/what-is-quality-assurance.html

[6]   Editorial. Dengue in the context of "safe blood" and global epidemiology: to screen or not to screen? Lanteri, M. C. and Bush, M. P. *Transfusion* 2012;52:1634-1639

[7]   http://en.wikipedia.org/wiki/Human_Development_Index

[8]   Guide to the Preparation, Use and Quality Assurance of Blood Components. Annex to Recommendation No. R(95)15, Committee of Ministers of the Council of Europe. Latest edition, Strasbourg, F Council of Europe Publishing.

[9]   www.cec.health.nsw.gov.au/documents/programs/blood-watch/better-safer-transfusion.pdf

[10] http://www.ehow.com/about_5377881_importance-quality-management.html

[11] www.who.int/bloodproducts/quality_safety/.../AM_quality_system.5

[12] http://www.transfusionguidelines.org.uk/index.aspx?Publication=rbandSection=25andpageid=743

[13] WHO Editorial team. 2005. Quality Management Training for Blood Transfusion Services.

[14] *Ecological psychology*, 3(4), 317-348 Copyright c 1991, Lawrence Erlbaum Associates, Inc.

[15] Barr, P. J., Donnelly, M., Cardwell, C. R., Parker, M., Morris, K., Bailie, K. E. M. The appropriateness of red blood cell use and the extent of over transfusion: right decision? Right amount? *Transfusion* 2011;51: 1684-1694

[16] Hofmann, A., Farmer, S., Shander, A. Five Drivers Shifting the Paradigm from Product-Focused Transfusion Practice to Patient Blood Management. *The Oncologist* 2011;16(suppl. 3):3–11.

[17] Newman, R. J., Podolsky, D., Loeb, P. *Bad Blood* in: US News and World Report. 19 June 1994.

[18] *Guidance for Industry Formal Dispute Resolution: Scientific and Technical Issues Related to Pharmaceutical CGMP.* US Department of Health and Human Services, Food and Drug Administration, Center for Drug Evaluation and Research (CDER), Center for Biologics Evaluation and Research (CBER), Center for Veterinary Medicine (CVM), Office of Regulatory Affairs (ORA), Pharmaceutical CGMPs. Washington, D.C. January 2006 OMB Control Number 0910-0563.

[19] Finding the Right Consultant for dealing with an FDA Injunction. May 2003. Available from http://mdiconsultants.com/Section_NI/Insights/ insight_V6_is3.htm

[20] American Red Cross Agrees to Revised Consent Decree to Improve Blood Safety. April 2003. Available from http://www.scienceblog.com/community/older/archives/M/2/fda 1398.htm.

[21] Bonnin, E. *United States* v. *American National Red Cross,* Civil Action No. 93-0948 (JOP). Baltimore, MD. March 2012.

[22] http://www.cbc.ca/archives/categories/health/public-health/the-krever-report-canadas-tainted-blood-disaster/topic---the-krever-report-canadas-tainted-blood-disaster.html

[23] Stoto, M. *HIV and the Blood Supply: An Analysis of Crisis Decision making.* Washington, D.C. October 30, 1997

[24] Implementation Guide for The Joint Commission Patient Blood Management Performance Measures The Joint Commission, Chicago, IL Available from http://www.jointcommission.org/patient_blood_management_performance_measures_project/

[25] Carr-Greer, M. A. Considerations for Options to Further Reduce the Risk of Bacterial Contamination in Platelets. Rockville, M. D. September 2012. Available from http://www.aabb.org/pressroom/ statements/Pages/statement092112.aspx.

[26] Oh, J. National Association for Healthcare Quality Offers 5 Recommended Practices for Quality. October 2012. Available from 5-recommended-practices-for-quality.html

In: Quality Management in Transfusion Medicine
Editor: Cees Th. Smit Sibinga

ISBN: 978-1-62618-665-1
© 2013 Nova Science Publishers, Inc.

Chapter III

Quality and Quality Management Systems Applicable in Transfusion Medicine

Cees Th. Smit Sibinga[1], Christian Seidl[2],
Eduardo Nunes[3] and James P. AuBuchon[4]*

[1]International Development of Transfusion Medicine,
ID Consulting for International Development of Transfusion Medicine (IDTM),
University of Groningen, Zuidhorn, NL
[2]Experimental Haematology, Johann Wolfgang Goethe University Hospital and
Vice Medical Director Institute of Transfusion Medicine and Immunohaematology,
Red Cross Blood Donor Service Baden-Württemberg – Hessen,
Frankfurt am Main, DE
[3]Policy, Standards, and Global Development, AABB, Bethesda
[4]President and CEO Puget Sound Blood Center, Seattle, WA, USA

Abstract

The vein-to-vein transfusion chain contains two distinct elements – 1) the procurement part, focused on the manufacturing of blood components from blood donated by voluntary blood donors; and 2) the clinical prescription and use of blood components in the hospitals.

To allow consistent preparation and use of blood components that are safe and clinically efficacious, an appropriate quality system should be put in place that covers both the administration as well as the technical operations of facilities involved in the chain.

This chapter describes and discusses the different managerial and operational systems available and their applicability in transfusion medicine.

* Tel: +31-6-2223.4325; E-mail: c.sibinga@planet.nl.

Keywords: Quality system, Quality management, ISO, GMP, ISQua, EFQM, DOMAINE, EuBIS, Optimal Blood Use

1. Introduction

There are several good reasons for a Blood Establishment to develop and implement a quality management system. Quality management systems are an important aspect of standardizing the Blood Establishment's performance of critical tasks. In implementing a quality management system framework, it is important for the Blood Establishment's leadership to understand how existing quality systems such as Good Manufacturing Practice (GMP) and ISO 9000 are complementary, with slightly different areas of emphasis. Whatever system is introduced, it will need active involvement and support from the Blood Establishment's management team to make it work.

Under a quality management system, the Director of the Blood Establishment will be able to demonstrate that the components that are made and the services that are offered under his final responsibility are of a good, consistent and reliable quality and safety. To accomplish this, a Quality Manual is needed. The Quality Manual describes the Quality System and Management in such a way that others (outsiders) will be able to evaluate the reliability of the Blood Establishment. The legal principle of product liability applies although in some countries this is being covered by so called Blood Shield Acts. The clinicians prescribing and using the various blood components want to achieve demonstrable clinical improvement of their patients (clinical outcome).

These improvements in clinical condition are observable (organ function) and measurable (Hb, platelet count or Ht). To achieve predictable improvements the quality of the products must be of a specified and consistent level of quality and efficacy, and should have a minimum risk of adverse events. For this reason clinicians receiving units from the Blood Establishment will also rely on the quality management system used by the Blood Establishment.

When the results of a blood transfusion are predictable there will be a much more efficient and appropriate use of these products. Here legally the principle of the Hippocratic medical ethics *primum est non nocere* or 'first do no harm' apply. That means in essence the moral-ethical and professional protection of the rights of the ultimate 'customer', i.e., the patient.

The Ministry of Health is ultimately responsible for the wellbeing of the citizens and would like to assure the community that the blood supply is optimally safe, presenting minimum risk of adverse events and a reliable beneficial effect of blood transfusion. Also it would like to promote optimal accessibility and affordability. The international legal principles of the UN Declaration of Universal Human Rights apply. [1]

The patient, who is ultimately the most important party in this matter, will not be fully able to judge the quality and safety of blood products provided, and must therefore rely on the Blood Establishment, the clinician, and the Ministry of Health. Legally the principles of consumer rights and consumer protection apply.

1.1. Quality Systems

There are a number of quality and quality management systems available which can be applied to the procurement and clinical use of blood. Some are more process- and operations-oriented and others deal more with the management aspects, securing a quality environment and culture necessary for consistency and reliability of the operational processes.

1.1.1. HACCP

HACCP is product oriented.

The most simple system is the Hazard Analysis and Critical Control Points System (HACCP). [2] This system is often used in the food sector. It describes the hazard analysis and defines the points where special attention must be paid to avoid the production of unsafe or even dangerous products.

1.1.2. Good Practice (GP)

GP is production or process oriented.

The most appropriate system for a Blood Establishment is Good Manufacturing Practice (GMP). This system was developed in the USA after the so called Thalidomide affair. It was first published as part of the Food, Drug and Cosmetics Act Amendments in 1962, and was implemented for the manufacture of human drugs in 1963. The U.S. Congress amended the Biologics Act in 1970 to include blood and blood components or derivatives, and in 1975, FDA published GMP regulations for the collection, processing, and storage of human blood and blood components. [3] It took some time to establish the first GMP rules in Europe and since 1992 there is the EU Directive about the *"GMP for Proprietary Medicinal Products for Human and Veterinary Use"*. [4]

Blood products have a therapeutic purpose and should therefore be considered to be produced in accordance to pharmaceutical principles. Because in many cases a regulatory framework for biologics came into existence after regulations for pharmaceuticals, approaching GMP rules requires understanding the similarity and differences between blood products and pharmaceuticals. The procurement of the active starting material – whole blood, a living tissue – is completely different from the purchasing of active ingredients for medicinal products. Human blood or plasma is collected under aseptic conditions and these have to be guaranteed during processing. The batch size of blood components is limited to each whole blood donation and the production of a few blood components thereof. In the pharmaceutical industry the starting materials are raw and need to be processed into aseptic finished products through usually large batch sizes.

GMP for pharmaceuticals do not provide requirements for storage and transport of the product, where these requirements are critical for blood and blood components. For this reason the EU Commission Directive 2005/62/EC contains the GMP for blood components. This Directive is mandatory for EU Member States since August 31, 2006. [5] The GMP for medicinal products mostly concerns the purchasing, production and quality control (procurement) of the various components. This implies the involvement of a restricted number of departments within the organization.

1.1.3. PIC/S

The Pharmaceutical Inspection Convention and Pharmaceutical Inspection Co-operation Scheme (jointly referred to as PIC/S), based in Geneva, are two international instruments between countries and pharmaceutical inspection authorities, which provide together an active and constructive co-operation in the field of GMP.

PIC/S' mission is "*to lead the international development, implementation and maintenance of harmonised Good Manufacturing Practice (GMP) standards and quality systems of inspectorates in the field of medicinal products.*"

This is to be achieved by developing and promoting harmonised GMP standards and guidance documents; training competent authorities, in particular inspectors; assessing (and reassessing) inspectorates; and facilitating the co-operation and networking for competent authorities and international organisations. There are currently 40 participating Authorities in PIC/S (Convention and Scheme taken together).

In 2001 PIC/S developed and entered in force a GMP Guide for Blood Establishments. [6] The document gives an insight into the thinking and concerns of inspectorates and could provide useful information for Blood Establishments relating to the collection, processing, storage and distribution, and the quality control and quality assurance of blood and blood components.

The purpose is to provide guidance for GMP-inspectors to use during inspections of blood establishments. It is intended that guidelines already in place or intended to be used by a Competent Health Authority, the European Commission, Council of Europe and WHO or any other authorized body would be used in conjunction with the PIC/S GMP guide. The GMP guide for Blood Establishments intends only to provide guidance that is specific for blood establishments including apheresis establishments, and for blood components for immediate clinical use.

1.1.4. ISO

ISO is quality management and leadership oriented.

ISO as an abbreviation of the International Organization for Standardization, has developed a series of quality standards for management and leadership –

- ISO 26000 - Social responsibility;
- ISO 31000 - Risk management;
- ISO 50001 - Energy management;
- ISO 9000 - Quality management;
- ISO 14000 - Environmental management.

These are actually the best known of what ISO is offering. Most of them are modelled on the management system structure of ISO 9001 and ISO 14001, which are requirements and thus certifiable, where the others provide guidance and are not certifiable, e.g., ISO 26000 giving guidance on social responsibility, and ISO 31000 of which the ISO 31000:2009 (*Risk Management – Principles and guidelines*) provides principles and generic guidelines on risk management that can be used by any organization or institution in any sector. The ISO norms are global standards for a quality management system. However, the certificate does not guarantee the quality of the products produced.

ISO 9001:2008 –

The current ISO 9001:2008 edition [7] has more clear standards and a better alignment with the ISO 14001 (published in 2000) standards for environmental management. [8]

Although ISO 9000 series was first published in 1987, it is in origin older than GMP. It was originally developed in 1969 by NATO after the second World War and named: Allied Quality Assurance Publications (AQAP). AQAP is an American standard for quality assurance specially developed for the war industry where it is impossible to have any inside information about the production and quality control. [9]

ISO 9000 series is the civil version of the AQAP and is therefore organization and management oriented. It involves all departments of the organization, including the top management. The ISO 9000 series consisted of 4 elements and originally contained 20 separate clauses. The second edition of ISO 9000 (ISO 9000:1994) introduced the 'supplier chain' and quality is defined as the level of satisfaction of the customer.

The system assures the consistency and reliability of the product quality and has been restructured in 4 major chapters clustering and consolidating the original 20 clauses. The current 2008 edition is largely focused on the environment with emphasis on customer satisfaction and therefore demand driven rather than supply (production) driven. [7]

1.1.5. EFQM

EFQM or Total Quality Management provides an approach to manage all aspects of quality. In Europe the European Foundation of Quality Management (EFQM) has been developed and has introduced a few new aspects of quality [10] –

- the customer,
- the employees and
- the results or outcomes.

EFQM describes 5 levels of development –

- product orientation (QC),
- process orientation (QA,GMP),
- system orientation (GMP, ISO9001:2000),
- chain orientation and
- total quality management (EFQM).

It also contains a new approach to self-inspection to allow analysis of the level of the quality and quality management system from a simple level up to Total Quality Management or TQM.

1.1.6. ISQua

ISQua is quality management and leadership oriented.

The International Society for Quality in Health Care (ISQua) offers a unique opportunity to share expertise via an international multidisciplinary forum. The focus is on management of the care processes. [11]

ISQua is supported and funded by members, including leading quality health care providers and agencies in over 70 countries, and additional funds from the Irish Government. ISQua is formally recognized by the World Health Organisation as being in 'Official Relations' with WHO. ISQua is assisting with technical and policy advice based on evidence and best practices and contributing to knowledge sharing as part of WHO initiatives.

ISQua has developed international principles for health care standards and an accreditation system to assess compliance. The first edition was published in 1997 with a second edition implemented in 2004. These two editions followed five principles.

Since 2008 there is a revised third edition. This third edition shows an increased emphasis on safety and has six principles –

- Quality Improvement:
- Patient/Service User Focus;
- Organisational Planning and Performance;
- Safety;
- Standards Development;
- Standards Measurement.

The common approach is a document with four elements, consisting of Leadership; Resource Management; Safety Management; Patient Care, containing the relevant quality management standards for a Health Care Institution.

The Canadian Society for International Health has designed an ISQua based quality management system for the blood supply and clinical treatment of patients with blood and blood components. This variant consists of five elements - Leadership; Resource Management; Safety Management; Donor and Recipient Care; and Process Control.

1.1.7. ASQ

The American Society for Quality is staff-oriented.

ASQ offers a number of different certification programmes for professionals in almost any industry. ASQ certification is becoming more common in the transfusion medicine community among individuals who work in the quality assurance. [12]

Many of the certifications offered by ASQ are based on quality management systems described in this chapter; for example, through ASQ an individual may become a certified HACCP auditor. ASQ also offers certification in other well-known quality management oriented frameworks, such as Lean and Six Sigma.

1.1.8. No Quality System

An organization without a system for quality (QS) and quality management (QMS) has no control over the quality of the products. Much attention will have to be paid to quality control (QC) and quality assurance (QA) to avoid the distribution of products that might cause any damage to the user. This will result in repair or rework activities, with consequently can result in the following:

- Extra costs: money and man power
- The risk of loss of confidence and trust

- Prosecution by customers that are injured by a product, and
- Claims for the cost for medical care and financial compensation.

Development and implementation of a quality system and quality management may seem to cost much money. However, as an important investment on the long run it will save even more money. These costs are likely to be repaid many times over in avoiding the even greater costs associated with rework and dealing with dissatisfied customers and regulators.

2. Management Oriented Quality and Quality Management Systems

2.1. ISO 9001:2008

2.1.1. Introduction

The ISO 9000 family addresses quality management, which means that the organization shall fulfil the customer's quality requirements and the applicable regulatory requirements, while aiming to enhance customer satisfaction and achieve continual improvement of its performance in pursuit of these objectives.

ISO 9001 is a system and management oriented quality system. It is universally applicable to all small and large organizations and industries. In the course of the development of the first three versions the supplier chain plays a more and more important role. In the last version of 2008, however, environment with customer satisfaction became dominant. The entire vein-to-vein blood transfusion chain is divided over two different organizations with different legal obligations and responsibilities: the blood establishment (procurement institution) and the hospital (consumer).

The responsibilities of both parties must be agreed upon at top management levels and must be documented in the contract between both parties. The management will, while taking into account the customer product or service requirements, set-up the resource management so that the product(s) or services can be made and offered. Customer satisfaction must be measured and together with internal measurements and analysis this must result in the implementation of improvements. This is an ongoing process that has to be covered by a continuously improving Quality Management System.

The 9001:2008 edition of the ISO system consists of 9 chapters of which the ultimate standards are captured in 4 major chapters [7] –

- Chapter 5 - Management Responsibility
- Chapter 6 - Resource Management
- Chapter 7 - Product Realization
- Chapter 8 - Measurement, Analysis and Improvement

The original 20 clauses of the previous versions have been clustered in the current 9001:2008 edition.

2.1.2. Quality Management

A quality system not only should be developed and implemented, it also has to be maintained and continuously improved. In other words, it has to be managed.

All processes throughout the entire organization and their sequence and interaction must be analyzed and described. These processes are not limited to the core business but include the processes from the supportive and managerial or steering departments, including the Director and resources (materials, consumables, means, human, finance, etc).

Special attention must be paid to the Critical Control Points (CCPs) and Quality System Essentials (QSEs) to ensure that processes are performed continuously in the same way resulting in outcomes that meet customer requirements (fit for purpose).

An essential part of the quality system is the monitoring and evaluation of all processes in order to detect needs for improvement of processes, procedures, equipment, people etc.

The four key elements of the Quality Management System are:

- Mission Statement and Quality Policy and Strategy, and Quality Plan;
- Process descriptions; Job descriptions (1)[1]
- Job descriptions (2) and work instructions (SOPs), including effective planning, operations and control of the processes;
- Forms, records, reports needed to document all activities.

The first two elements together represent the Quality Manual.

The Quality Policy and Strategy must describe the interrelationships of the various processes and if applicable why certain element(s) is / are excluded from the quality management system. All documents as mentioned in the four elements must be controlled.

This implies that all documents have to be carefully developed, approved and authorized, implemented, reviewed regularly, legible and readily identifiable. They have to fit into a clear though simple identification or numbering system, starting at the top. This will allow easy traceability and identification of any document in use. Changes in documents must be clear and staff must be informed (trained) about them. Documents (from external origin) must be controlled, that is to say only current versions must be available where they are needed. One copy of each superseded version must be archived for at least 10 years.

2.1.3. Management Responsibility

Any Quality System not adequately and/or sufficiently supported by Top Management is doomed to fail. Therefore it is required that Top Management proves its involvement in the Quality Management by:

- set–up and maintenance of a Mission Statement of the organization that makes clear the need to fulfil customer, statutory and regulatory requirements;
- set-up and maintenance of a Quality Policy and Strategy;
- having monitored and evaluated the quality objectives;
- performing periodic management reviews;
- providing sufficient resources (money, materials, personnel, etc.).

---

[1] Job descriptions at level 2 represent the hierarchical need for positions in order to implement processes.

Sub a) - Customer requirements or expectations must be met and this must be regularly checked by analyzing customer satisfaction. This is not limited to product or service characteristics but concerns also (post)-delivery activities, intended use, and where applicable statutory and / or regulatory requirements.

Sub b) - The Mission Statement must be worked out by Top Management in the Quality Policy and Strategy (QPandS). This QPandS proves the commitment to meet all necessary requirements and the continuous improvement of the quality and efficiency of the products, services and organization *per se*. It describes all measures taken to maintain and improve the quality objectives. The QPandS must be maintained and reviewed regularly by Top Management and consequently implemented in the organization.

Sub c) - All CCPs and QSEs as analyzed, detected and/or recognized must be monitored.

The results of these monitoring procedures must be evaluated resulting where appropriate in improvement(s). The activities mentioned under 'Quality Management' must be carefully planned in order to be continuously developed, maintained, reviewed and implemented. Also authorities and responsibilities must be monitored and evaluated. These activities are performed by the management representative (the Quality Manager.)

Sub d) - Regularly, at least once a year, planned management review must be performed. The review input aspects must be described including the expected review output.

Sub e) - see Resource Management

2.1.4. Resource Management

To meet all the quality aspects there must be sufficient resources available, within a good infrastructure and a good working environment. The resources include personnel, starting materials and reagents. The infrastructure includes premises, equipment and supporting services like technical and civil service, (internal) transport and communication. A good work environment is needed to meet the product requirements and specifications.

2.1.5. Product Realization

General – Planning for product realization in transfusion medicine is somewhat different from other organizations and industries. The basis for this planning is donor management.

A good and stable population of reliable, regular and non-remunerated donors is the best guarantee for a continuous input of quality whole blood and thus a continuous availability of blood products.

In addition to donor mobilization, this requires a good degree of planning e.g. the Blood Establishment must have an adequate stock of materials such as blood bags and sufficient reagents to test the collected whole blood units.

Measures must have been taken to guarantee e.g., continuous power supply.

New product – If new processes or procedures will be developed, or if current processes or procedures will be changed, the new or changed procedures need to be validated.

Validation is the comparison of the results of the design and development output with the design and development input. If a Blood Establishment wants or needs to introduce a new product or service, the product or service has to be well designed. A design should be reviewed, verified and validated.

This implies the testing of the processes used to produce and deliver the new product (e.g., comparison of performance to specifications defined by the manufacturer or in the literature) as well as fulfilment of statutory and regulatory requirements. Where possible comparison of new product to the same product made by other Blood Establishment(s) can be performed.

Purchasing – The most critical starting material is the collected whole blood. Therefore all units must be collected and tested as required by national and/or international law.

Specifications of all other critical goods must be known and tested so as to achieve continuous quality of the final product(s). These products may only be purchased from qualified suppliers. The qualification process is based on supplier specifications and a supplier audit.

Production – All production processes must be described. Work instructions (SOPs), equipment manuals (EOPs) must be available in order to prove that products are continuously produced in the same way. As the processes and procedures are validated this will result in a constant quality of the products.

A Batch Manufacturing Record (BMR) or Manufacturing Formula and Processing Instructions (MFPI) must be completed for every production run[2] for identification and traceability reasons. Production includes the labelling, handling, packaging, storage of the constituting parts and the final product.

Control of measuring devices – Final products must meet set specifications or standards.

To be sure that the measuring devices, monitoring tools and/or computers are reliable they must be tested by means of validation, calibration, proficiency testing.

This includes ongoing evaluations of the competence of personnel performing these tests.

2.1.6. Measurement, Analysis and Improvement

General – Each organization must be able to demonstrate the conformity of the products. Records of quality management activities should provide evidence that the establishment's processes are in control and that the quality management system is continually improving.

For this reason, results of monitoring activities, including customer satisfaction, internal audits, and tracking and trending of non-conformances must be reviewed. The results of these activities must be analyzed and translated into corrective and preventive actions.

Customer satisfaction – Organizations must be informed about the level of satisfaction of customers. This can be achieved by active questioning or more passively, via complaints.

Internal audits – Part of the Quality Plan is the planning of internal audits. Audits are to be performed and documented against the Quality Plan and any applicable specified requirements (such as ISO articles, or requirements of other accrediting bodies.)

The purpose of internal audits is to investigate the level of compliance with the Quality System. All departments, including the Quality Department, must be audited at planned intervals though internal audits may be planned and conducted in phases to ensure that individual departments are not auditing activities for which they are responsible.

Monitoring of processes and products – Each organization must have a system for monitoring and evaluating processes and products to ensure the continuous conformity of the processes and products. Where necessary, the evaluation might result in improvement of processes, procedures and/or training of personnel.

Monitoring of product characteristics can be performed through the definition of key quality indicator data, and may be accomplished by inspection of every product or through sampling of a subset of products.

---

[2] Each organization should define the term 'run' depending on the production organization or planning.

Non-conformance policy – There must be a policy to report all non-conformances in order to re-work products where possible and to improve the quality of products and the Quality System and Management. The system must be anonymous and non-punitive in order to promote the identification and reporting of non-conformances.

Improvement – The results of the evaluations of internal audits, monitoring, complaints and non-conformance reporting must result in corrective and/or preventive actions (CAPA) in order to improve the Quality System and Management. Corrective and preventive actions should be designed to address the observed non-conformance as well as, whenever possible, the root cause of the non-conformance, in order to prevent recurrence.

2.2. EFQM

2.2.1. Introduction
The European Foundation for Quality Management has developed a quality management system based on nine criteria as shown in the scheme below. [10]

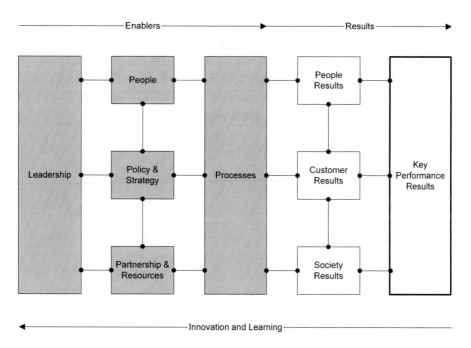

Figure 1. EFQM Quality Management Scheme. Quality Processes (centre) depend on Leadership (left) steering Policy and Strategy, People (human resource) and Partnerships and Resources. Quality Processes lead to Key Performance Results through Customer Results (satisfaction), People Results (competent and satisfied human resource) and Society Results (embedding and full acceptance).

2.2.2. The Concept of Excellence
The EFQM system is based on fundamental concepts of excellence.
Excellence is:

- achieving results that delight all the organization's stakeholders (*results orientation*);

In the fast changing environment of today's world, excellent organizations are agile, flexible and responsive as stakeholders needs and expectations change, often frequently and quickly. Excellent organizations measure and anticipate the needs and expectations of their stakeholders, monitor their experiences and perceptions, and monitor and review the performance of other organizations. Information is gathered from both current and future stakeholders. This information is used in order to set, implement and review their policies, strategies, objectives, targets, measures and plans, for short, medium and longer term. The information gathered also helps the organization to develop and achieve a balanced set of stakeholder results.

- creating sustainable customer value (*customer focus*);

Excellent organizations know and intimately understand their customers. They understand that customers are the final arbiters of product and service quality. They also understand that customer loyalty, retention and market share gain is maximized through a clear focus on the needs and expectations of both existing and potential customers. They are responsive to present needs and expectations of those customers. Where appropriate they segment their customers to improve the effectiveness of their response. They monitor competitor activity and understand their competitive advantage. They effectively anticipate what customer's future needs and expectations will be and act now in order to meet and where possible to exceed them. They monitor and review the experiences and perceptions of their customers and where things go wrong they respond quickly and effectively. They build and maintain excellent relationships with all their customers.

- visionary and inspirational leadership, coupled with constancy of purpose (*leadership and consistency of purpose*);

Excellent organizations have leaders who set and communicate a clear direction for their organization. In doing so they unite and motivate other leaders to inspire their people. They establish values, ethics, culture and a governance structure for the organization that provides a unique identity and attractiveness to stakeholders. Leaders at all levels within these organizations constantly drive and inspire others towards excellence and in so doing display both role model behaviour and performance. They lead by example, recognizing their stakeholders and working with them on joint improvement activity. During times of turbulence they display a constancy of purpose and steadiness that inspires the confidence and commitment of their stakeholders. At the same time they demonstrate the capability to adept and realign the direction of their organization in the light of a fast moving and constantly changing external environment, and in so doing carry their people with them.

- managing the organization through a set of independent and interrelated systems, processes and facts (*management by processes and facts*);

Excellent organizations have an effective management system based upon and designed to deliver, the needs and expectations of all stakeholders. The systematic implementation of policies, strategies, objectives and plans of the organization are enabled and assured through a clear and integrated set of processes. These processes are effectively deployed, managed and improved on a day-to-day basis. Decisions are based on factually reliable information relating to current and projected performance, process and systems capability, stakeholder needs, expectations and experiences, and the performance of other organizations, including, where appropriate, that of competitors. Risks are identified based on sound performance measures and effectively managed. The organization is governed in a highly professional manner, meeting and exceeding all corporate external requirements. Appropriate prevention measures are identified and implemented, inspiring and maintaining high levels of confidence with stakeholders.

- maximizing the contribution of employees through their development and involvement (*people development and involvement*);

Excellent organizations identify and understand the competencies needed, both now and in the future, in order to implement the policies, strategies, objectives and plans of the organization. They recruit and develop their people to match these competencies and actively and positively support them throughout.

Personal development is promoted and supported allowing people to realize and unlock their full potential. They prepare people to meet and adapt to the changes required of them both in terms of operational changes and personal capabilities.

They recognize the increasing importance of the intellectual capital of their people and use their knowledge for the benefit of the organization. They seek to care, reward and recognize their people in a way that builds their commitment and encourages their loyalty to the organization. They maximize the potential and the active involvement of their people through shared values and a culture of trust, openness and empowerment. They utilize that involvement to generate and implement ideas for improvement.

- challenging the *status quo* and effecting change by utilizing learning to create innovation and improvement opportunities (*continuous learning, innovation and improvement*);

Excellent organizations continuously learn, both from their own activities and performance and from that of others. They rigorously benchmark, both internally and externally. They capture and share the knowledge of their people in order to maximize learning across and within the organization. There is an openness to accept and use ideas from all stakeholders. People are encouraged to look beyond today and today's capabilities. They are careful to guard their intellectual property and to exploit it for commercial gain, where appropriate. Their people constantly challenge the status quo and seek opportunities for continuous innovation and improvement that add value.

- developing and maintaining value adding partnerships (*partnership development*);

Excellent organizations recognize that in today's constantly changing and increasingly demanding world, success may depend on the partnerships they develop.

They seek out and develop partnerships with other organizations. These partnerships enable them to deliver enhanced value to their stakeholders through optimizing core competencies.

These partnerships may be with customers, society, suppliers or even competitors and are based on clearly identified mutual benefit. Partners work together to achieve shared goals, supporting one another with expertise, resources, and knowledge and build a sustainable relationship based on mutual trust, respect and openness.

- exceeding the minimum regulatory framework in which the organization operates and to strive to understand and respond to the expectations of their stakeholders in society (*corporate social responsibility*).

Excellent organizations adopt a highly ethical approach by being transparent and accountable to their stakeholders for their performance as a responsible organization. They give consideration to, and actively promote, social responsibility and ecological sustainability both now and in the future. The organization's Corporate Social Responsibility is expressed in its values and integrated within the organization.

Through open and inclusive stakeholder engagement, they meet and exceed the expectations and regulations of the local and, where appropriate, the global community.

As well as managing risks, they seek out and promote opportunities to work on mutually beneficial projects with society inspiring and maintaining high levels of confidence with stakeholders. They are aware of the organization's impact on both the current and future community and take care to minimize any adverse impact.

2.2.3. The Nine Model Criteria (figure 1)

Leadership – Excellent leaders develop and facilitate the achievement of the mission and vision. They develop organizational values and systems required for sustainable success and implement these via their actions and behaviours. During periods of change they retain a constancy of purpose. Where required, such leaders are able to change the direction of the organization and inspire others to follow.

- Leaders develop the mission, vision, values and ethics and are role models of a culture of Excellence
- Leaders are personally involved in ensuring the organization's management system is developed, implemented and continuously improved
- Leaders interact with customers, partners and representatives of society
- Leaders reinforce a culture of excellence with the organization's people
- Leaders identify and champion organizational change

Policy and strategy – Excellent organizations implement their mission and vision by developing a stakeholder focused strategy that takes account of the market and sector in which it operates. Policies, plans, objectives and processes are developed and deployed to deliver the strategy.

- Policy and strategy are based on the present and future needs and expectations of stakeholders
- Policy and strategy are based on information from performance measurement, research, learning and external related activities
- Policy and strategy are developed, reviewed and updated
- Policy and strategy are communicated and deployed through a framework of key processes

People – Excellent organizations manage, develop and release the full potential of their people at an individual, team-based and organizational level. They promote fairness and equality and involve and empower their people. They care for, communicate, reward and recognize in a way that motivates staff and builds commitment to using their skills and knowledge for the benefit of the organization.

- People resources are planned, managed and improved
- People's knowledge and competencies are identified, developed and sustained
- People are involved and empowered
- People and the organization have a dialogue
- People are rewarded, recognized and cared for

Partnership and resources – Excellent organizations plan and manage external partnerships, suppliers and internal resources in order to support policy and strategy and the effective operation of processes. During planning and whilst managing partnerships and resources they balance the current and future needs of the organization, the community and the environment.

- External partnerships are managed
- Finances are managed
- Buildings, equipment and materials are managed
- Technology is managed
- Information and knowledge are managed

Processes - Excellent organizations design, manage and improve processes in order to fully satisfy and generate increasing value for customers and other stakeholders.

- Processes are systematically designed and managed
- Processes are improved, as needed, using innovation in order to fully satisfy and generate increasing value for customers and other stakeholders
- Products and Services are developed based on customer needs and expectations
- Products and Services are produced, delivered and serviced
- Customer relationships are managed and enhanced

Customer results - Excellent organizations comprehensively measure and achieve outstanding results with respect to their customers.

- Perception Measures
- Performance Indicators

People results -Excellent organizations comprehensively measure and achieve outstanding results with respect to their people.

- Perception Measures
- Performance Indicators

Society results - Excellent organizations comprehensively measure and achieve outstanding results with respect to society.

- Perception Measures
- Performance Indicators

Key performance results - Excellent organizations comprehensively measure and achieve outstanding results with respect to the key elements of their policy and strategy.

- Perception Measures
- Performance Indicators

2.2.4. The Five Development Stages

The five development stages mentioned are symbolized with pictograms –

1. Activity or product oriented

Each and every employee strives to do his work optimally. Craftsmanship is highly appreciated and supported by education and training. In case of any complaint the organization shall try to correct. The focus is on the product as an outcome without really observing the need for an input and the process leading to the product as an output.

2. Process oriented

The production or primary process is controlled. The mutual dependence of the successive steps or procedures is getting clear. The single process steps from input to output are identified; tasks and responsibilities are laid down. Achievement indicators serve as guidance. Processes are improved based on noticed non-conformances.

3. System oriented

Improvement of the total organization is a matter on all levels. The Deming cycle (Plan, Do, Check, Act) is applied in primary, supporting and guiding processes. The supplier-customer principle is built in and the focus on satisfaction and complaints is dominant for the policy that is focused to prevent problems rather than correction.

4. Chain oriented

The organization strives together with partners in the production chain to maximum additive value. The organization is embedded in its environment and has developed a continuous interaction in a question and answer (QandA) principle.

5. Recognized for Excellence or Total Quality Management

In its market segment the organization is on the top. The process of continuous improvement in anchored in the organizational structure and culture. Based on long term vision, changes are implement in time to start new activities and to prepare the organization. The organization is customer oriented and has become a major partner in its environment.

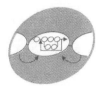

2.2.6. Self Assessment

To advance from activity orientation to *Recognized for Excellence* self-assessment is needed from time to time. For this purpose EFQM has developed a special system of assessment.

For the first five of the nine criteria it must be determined how of the five stages the various sub-ranges can be classified.

The average stage is plotted in a 'spider net'. For the last four criteria (customer result, people result, society result and key performance results) matrices are developed to calculate the score of these criteria.

Leadership	Orientation
	Organization
	Performance

Strategy and policy	Orientation
	Creation
	Implementation
People	Organization
	Invest
	Respect
Partnership and resources	Money
	Knowledge and technology
	Materials and services

Processes	Design
	Control
	Improvement and renewing

The scores are also plotted in a 'spider net' or 'radar' chart:

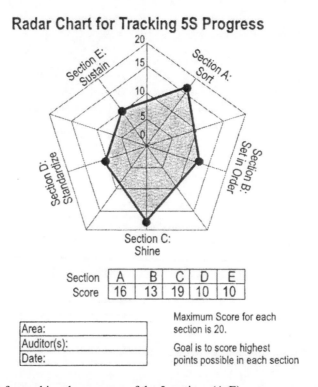

Figure 2. Radar chart for tracking the progress of the 5 sections (A-E).

This example illustrates in the 5 sections a progress tracking of a specific 5S progress system for cleaning (Sort, Set in Order, Shine, Standardize and Sustain) where the weak points are that need improvement: sections B, D and E.

The average stages and scores can also be plotted in the following table:

Table 1. Table to record the average stages and scores of a radar chart

	stages	I activity oriented	II Process Oriented	III system oriented	IV chain oriented	V Recognized Excellence
Leadership	Orientation					
Leadership	Organization					
Leadership	Performance					
Strategy and Policy	Orientation					
Strategy and Policy	Creation					
Strategy and Policy	Implementation					
People	Organization					
People	Invest					
People	Respect					
partnership and Resources	Money					
partnership and Resources	Knowledge and technology					
partnership and Resources	Materials and services					
Processes	Design					
Processes	Control					
Processes	Improvement and renewing					
		1	2	3	4	5
	Customer result					
	People result					
	Society result					
	Financial results					
	Key performance result					

2.3. ISQua

2.3.1. Introduction

The dimensions of quality are no longer grouped within one Principle as in the previous second edition, but are now addressed in four of the Principles. The increased emphasis on safety is reflected by a Principle devoted to that dimension. The revised Principles are (see also annex 1):

1. *Quality Improvement*: Standards are designed to encourage healthcare organisations to improve quality and performance within their own organisations and the wider healthcare system
2. *Patient/Service User Focus*: Standards are designed with a focus on patients/service users and reflect the patient/service user continuum of care or service
3. *Organisational Planning and Performance*: Standards assess the capacity and efficiency of healthcare organisations
4. *Safety*: Standards include measures to protect and improve the safety of patients/service users, staff and visitors to the organisation

The two complementing Principles relate to the development of standards and the monitoring of the implementation –

5. *Standards Development*: Standards are planned, formulated and evaluated through a defined and rigorous process
6. *Standards Measurement*: Standards enable consistent and transparent rating and measurement of achievement.

The dominant philosophy for the ISQua principles for standards is in improvement of quality of care. [11] Quality improvement implies such things as: patient centred care (emphasis on the patient care process), team delivery of care to the patient, quality improvement activities throughout the health care facility, documentation and measurement of improvements, and strong leadership for quality and quality improvement from senior facility officials.

The most fundamental characteristic of quality care is that it is safe care for the patient and that staff are able to provide that care in a safe way. Unsafe care cannot be quality care. Thus, there is enhanced emphasis on safety in the upgraded 2008 edition of the ISQua standards.

2.3.2. ISQua Accreditation Standards

Accreditation standards are complementary to, and supportive of, operational standards for procurement and clinical transfusion practice.

Production and processing of blood and blood components are governed by technical standards and guidelines to ensure quality. These standards and guidelines are required to be in place to support the overall quality of blood services and are in generally based on cGMP. An effective relationship between operational standards and guidelines and accreditation standards results in an effective evaluation process for blood banks and transfusion services.

Canadian Society for International Health (CSIH) used the common ISQua format and principles in use for all sets of accreditation standards, for the design of accreditation standards for blood establishments (procurement and supply) and hospital blood banks (patient care). To accommodate the uniqueness of the blood establishments and hospital blood banks appropriate modifications to the format have been made. One of these unique aspects is that in principle the procurement part, producing blood components, is liable for the quality and efficacy of the blood components, where the consumer (recipient) needs to be protected against faulty products – consumer rights protection. It has been assumed that quality improvement will be the underlying basis for the upgraded standards. This basis is also reflected in the dominant philosophy for the ISQua principles for standards – quality improvement. Quality improvement implies such things as: donor/recipient focus, quality improvement activities throughout the blood establishments and hospital blood banks, documentation and measurement of improvements, and strong leadership for quality and quality improvement from senior service officials. The most fundamental characteristic of quality service is that it is safe for all those who participate in the provision of service [collection, processing, testing (QC), storage and/or distribution of blood and blood components] or receive service (donors and recipients). Unsafe service cannot be quality service. Thus, there is a strong emphasis on safety in the upgraded 2008 ISQua standards.

2.3.3. Design of ISQua Standards for Transfusion Medicine
Based on the principles and the common format, CSIH created the following design –

SECTION A.   LEADERSHIP

1. Organization Mandate
2. Governance
3. Strategic and Operational Planning
4. General Management
5. Risk Management and Quality Improvement

SECTION B.   RESOURCE MANAGEMENT
1. Financial Management
2. Information Management
3. Human Resources Management

SECTION C.   SAFETY MANAGEMENT
1. Safe facilities
2. Disaster and Safety Management
3. Safe Equipment and Supplies
4. Healthy Work Environment
5. Infection Control

SECTION D.   DONOR AND RECIPIENT
1. Informed consent
2. Documents and Records
3. Non-conformances and Adverse Event Reporting

SECTION E.   PROCESS CONTROL
1. Collection of Blood.
2. Manufacturing of components
3. Transfusion Related Activities

As can be seen, these elements follow largely the quality management systems of ISO and EFQM, with an underlying structure of cGMP with its ten key elements. A set of standards focused on the recipients of blood and blood components has also been designed (Annex 2) that largely follows the in-hospital transfusion chain of events (Figure 2.3.1) with an emphasis on policies and procedures, and consistent documentation.

2.4. PIC/S GMP Guide for Blood Establishments

The Pharmaceutical Inspection Co-operation Scheme as designed and entered into force in 2001 by the Pharmaceutical Inspection Convention, Geneva, is a Good Manufacturing Practice guide focused on blood establishment and the collection, processing, testing, storage and distribution of blood and blood components. [6] It also covers the operations of apheresis establishments for the collection of plasma and cells from donors. Besides the general introductory chapters describing purpose and scope, there are eleven chapters that provide the managerial standards for the operations in blood establishments. The current third edition is from 2007 [6].

1. Quality Management – the aspects covered are general standards, quality assurance, corrective and preventive actions, change control and self-inspection;
2. Personnel – opens with the important statement that *"the collection of blood and preparation of safe and efficacious blood components is dependent on the availability of sufficient and appropriately qualified and trained personnel"*. It covers the aspects of responsibilities, training and hygiene;
3. Premises – provides general guidelines, and guidelines for production areas, environmental control, storage conditions, and mobile sites for donor sessions;
4. Equipment – lists general guidelines and covers maintenance and calibration;
5. Documentation – opens with the statement *"the documentation of procedures and records is essential to a quality assurance system. It ensures that work performed is standardised, and that there is traceability of all steps in the manufacturing of blood and blood components – i.e., donor selection, collection, preparation, storage, dispatch/distribution, quality control and quality assurance"*. Besides general guidelines the chapter also focuses on the use of computers;
6. Donor Sessions – special attention is given to proper and standardized donor selection based on selection criteria to ensure that both the donor and the potential recipient are protected. The chapter is pretty detailed and covers donor selection, whole blood collection and collection by apheresis;
7. Component Preparation – provides general guidelines, and standards for starting material, preparation of components, irradiated components, labelling and the important aspect of release of components from quarantine;
8. Storage and Dispatch/Distribution – covers storage and dispatch/distribution of blood and blood components to hospitals;
9. Quality Monitoring – underlines the need for validation of each process of preparation of blood components to ensure that these meet set specifications, demonstrating that the process is under control. The compliance is to be established by the relevant Competent Health Authority. Aspects covered are quality monitoring,

microbiological monitoring and specifications of blood and blood components stating that *"acceptance criteria should be based on a defined set of specifications for each blood and blood component"*;

10. Laboratory Testing – provides a number of general guidelines and sets standards for screening tests for infectious disease markers and for blood group serology testing of each donation;

11. Complaints and Recalls – focuses on protection of the recipient from defective blood components (consumer rights protection) and sets standards for notification of the Competent Health Authority.

The goals of PIC/S for the next period of time are to improve PIC/S position as a 'global player' in the GMP field for Regulatory Authorities.

This being done by attracting non-EU Agencies having an equivalent GMP inspection and quality system and integrating at least 10 – 12 new Agencies by 2015.

3. Operational Quality Systems

3.1. Introduction

Besides the management oriented quality systems there are also the process oriented systems, focused on the chain or processes and procedures in production or manufacturing of products. There is a sliding interrelation between these process oriented systems and the management oriented systems as discussed in part 2 of this chapter. This is particularly clear in the EFQM structure which starts with the simple product orientation and develops in five phases into total quality management, the comprehensive and complete final stage. The EFQM phases or stages – product, process, system, chain and total QM – represent the managerial structure of the underlying quality systems. In the development they build up like the rings of an onion (Figure 3). Quality control or QC is the basic technical control of a product focused on the set product specifications. Quality assurance or QA focuses on the process with its procedures and assures the quality of the described process with its procedures. Good Practice or GP oversees the system of processes and their procedures to control the quality of the outcome, from input through the processes to the output (product or service). The Quality System of preference in the procurement of blood components is GP for manufacturing or GMP. There are equivalents for the laboratory aspects – Good Laboratory Practice or GLP, and the clinical aspects – Good Clinical Practice or GCP. Similarly one could apply the principles to office practices, named Good Office Practice or GOP.

3.2. Good Manufacturing Practice (GMP)

GMP is also called cGMP indicating the current Good (pharmaceutical) Manufacturing Practice. The system is process oriented and all versions contain the same key elements or quality system essentials (QSE), which are:

- Quality Management or Organisation and Structure
- Personnel
- Contracts or Agreements
- Purchasing
- Premises and Equipment
- Documentation
- Production
- Quality Control
- Complaints and Recall (Deviations and Non-Compliances)
- Self-inspection

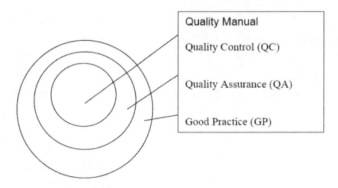

Figure 3. The onion ring relation of quality systems for the manufacturing of a product.

3.2.1. Quality Management

A Blood Establishment collects whole blood, processes whole blood into blood components, stores and distributes the finished blood components to the hospitals it serves. The purpose is to ensure that the products and related services are

- fit for their intended use (fit for purpose),
- comply with agreed requirements and specifications (e.g. in Annex V of the EU Commission Directive 2004/33/EC [13] or the AABB Technical Manual [14]),
- do not put donors, patients and staff at risk due to inadequate safety, quality and/or efficacy.

The achievement of this quality objective is the responsibility of the senior management and requires participation and commitment of all staff in all departments (operational and supportive/administrative) and at all levels within the establishment.

To achieve the quality objective reliably there must be a comprehensively designed and correctly implemented system of current Good Manufacturing Practice incorporating Quality Assurance and thus Quality Control. It should be fully documented and its effectiveness monitored and evaluated. All parts of the GMP system should be adequately resourced with competent personnel, suitable and sufficient premises and equipment.

The basic concepts of current Good Manufacturing Practice, Quality Assurance and Quality Control are interrelated. Assurance can only function if based on control. They are described here in order to emphasize their relationships and their fundamental importance to the production and control of medicinal products[3].

There are various systems to manage the Quality System. For small organizations this can be a self developed data base system, or a simple document management system. In both cases the documentation is not structured and it is almost impossible to prove that all needed documents are available. Additionally it will be very difficult to write the necessary Quality Manual.

The Quality Manual Preparation Workbook for Blood Banks by Lucia M. Berte [15] might be helpful.

There is, however, a structured way to design and implement Quality Management which is called the Pyramid model which consists of 4 levels (Figure 4): Two managerial levels and two operational levels. The essence of the model is in documentation – write up what you do, so that you can do what has been written.

This means that at the managerial level the policy and strategies have to be documented, based on a mission statement, a vision and a careful analysis of the processes, both the primary processes or operations and the secondary supportive or managerial processes.

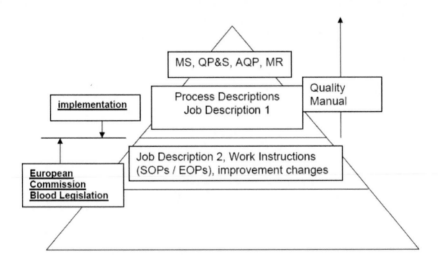

Figure 4. The Pyramid model. MS = Mission Statement; QPandS = Quality Policy and Strategy; AQP = Annual Quality Plan; MR = Management Review

3.2.1.1. Managerial Levels

Top level – The top level contains the Mission Statement and the Vision, describing in 1 or 2 sentences the ultimate objectives of the Blood Establishment: *What the Blood Establishment wants to achieve.*

These objectives form the core business of the organization and must be reflected in the organogram (see annex 3 for an example).

This Mission Statement and Vision must be written by Top Management and in many countries it has to be authorized by the Ministry of Health. Once the Mission Statement and Vision are authorized, these must made known and familiar to all employees.

---

[3] Text based on the European GMP for Medicinal Products for Human and Veterinary Use

The top level also contains the Quality Policy and Strategy and the Annual Quality Plan. The Quality Policy and Strategy has to be written by Top Management and the Quality Manager assisted by some Heads of Departments. It describes how the objectives in the Mission Statement and Vision will be achieved: *How the processes will happen.*

The Director's tasks, authority, responsibilities, and accountability must be described. The organization showing the lines of command or accountability must be described and captured in the organogram. The financial structure must be explained.

The Annual Quality Plan must be written by the Quality Manager and will explain which of the quality objectives will have to be achieved over the next year and must give reasons why objectives of the previous year were not completely or not at all achieved. Annually top management has to review the management processes and their achievements based on the Quality Plan – Management Review.

Second level – An important part of the second level contains Job and Process descriptions of all processes mentioned in the Quality Policy and Strategy.

All processes identified and needed to achieve the goals described in the Mission Statement and Vision must be listed and described, including the identified procedures of each process. Each Process Description or PD should be written by the Head of the Department that has to perform the process and should contain the following chapters:

1. Introduction
2. Scope
3. Definitions and Abbreviations
4. Tasks, responsibilities, authorizations and accountability
5. References
6. Attachments
7. Detailed description of the process mentioning all classifications of staff with JDs, procedures with SOPs and equipment with EOPs
8. Related processes to analyze the interfaces between processes and Departments

The core of a PF is the number 7. This level also contains the indications of the jobs needed to perform the various processes and mentioned in the organogram. Job Description 1 (JD-1) describes the hierarchical position of a function in the organization, should contain the authorizations, responsibilities and accountability of all functions mentioned in the organogram and should as a minimum contain the following information:

1. Name of the organization
2. Department
3. Title of function
4. Educational or vocational requirements or level
5. Salary indication/scale
6. Short description of the organization, department and function
7. Authorization(s), responsibilities and accountability (TARA).

A Job Description 1 (JD-1) should be written by those responsible for the job. So, the Director in case of the jobs for Quality Manager and Head of Departments, and the Heads of Departments for the identified functions in their respective Departments. The detailed task and related performance requirements should be in Job Description 2 (JD-2) which is part of the next level (operational). The two upper levels of the pyramid form together the Quality Manual and reflect the managerial part of the organization. At this level top-down changes are changes in the system and bottom-up changes are improvements in the operations.

3.2.1.2. Operational Levels

Third level – The third level contains all work or performance instructions as mentioned in the Process Descriptions:

- Job Description 2
- Standard Operating Procedures (SOPs)
- Equipment Operating Procedures (EOPs)

It reflects the question: *How are the processes and procedures done?*
Job Description 2 should be written by the supervisor of that particular function:

- Specific tasks to be performed
- Performance requirements

The SOPs and EOPs must be written by the persons who perform the activities (operators / technicians / analysts).
Each SOP should contain the following chapters:

1. Introduction
2. Scope
3. Responsibilities
4. Definitions and abbreviations
5. Work instructions
6. Related SOPs to analyze the interfaces between SOPs
7. Forms and/or records to document the outcome

The core of any SOP is the number 5 – Work Instructions, which should also contain the consumables and supportive utensils needed.
Each EOP should contain the following chapters:

1. Introduction containing the principle of the machine
2. Scope
3. Responsibilities
4. Work instructions
5. Maintenance scheme (cleaning, maintenance and calibration)
6. Name and address of the supplier or manufacturer
7. Forms and/or records to document the performance

Here the number 4 – Work Instructions, is the core of any EOP.

Fourth level – Finally the fourth level contains all forms, records to document the outcome, attachment, operating manuals etc. that are addenda to the process descriptions or SOPs and EOPs.

They reflect the question: *What are the results and outcomes of the processes and procedures*

3.2.2 Quality Management Department

The Department of Quality Management is a supportive department to the all core departments of the Blood Establishment. The most important tasks of Quality Management are:

- Control of Documents, Equipment, Validation and Education (teaching and training) of staff
- Release of incoming, critical goods (consumables, reagents etc.) and of final/finished products
- Release
- Non-conformance policy (error detection, correction and prevention)
- Proficiency testing
- Monitoring and Evaluation (MandE), which includes quality control (QC)
- Primary purchasing
- Stock control of resources (supplies) and final products
- Complaint handling and Recall
- Haemovigilance reporting to the Competent Authority
- Internal Auditing/Assessments

3.2.2.1. Document Control

From the Pyramid model it will be clear that the Quality Management Department is not writing the necessary documents except the Annual Quality Plan and the documents regarding the Quality Management Department. However, the Quality Manager is responsible for the presence of all documents. He must be authorized to make heads / managers of the various departments aware of incomplete documentation.

The original documents are archived by Quality Management. Authorized copies are issued by Quality Management to assure that when issuing a new version all existing copies will be retrieved and destroyed. No obsolete copies of documents should circulate in the organization.

Documents have to be authorized and released by the Head or Manager of the respective Department and the Quality Manager. Prior to release the Quality Manager should assure that the document is in compliance with cGMP, Laws and Regulations and not conflicting with other documents within the organization.

All change requests must be judged by the Head of the Department on technical aspects and by the Quality Manager on cGMP and legal aspects.

After approval by these two persons the change may be made in the document and the version indication will be raised one level. The released new version will only become in force following training and assessment of all personnel involved.

All documents must be revised periodically (once every two years at least). The original of obsolete documents must be archived (in hard copy or electronically) during the period of time as required by National law or regulation. This must be a period of at least 5 years, but usually 10 years and within the European Union even 30 years.

3.2.2.2. Equipment Control

All equipment used in the primary process departments must be validated and released for use prior to operation. This release is based on the results of the validation procedure performed upon arrival in the organization and after release of the EOP.

Quality Management issues a 'label' that is attached to the equipment indicating for which period of time the equipment is released for operation. The department owning the equipment is responsible for the cleaning, maintenance and calibration of the equipment.

Cleaning forms/records must be completed after each cleaning of the equipment and Quality Management will check this regularly for compliance. Each time the release period has expired or after each maintenance or repair, the equipment must be re-validated and released by Quality Management.

All described actions must be carefully documented and controlled by Quality Management

3.2.2.3. Validation Control

All equipment, processes and procedures must be validated. Prior to performing each and every validation the Validation Protocol must be approved for validity by Quality Management.

Prior to starting training people to perform, the Validation Report must be approved by Quality Management. Validation must be performed on all new equipment, procedures and processes, after maintenance or repair of equipment and after any change in processes and procedures.

Quality Management is responsible for the validation policy, but not for the performance of the validation itself.

3.2.2.4. Education (Teaching and Training) Control

Equipment may be operated and processes and procedures should be performed only by authorized (competent) personnel. People are authorized after (re)training and (re)assessment of competency. There shall be a continued education programme focused on maintenance and continued development of competence in the profession – CPD or continued Professional Development.

Quality Management is responsible for the training policy and strategy, but not for the training itself.

3.2.2.5. Release of Critical Incoming Goods

Critical goods are those consumables, reagents etc. that may influence the quality of the final product and/or are part of the final product. Critical goods must be placed in quarantine by the Blood Establishment upon receipt from the supplier.

Quality Management makes a decision about the release based either on laboratory results (reagents and test kits) or on general and documented information from the

Manufacturer and/or Supplier, the Competent Authority (rapid alert system), or other Blood Establishments.

Release must be documented per batch and products must be recognized as such (label). If a batch will be refused, the products must be segregated and they should be recognized as *refused* or *rejected* (label). In case of any doubt products and/or batches should be put *'on hold'* until final decision is made.

3.2.2.6. Release of Final Products

Although Quality Management is responsible for the critical procedure of release of the final or finished products or blood components, usually personnel from the operational department do perform the release procedure.

The release is based on the conformity of the results of e.g., the blood group determination with the historic data of the donor and on the negative results of the mandatory infectious disease marker tests.

3.2.2.7. Non-conformance Policy

It is of paramount importance to have a non-repressive non-conformance or error policy. When implementing the quality system, the system might lead to non-conformances and people may cause non-conformances, deviations from the standards or errors. To improve the system and to further train employees it is important to have all non-conformances reported to Quality Management for root-cause analysis of the reports and trend analysis.

Non-conformance caused by the system must initiate corrective actions and preventive actions (CAPA) to improve the system. Non-conformances caused by people should lead to further education of the person(s) involved. Punishing people for non-conformances or errors will cause reduction of reports and finally in getting out of control as the quality system would not function any longer.

Quality Management should have a monthly meeting with representatives of all core departments to discuss the reports.

The representatives shall report the results of such meetings to the business meeting of their Departments in order to generate a good feed-back from reporting non-conformances to the conclusions from Quality Management and the Non-Conformance or Error Committee.

3.2.2.8. Proficiency Testing

Proficiency testing is organized by a reference laboratory. They prepare the samples that are sent to the participating laboratories. All samples are equal. The participating laboratories perform the test and send the results to the organizing (reference) laboratory. Here all results are analyzed and accompanied with appropriate statistical analyses. All result are anonymously sent back to the participant and they can compare or benchmark their results with those of other laboratories (without revealing the identity of the other participants). To get an idea about the reliability the results of biological tests it is essential to participate in regional, national or international proficiency test programmes or external quality assurance schemes (EQAS).

Proficiency tests are organized for blood grouping AB0 Rhesus(D), immunohaematology tests, infectious disease marker screening tests, NAT/PCR tests, blood coagulation tests and cell counts.

3.2.2.9. Monitoring and Evaluation (MandE), Including Quality Control (QC)

Critical control points (CCP) must be measurable and may therefore be monitored. Monitoring is only useful if the results are evaluated (analyzed) and conclusions drawn. Regularly the results must be analyzed and discussed in the presence of Quality Management.

The information is important for the release policy and strategy of final products.

3.2.2.10. Primary Purchasing

When a critical product has to be purchased for the first time usually a group of at least three people form the committee to decide what product shall be bought. The Head of the Department is responsible for the functionality (efficiency, effectiveness, etc.) of the good. The Administrator is responsible for the price (cost-effectiveness) and the contract. The Quality Manager is responsible for the observing the quality of the products and the manufacturer and/or the supplier. This can be investigated through a supplier audit.

3.2.2.11. Stock Control Resources (Supplies)

Quality Management is of course not the department that keeps control over the stock of the supplies. This is the responsibility of the warehouse manager. However, the warehouse manager shall regularly inform Quality Management about the stock and Quality Management might inform the warehouse manager which products will expire within the next period of time. So the warehouse manager has to control whether these goods are still on stock and inform Quality Management about the youngest batches on stock. The warehouse should have a system that prevents distribution of outdated supplies, and Quality Management should ensure that the warehouse's system works.

3.2.2.12. Stock Control Final Products

The Head of Distribution is responsible to regularly count the available stock. This can be done by physical counting, review of the output of a validated computer system, or even by a simple programme in MS Excel. The inflow and outflow can be put in the programme and a perfect control could be introduced if one or two warning levels automatically change colour. Daily Quality Management must be informed about the stock of the blood components.

3.2.2.13. Complaint Handling

There are three different types of complaints in a Blood Establishment:

Complaints from donors – these are usually handled by the employees from the Donor Department. Each donor complaint shall be documented and forwarded immediately to Quality Management and shall be analyzed and handled in a timely manner. It is the task to Quality Management to assure a correct and timely reply to the complaining donor.

Complaints from customers – these usually are oral complaints from the Hospital Laboratory to the driver who delivers the products. Complaints have to be in writing and must be forwarded immediately to Quality Management. Where necessary more information may be collected and the complaint must be analyzed.

As soon as possible the results must be reported to the complaining customer. Where appropriate corrective and preventive actions shall be initiated. A complaint may lead to a non-conformance report.

Both type of complainers must have the feeling to be taken seriously even in case it is obvious that the complaint will not be followed up.

Complaints from the Blood Establishment about supplied goods – usually the various suppliers have their own complaint form that should be completed. It is important to describe the complaint as detailed as possible and to contact the supplier about possible remuneration of the refused/rejected goods. All complaints must be well documented.

Internal complaints are complaints from employees about other employees or work situations. This is often about undesired behavior of an employee. Some accrediting bodies (e.g., AABB, CAP) require posting of information to allow complaints to be directed anonymously to them, bypassing an internal system that the employee may not trust for lack of punitive action. However, usually a confidential committee handles these complaints and report (anonymously) to the Quality Manager.

3.2.2.14. Recall

There are several good reasons to recall one or more blood components:

- Positive result of bacteriology testing after issue of one or more blood components
- Customer complaint(s)
- Test results in the quality control of blood components
- Information from the Competent Authority
- Haemovigilance reporting

Usually the Quality Manger is authorized to start a recall procedure. It must be possible to start a recall at any time of the day or the week. Returned blood components must be segregated from all other components and re-entry is prohibited and must be prevented. If the recall was necessary due to a report of a serious adverse reaction or event, it must be reported immediately to the Competent Authority.

3.2.2.15. Haemovigilance Reporting to the Competent Authority

Once the Blood Establishment produces continuously blood components of a reliable quality and safety, the clinician might expect a certain outcome of blood transfusion. When verifying the clinical outcome also adverse reactions or events may be seen and must be documented and reported to the Blood Establishment. Serious adverse reactions or events must be reported to the Competent Authority.

NB: A way of reporting is described in the EU Commission Directive 2005/61/EC [16]

3.2.2.16. Internal Audits

Quality Management should compile a scheme for internal audits of all core departments including all locations for mobile blood collection sessions. Each audit must be performed preferably by 2 auditors of whom at least one is an experienced auditor. It is not necessary that one or both auditors are employees of Quality Management. Both auditors, however, must be independent from the department to be audited. Quality Management shall archive the audit reports and will assure that recommendations by the auditors result in measurable improvements. Inspectors of the Competent Authority may ask to see the scheme of internal audits, but are not allowed to require to see the audit reports. Especially when starting to develop a quality system and management it would be wise to ask colleagues from another Blood Establishment in the country or abroad to perform a peer audit.

Peer audits differ from internal audits in such a way that the auditor is more or less obliged to advice the Blood Establishment in case of a major deviation of the cGMP rules. Where appropriate such situations should be discussed extensively with the peer auditor, which might result in ideas or proposals for improvement.

Internal audits result in recommendations and inspection by the Competent Authority results either in an authorization to continue the operations or to improve the operations of one or more departments, processes or procedures within a set period of time.

3.2.3. Personnel

The Dutch GMP for Blood Banks provides in article 3.2.1 a most important statement:

> *"The blood bank must have sufficient personnel with the necessary qualification and experience. Sufficient personnel means such a quantity of people that in view of the requirements of the operations, the work can be performed easily without continuous pressure of time. The tasks and responsibilities placed on any one individual should not be so extensive as to represent a risk to the quality of a product, or service and advice."*

Personnel must have the right vocational education, training and experience. Tasks, authorities, responsibilities and accountability (TARA) must be described clearly in each job description. The hierarchic structure (accountabilities) must be laid down in the organogram.

Usually the Blood Establishment has distinct core departments related to the primary process:

- Blood Collection,
- Blood Processing including Storage and Distribution,
- Quality Control (Laboratory),
- Medical Advice and Clinical Consultation,
- Quality Assurance/Management.

These departments shall have a (preferably) full time employed responsible head or manager.

Blood Collection – the Head or Manager generally has the following responsibilities:

- To ensure, in cooperation with the blood establishment physician, that donors are selected conform the guidelines;
- To ensure, in cooperation with the blood establishment physician, that blood and plasma are collected conform the guidelines;
- To ensure, in cooperation with the blood establishment physician, that the safety of donors during the collection of blood or plasma is guaranteed;
- To ensure, in cooperation with the blood establishment physician, that donors are treated with care, their rights are respected and their interests protected;
- To ensure the validation of collection methods and processes;

- To ensure that intermediate storage and transport of collected blood and plasma is performed conform the guidelines;
- To authorize together with others the instructions and protocols for donor selection, and blood and plasma collection and to ensure proper implementation.

Blood Processing Department - the Head or Manager generally has the following responsibilities:

- To ensure that components are produced according to the appropriate documents;
- To ensure that the various processing methods are validated;
- To ensure that the storage of starting materials, intermediate products, packaging and final products is in accordance with the guidelines;
- To ensure that the release of final products (including such steps as verification of all data per product) is in accordance with the guidelines;
- To authorize together with others the instructions and protocols for processing and issuing and to ensure proper implementation.

Quality Control or Testing Department (Laboratory) – the Head or Manager generally has the following responsibilities:

- The control of test kits and reagents;
- To ensure that laboratory tests are performed according to the applicable documents;
- To ensure that the validation of laboratory tests, equipment and processes takes place;
- To make the test results necessary for the release of the blood components available;
- To ensure that test kits and reagents are stored according to the relevant guidelines;
- To authorize together with others the instructions and protocols for quality control and to ensure the proper implementation.

Quality Management Department – the Head or Manager is generally responsible for:

- Authorization of all procedures, instructions and protocols for blood and plasma collection, blood processing and quality control of blood components;
- Authorization of all instructions for quality control of collected blood and plasma;
- Responsibility for the release of all product and critical materials;
- Approve or reject on his own authority starting materials, packaging materials, intermediate products or final products, in case it is necessary in terms of quality;
- (supervising) document control and organizing internal audits;
- ensuring that the proper validations are carried out;
- ensuring that the proper procedures are carried out for handling complaints and non-conformances;
- To assure that there are proper training and up-to-date teaching programs.

Additionally, the Head or Manager of Quality Management jointly with other key personnel has the following tasks:

- Supervision over the conditions for blood collection;
- Supervision over the conditions for blood processing;
- Supervision over laboratory/testing conditions;
- Validation of the methods and processes used in the various departments.

The previously mentioned key managerial personnel also have the following tasks:

- Supervision over the responsible personnel;
- To ensure that personnel receive the appropriate training and refresher courses;
- Supervision over the areas and equipment used by personnel.[4]

Each department is responsible for vocational training on the job and assessment of its employees to assure continued competency. All personnel of core departments must have adequate knowledge of microbiology, hygiene and cGMP. Employees of the core departments should pay adequate attention to personal hygiene and strictly follow the instruction concerning hygiene.

Employees involved in blood collection or blood processing should be free of any infection or open wounds of uncovered skin. If necessary the use of disposable gloves is allowed.

Consumption of food, drinks, sweets and smoking is strictly prohibited in all core departments.

To avoid any damage to blood bags each Blood Establishment must have rules concerning wearing rings, bracelets and wrist watches (sharp edges). There must be rules for wearing personal protective equipment. (Dressing Codes, including clothing, shields, goggles and gloves)

3.2.4. Contracts

All activities concerning the core business performed by third parties (e.g. irradiation of blood components, laboratory tests etc.) must be described in details in a contract or agreement.

The Blood Establishment must investigate – by performing an audit - the competency and quality of work of the third party. The third party must work according to cGMP/cGLP. The Blood Establishment must ensure that the products, including services delivered by the third party are in accordance with the quality specifications and standards. The Blood Establishment must provide the third party with all necessary information to perform the activities properly and in accordance with the applicable laws and regulations. The third party – working conform cGMP/cGLP – must have enough well trained personnel and validated equipment. The starting materials must be fit for use.

Without the Blood Establishment's permission the third party may not outsource the work to be done to another company. The contract should contain:

---

[4] Translation of the Dutch Guideline GMP for Blood Banks articles 3.3.5 to 3.3.10

- The tasks, authorities, responsibilities and accountability of the both parties;
- All necessary technical information, test methods and GMP;
- Specifications about the release of products by the qualified person of the third party;
- The responsibility for the procurement of starting materials, including the release of them;
- Performance of quality control including the sampling methods and evaluation;
- The way the Blood Establishment has access to documents and samples;
- The frequency of auditing by the Blood Establishment;
- Information about the requirement that the third party must allow inspectors from the Competent Authority to perform inspections at all times.

3.2.5. Purchasing

Purchasing of critical goods can be divided in two procedures:

- Primary purchasing is the determination of the specifications and the authorization of the supplier. Critical goods may only be purchased from authorized suppliers. Suppliers can be authorized by the Quality Manager of the Blood Establishment after having performed a supplier audit.
- Routine purchasing will be performed by the warehouse Manager or any therefore assigned person after the primary purchasing is finished and documented.

Critical goods are those goods that can influence the quality of the final product and/or are part of the final product.

Purchasing relates to both consumables and equipment as well as to the collection of whole blood and plasma from donors. Although the 'purchase' of blood and plasma should be done on a voluntary non-remunerated basis, there is certainly a situation of mutual agreement between the Blood Establishment and the donor offering the invaluable source material – human blood.

The procurement of the most important starting material – whole blood – is performed by the Donor Department. Whole blood may only be collected from voluntary, non-remunerated donors after being accepted as donor following the donor suitability and selection procedure, and following informed consent. The Blood Establishment must provide each donor appropriate information (e.g. Annex II, part A, of Directive 2004/33/EU [13]or the AABB Technical Manual current edition [14]). Donors must provide the Blood Establishment with life style and health information (e.g. Annex II, part B of Directive 2004/33/EU [13]or AABB Technical Manual current edition [14]). Acceptance and deferral criteria, including the duration of the deferral period for donors should be listed (e.g. Annex III of Directive 2004/33/EU [13] or the AABB Technical Manual current edition [14]).

At all times donor privacy must be guaranteed. Strict hygiene precaution must be taken during blood collection both in fixed locations as in mobile sessions.

3.2.6. Premises and Equipment

Premises must have the right dimensions and floor plan for a proper performance of the various activities. Sizes are difficult to mention as they depend on the number of blood collections to be performed per day and the number of units that have to be processed and tested.

The order of the various rooms must be logical to perform the various activities. The floor plan should allow the right flow and sequence without the risk of cross contamination or crossing lines to avoid mix-up of products in different stages of production. Premises and equipment must be constructed in such a way that they can be cleaned and maintained efficiently and effectively.

Equipment must be fit for use.

Premises and equipment must be cleaned and maintained regularly conform written requirements. Cleaning and maintenance must be documented. Illumination, temperature, humidity and air refreshment must be monitored and must not have any negative or deleterious effect on blood and blood components, equipment or processes.

All areas and rooms must have entrance criteria restricting access to authorized persons only. Working areas may not be used as a shortcut to other areas. All areas for the core activities must be clearly separated and marked.

3.2.6.1. Blood Collection Areas

There must be separate rooms in the blood collection area for donor selection in order to guarantee privacy. Domestic animals, plants and flowers (natural and artificial) are not allowed in these areas. This applies also for guide dogs.

The tasks of the guide dog must be taken over by blood collection employees. There must be a special room for treatment of donors with an adverse reaction during or after blood donation.

3.2.6.2. Blood Processing Areas

There must be enough space or rooms to perform the different activities separately from each other. Crossing lines must be avoided unless the crossing takes place controlled and at different points in time. For areas where processing takes place only in closed systems no special precautions other than normal hygiene have to be taken. Areas where opening takes place should be of class D (see Annex 1 of Directive 91/365/EEC [4]). Areas where blood or blood components are coming into contact with air should be of class A (see Annex 1 of Directive 91/365/EEC [4]).

Walls, floors and ceilings must be smooth and easy to clean and disinfect. Working benches must be of a light colour and smooth to be cleaned daily, inert and not affected by chemicals or alcohol.

3.2.6.3. Storage and Distribution Areas (Cold Chain)

(Starting) materials and final products, including intermediate products must be stored separately. For both enough space must be available. All storage areas must have the appropriate conditions for the products that are stored. Where special temperatures with lower and upper limits are required an independent alert system must be in place in order to warn personnel when limits are passed.

Special attention should be paid to the area(s) where labels are stored and/or where the release procedure is performed including the final labelling. There must be special, defined areas for returned components after a recall and for components of which results of infectious disease markers is unacceptable (to be discarded as bio-hazardous).

3.2.6.4. Areas for Laboratory Investigation and Quality Control

There must be enough space to avoid mix-up or cross-contamination of samples, products, equipment or materials. There must be enough space for sample storage and reagent storage. If applicable, special attention should be paid to equipment sensitive to vibration, electric interference, humidity etc. Separated rooms must be used when infectious samples, samples sensitive for contamination are processed (e.g., samples for nucleic acid amplification tests).

3.2.6.5. Areas for Irradiation of Blood Components

The room where the gamma irradiator is placed must meet the access and security requirements of the authorizing governmental agency. The irradiator must be used only for irradiation purposes. This room must fulfil national requirements for capsulated radioactive sources.

3.2.6.6. Other Areas

Separated from all other areas there must be rooms for rest, canteen, dressing, toilets, cleaning of transport containers and other materials, maintenance and repair of equipment.

3.2.6.7. Equipment

Equipment must be designed, placed and maintained as to be fit for use. Maintenance and repair should not have any influence on the quality of the performance or contaminate the equipment. There must be a schedule for periodic maintenance. There must be a schedule for calibration of weighing, measuring, control and registration equipment. Expired and/or defect equipment must be clearly indicated as such and removed from the working area if possible. Equipment may not negatively influence the quality of the products; physical damage must be avoided to containers as well, so sharp points or edges on equipment that comes into contact with plastic blood bags should be avoided. All parts of equipment that come into contact with the plastic of blood bags must be cleaned daily and regularly disinfected.

Equipment must be validated and re-validated periodically or after each repair or maintenance. Equipment coming into contact with donors must have special precautions to avoid electrocution of donors.

3.2.7. Documentation

Appropriate documentation is an essential part of the quality management system. Clearly written documentation prevents errors from verbal communication and is crucial in the traceability of blood collection, processing and control, with additional data that are of importance for the quality of the product, from donor to recipient. Specifications, manufacturing protocols, instructions, procedures, records and labels must be free of errors and available in writing. The legibility of documents is of paramount importance.

3.2.7.1. General

Documentation consists at least of:

- Policies and plans, e.g. the Quality Policy and Strategy and Annual Quality Plan
- Standards and specifications/requirements

- Description of processes
- Specifications of starting materials and final products, including intermediates
- Description of equipment, including computer hardware and software
- Description of procedures (SOPs) and EOPs
- Job descriptions
- Registration of performed activities and outcomes

Documents must be carefully designed, set-up, controlled and distributed. They must be authorized, signed and dated by authorized persons. Documents must be clear not only in terms of legibility but also in terms of language. Documents must be regularly revised with a minimum frequency of every 2 years. Documents should be typed; manual corrections are allowed unless when duly dated and signed and must be worked out in the next version as soon as possible. The date a document is coming into force is always later than the authorization date as there must be time to instruct and train all personnel involved. In case of electronic document control only authorized persons can make new documents or changes in existing document. This electronic system must be validated and regularly checked.

3.2.7.2. Specifications

There should be appropriately authorized and dated specifications for starting materials and packaging materials. When appropriate they should contain a description of the materials, including:

- The designated name and internal reference code;
- The reference, if any, to a pharmacopoeia monograph;
- The approved suppliers and, if possible, the original producer of the products;
- A specimen of printed materials;
- Directions for sampling and testing or reference to procedures;
- Qualitative and quantitative requirements with acceptance limits;
- Storage conditions and precautions;
- The maximum period of storage before re-examination.

Specifications for intermediate products should be available if they are purchased or dispatched, or if data obtained from intermediate products is used for the evaluation of the finished product. The specifications should be similar to specifications for starting materials or for finished products, as appropriate. Specifications of the final product should contain:

- The designated name of the product and the reference code if applicable;
- The formula or the reference to a description of the pharmaceutical form and package details;
- Directions for sampling and testing or a reference to procedures;
- Qualitative and quantitative requirements with acceptance limits;
- Storage conditions , special precautions and special transport conditions when applicable;
- The shelf life.

3.2.7.3. Manufacturing Formula and Processing Instructions (MFPI)

There must be a document known as the Manufacturing Formula and Processing Instructions (MFPI) for each kind of blood component to be manufactured.

This document must be dated and signed by the persons responsible for manufacturing and quality assurance. The section of the MFPI document covering the composition of the product should contain the name and a description of the product, as well as a list of all starting materials, supplements and packaging materials to be used. This list should also indicate the acceptable upper and lower limits of the amount of starting material to be used and supplements to be added.

The section of the MFPI document covering the preparation of the blood component should contain at least the following:

- The location where the manufacturing process must take place and the equipment to be used;
- Instructions concerning all processing steps with an indication of the parts that need particular attention;
- Special precautions to be taken;
- The anticipated yield of each processing step and the acceptable upper and lower limits;
- The checks that must be carried out during or after each processing step and the acceptable limits;
- The storage of intermediate and final products;
- Labeling of intermediate and final products.

3.2.7.4. Processing Record

A processing record based on the MFPI document must be kept. For the manufacturing of a series of similar blood components, each prepared from one single donation, the processing record should consist of a list of all components produced on one day, or part of a day. A processing record consisting of a list of similar blood components should contain at least the following:

- Processing date;
- Product name;
- Processing method
- Number of units produced;
- Donation number of every unit;
- Nature and batch number of starting materials used and adjuvant added;
- Particular occurrences during processing;
- Results of checks carried out during processing;
- Initials of the person(s) responsible for the processing.

If blood components are prepared from more than one donation, a separate processing record should be made for each single product. After manufacturing each processing record must be signed by the Head of the Processing Department who assures that manufacturing has been carried out according to the MFPI document.

3.2.7.5. Packaging Instructions

There should be formally authorized Packaging Instructions for each product, with pack size and type listed. These instructions should contain:

- Product name;
- Description of the product and distinguishing specifications, when applicable;
- Description of the packaging and the number of packages per transport box;
- A complete list of all packaging materials required for a standard batch size, including quantities, sizes and types, with the code or reference number relating to the specifications of each packaging material;
- When appropriate, there should be an example or copy of the relevant printed packaging materials, and specimens indicating where to apply batch number references, and shelf-life of the product;
- Special precautions to be observed, including a careful examination of the area and equipment in order to ascertain the line clearance before operations begin;
- A description of the packaging operation, including any significant subsidiary operations and equipment to be used;
- Details of in-process controls with instructions for sampling and acceptance limits.

3.2.7.6. Procedures for Receipt and Storage

There must be written instruction for receipt and registration of each delivery of starting materials and primary and printed materials. This applies also for the receipt of collected units of blood from external locations.

Suppliers of starting materials and packaging materials must be on a designated list that is controlled by quality management. The registration of receipt should at least contain:

- Product name as given on the bill, including the number of packages and units;
- The in-house name and /or code for the material (if different from a);
- Date of receipt;
- Supplier's name and, if possible, manufacturer's name;
- Batch number or reference number;
- Total quantity and number of containers received;
- The batch number assigned after receipt;
- Relevant comments.

There should be written procedures for the internal labeling, the quarantine and storage of starting materials, packaging materials and other materials when appropriate.

3.2.7.7. Sampling, Tests and Release

There should be written procedures for sampling, which include the person(s) authorized to take samples, the methods and equipment to be used, the amount to be taken and any precaution to be observed to avoid contamination of the material or any deterioration in its quality. There should be written procedures for testing materials and products at different stages of manufacture, describing the methods and equipment to be used. The tests performed should be recorded.

Written release and rejection procedures should be available for materials and products, and in particular for the release of the finished product by the Qualified Person. It should record to whom each component is issued. There should be written procedures and the associated records of action taken or conclusions reached, when appropriate, for:

- Validations;
- Equipment assembly and calibration;
- Maintenance, cleaning and sanitation;
- Personnel matters including training, clothing, hygiene;
- Test control;
- Complaints;
- Recalls;
- Returns.

3.2.7.8. Instructions and Log Book for Equipment

Logbooks should be kept for major or critical collection, processing, or laboratory equipment. Use and maintenance instructions should be available. Logbooks should record the results of validation, and calibration, and the name of the person(s) who performed these activities (initials or any other identification) and the date on which it happened.

3.2.8. Production

3.2.8.1. General

The entire production process contains: donor selection, blood collection, processing and blood component issue. All production activities must be performed according to written and detailed procedures, that meet all cGMP and regulatory requirements and must be documented.

To ensure that products always meet the required specifications, all processes, procedures and equipment must have been validated before being operated in the (daily) routine. Each change in any procedure must be validated again. Re-validation must be performed regularly.

Regular in-process controls and controls on final product are necessary due to the variability of the biological starting material (whole blood or apheresis components) and the spread of the results of the measure techniques. Production must be performed by well trained, authorized and competent personnel.

3.2.8.2. Incoming Materials

Incoming materials must be checked for compliance with purchase order. Containers should be cleaned, when necessary, and labelled with the required data. Any damage or other problems that might compromise the quality of the final product must be reported to the Quality Department.

Until formal release, all critical goods are in quarantine. The manufacturer of plastic blood collection systems must be able to send a certificate about the tests performed on the blood bag systems.

Storage conditions in quarantine and stock must be in accordance with the manufacturer's requirements. Only critical starting materials and packaging materials released by the Quality

Department may be issued to the various departments for usage in the production processes. The released stock must be well documented. Rejected materials must be immediately segregated and appropriately labelled.

Production of different products in the same area at the same time is not allowed and products must be protected against (microbiological) contamination.

3.2.8.3. Blood Collection

As whole blood or a blood component is the most important starting material, donors must be carefully selected according to National or International selection criteria. The collected volume of whole blood or blood component must be measured and must meet the target volume within preset limits.

The collection time must be documented. As a minimum the following procedures must be available:

- Labelling donor selection form, blood collection bag, satellite bags and sample tubes and all other items related to the donation;
- Re-identification of the donor prior to vene puncture;
- Preparation and disinfection of vene puncture site;
- The use and storage of disinfectants;
- Vene puncture;
- Collection of blood or blood components;
- Sampling and termination of collection;
- Donor care during and after collection;
- Interim storage and transfer of the donation and samples to processing department or laboratory respectively.

3.2.8.4. Blood Processing

Most of the processing activities can be performed aseptic without opening the closed system of collection and satellite bags. The use of a proper functioning 'Sterile Connection Device' may be considered as aseptic. Spiking technique is only allowed under the following conditions:

- Work in special areas
- Use clean closed gowning
- Use hear and beard covers
- Use nose and mouth protection
- Disinfect hand and lower arms
- Use of gloves
- Disinfection of working benches
- Adjustment of expiry time: maximum 24 hours if stored at 2-6° C or 6 hours if stored at room temperature (20-24° C)

Starting materials and intermediate products must be labelled with a unique identification (donation) number and the status of the product must be clear, either electronically or visual, or both.

Part of the release procedure is the final labelling. For this purpose the bar code system ISBT 128 can be used. The following minimum information must be on the label:

- Unique identification (donation) number
- Blood group (ABO Rh(D))
- Name of the product
- Donation date
- Expiry date
- Storage conditions
- Status indication (released for issue to hospitals)

If the product is prepared from a donation of a donor who donated earlier, the present data should be compared with the historic data. If an earlier donation is still blocked the new product(s) can not be released. Both manual and automated release procedures must be validated.

Released products must be transferred to the available stock. The storage must be conform the FIFO (first-inn; first-out) principle. The issue of blood components must be performed by two persons; one takes the requested components and another will check this. During issue the components are visually checked.

3.2.9. Quality Control (QC)

Quality control relates to all activities on testing materials and (samples) of products to determine conformance with the set specifications. Quality control must be done independent from the Production Department.

Quality control employees have permanent access to the Production Department in order to be able to take samples. Regularly, the results of the routine tests must be summarized and discussed with Production Department and Quality Management. As a minimum the following documentation must be available:

- Specifications;
- Sampling procedure;
- Test procedures en registration (including registration forms and / or laboratory journals);
- Analytical reports and / or certificates;
- Data from environmental monitoring, when required;
- Registration of the validation of test methods, if applicable;
- Procedures for and registration of calibration of instruments and maintenance of equipment.

Detailed written instruction must be available for sample taking:

- Specifications;
- Sampling procedure, including labeling (date for sampling and product identification);

- Test procedures en registration (including registration forms and / or laboratory journals);
- Analytical reports and / or certificates;
- Data from environmental monitoring, when required;
- Registration of the validation of test methods, if applicable;
- Procedures for and registration of calibration of instruments and maintenance of equipment.

For repository reasons samples should be kept for at least 2 years.

Quality Control Laboratories should participate in local, regional, national and/or international programs of quality assessment [proficiency testing or external quality assessment schemes (EQAS)]. Each new or changed analytical procedure must be validated prior to perform the analysis in (daily) routine. Re-validation must be performed regularly. As a minimum QC performs the following tests:

- ABO Rh(D) blood group determination
- Rhesus phenotyping (only if necessary)
- Other blood group system (only if necessary)
- Irregular antibody testing
- HIV, HBV, HCV and syphilis antibody marker testing
- Quality Control of intermediate and final products
- Microbiological Control

By definition (sterility: risk of contamination is $< 10^{-6}$) blood components are not sterile. Therefore critical steps have to be sampled for microbial testing. Especially platelet concentrates should be sampled for this purpose, because of the risk of contamination (docking) and the storage conditions (room temperature). The testing method used must be in writing (SOP) and being validated. The sampling scheme and method as well as the results must be well documented.

3.2.10. Complaints and Recall

Complaints must be carefully investigated following the written procedures. In case of any doubt about the quality and / or safety of a component it must be recalled according to written instructions. A person must be assigned who will investigate donor complaints and who will report back to the donor. As a minimum the following procedures must be available:

- Investigation of reports of internal incidents;
- Investigation of customer's complaints;
- Investigation of donor's complaints
- Reporting of the various investigations

The Quality Manager must always be informed about complaints and internal incidents especially if he does not perform the investigation. Serious events or complaints must be forwarded by the Quality Manager to the Competent Authority

A person – usually the Quality Manager - must be assigned who has the authority to initiate a recall at any time. This person is also responsible for the correct performance of the recall conform the written, validated and re-validated instructions.

If more donations are involved in one recall the Competent Authority should be informed[5]. All returned components and the not issued components involved in the recall must be labelled as such and must immediately be segregated in a lockable special area. Reason, course and results of the recall must be documented in a separate report.

3.2.11. Self-inspection

Internal audits have to determine the level of compliance to the Quality System and must be performed from time to time by one or more experts on the quality system(s). Peer audits should be set up.

3.3. GLP and GCP

The principles of GMP with its 10 quality system essentials equally apply to the laboratory (GLP) and the clinical (GCP) part of the vein-to-vein transfusion chain. Good Laboratory Practice focuses on strict containment of hygiene and prevention of contamination.

Good Clinical Practice emphasizes the importance of rational and safe bedside practices, based on the principles of patient blood management. The right blood component at the right moment for the right patient – the Hippocrates addage *primum est non nocere*.

4. Adoption of Quality Management Systems in the USA

4.1. Introduction and Historical Background

As noted above, the use of Good Manufacturing Practices (GMPs) in the production of biologics was required by the Food and Drug Administration in 1975. [17] The GMP regulations that are applicable to blood and blood components are contained in Title 21, Part 606 of the Code of Federal Regulations, and are titled "*Current Good Manufacturing Practice for Blood and Blood Components.*" [18] Today, these regulations address:

- Organization and Personnel
- Plants and Facilities
- Equipment
- Production and Process Controls
- Finished Product Control
- Laboratory Controls
- Records and Reports

---

[5] This may depend on country regulations as well as the nature of the cause of the recall.

In keeping with the FDA's mandate and legal authority, the GMP regulations focus on sterility and ensuring that blood and components are accurately labelled. The regulations also introduced a number of new concepts and included a significant number of record retention requirements. Registration and licensure of Blood Establishments followed. In order to perform manufacturing steps, a Blood Establishment needs to be licensed by the FDA to manufacture these products. In 1974, the introduction to the 7th edition of the AABB *Standards for Blood Banks and Transfusion Services* included a statement in the introduction that the quality control of all activities was an inherent part of the definition of a blood bank [19]. The next edition, published in 1976, required that all blood banks and transfusion services *"utilize a program of quality control that is sufficiently comprehensive to ensure that reagents and equipment perform as expected."* [20] In 1978, requirements for participation in a proficiency testing programme were put in place, which established inter-laboratory comparability of results as a key aspect of blood banking [21]. The application of quality management systems to transfusion medicine took a significant step forward when, in 1988, the Clinical Laboratory Improvement Amendments (CLIA) were enacted, and required that *"each laboratory establish and follow written policies and procedures for a comprehensive quality assurance program."* [22]. Accordingly, in 1991, the 14th edition of *Standards* required that blood banks and transfusion services use a programme of *"quality assurance under the supervision of a designated person to ensure that policies and procedures are properly maintained and executed."* [23] The subsequent edition, published in 1993, included a requirement for 'quality management'. In 1997, the AABB published Association Bulletin #97-4, which introduced the Quality System Essentials (QSEs) to the membership. The QSEs consisted of 10 concepts – organization, resources; equipment; supplier and customer issues; process control; documents and records; nonconforming products and services; assessments; corrective and preventive action and facilities and safety. Also in 1997, the FDA published a proposed rule that would require extensive reporting of errors and accidents. The proposed rule also explicitly required that all Blood Establishments follow GMPs. [24]. The 10 QSEs were subsequently incorporated into the 19th edition in 1999, as the introductory chapter of the book. When the 20th edition was published, each QSE represented a chapter heading – a conceptual formatting change which remains in place today. [25]

4.2. Quality System Essentials: A Closer Look

The QSEs represent a structured way of understanding quality and technical requirements as a matrix. As such, they include high level requirements that are applicable to the executive management of a facility and specific technical standards that define operational issues at the level of a standard operating procedure. A summary of each QSE is provided below.

- *Organization*: The purpose of this essential is to identify key management positions who have defined responsibilities for actions related to the quality management system. This essential also requires that the facility have a defined structure that clearly identifies the individuals or positions that are responsible for the provision of blood, blood components, and related services. Policies, processes, and procedures must be in writing and must be followed.

- *Resources*: The facility must have sufficient resources. These include financial resources, human resources, and material resources. For example, there must be a process to ensure that there are enough employees to perform, verify, and manage critical tasks. This does not mean that the facility must always be fully staffed; however, the facility must have processes in place to seek out additional human resources when staffing levels are inadequate.

- *Equipment*: Equipment must be controlled. This means that the facility must have a process to select and acquire equipment. The facility must also have a process to calibrate measuring equipment. Equipment must be checked at defined intervals. Increasingly, this QSE is also applicable to computer systems and informatics, and has been expanded over the years to include validation and maintenance of computer systems used in critical tasks.

- *Supplier and Customer Issues*: This QSE defines how the facility enters into agreements and includes both situations where the facility is the customer and those situations where the facility is a supplier. Suppliers must be qualified through a defined process. Once specifications for a given product or service are identified, they must be incorporated into the agreement. Incoming products and materials are inspected. Failure by a supplier to meet agreed upon requirements is to be reported to management with contracting authority.

- *Process Control*: This QSE concerns most of the discipline-specific requirements. It includes general requirements that apply throughout the workflow of collecting, processing, storing, and transfusion blood and blood components, such as traceability and sterility. It also follows the chain of activities from donor qualification to transfusion.

- *Documents and Records*: Documents are items such as policies, processes, and procedures, as well as blank forms. The facility must have a document control system to ensure that only current documents are used. Similarly, documents such as operating procedures and forms must be readily available at areas where related tasks are performed. A record control system will ensure that records are created concurrently with the activity captured by the record. It will also ensure that records are complete, legible, and retrievable in a period of time appropriate to the circumstances.

- *Nonconforming Products and Services*: This QSE addresses incidents, errors, and accidents. It requires that the facility have a process to capture and investigate failures to meet requirements. The facility must also evaluate and determine the disposition of a nonconforming product or service. Non-conformances must be reported to regulatory or accrediting bodies.

- *Assessments*: Internal assessments must be performed with some regularity. The facility must also have a process to schedule and prepare for external assessments. It must have policies, processes, and procedures in place to act on the findings from internal and external assessments.

- *Corrective and Preventive Action*: Process improvement is achieved by correcting actual identified non-conformances and by taking pre-emptive measure to prevent the occurrence of non-conformances. Corrective and preventive actions taken must be monitored and evaluated to ensure that they have been effective.

- *Facilities and Safety*: The facility must have a plan in place to address hazards. Personnel must receive safety training, and the facility must have policies, processes, and procedures to ensure the safety of donors, patients, staff, volunteers, and visitors.

5. APPROACH AND DEVELOPMENT OF QUALITY MANAGEMENT OF THE EUROPEAN UNION (EU)

5.1. History and Challenges

In the early days of blood transfusion, the demand for blood was not high and enough donors were available. Apart from detailing their specific blood group, individual donor characteristics were not an issue, and donor eligibility was not a real problem. Those days are now behind us. Over the last decades many developments have taken place. Today in Europe, only a few countries are not able to supply enough red blood cell units to hospitals. [26, 27] WHO uses the number of 10 red cell concentrates per 1,000 inhabitants per year as a minimum requirement for adequate health care. [26] In 2004, the number of blood collections throughout Europe per 1,000 inhabitants per year was 42 and varied from 3 to 74. [27] Cultural differences and educational levels are likely factors to explain this variance [28]. Various groups of patients benefit from blood transfusions. Their needs arise from trauma, surgery, and blood diseases such as leukaemia, sickle cell anaemia or thalassaemia. Other patient groups, such as patients with haemophilia or immunoglobin deficiencies, benefit from blood derived therapeutic products. Blood Establishments throughout Europe now collect per year over 20,000,000 units of whole blood from 13,000,000 donors. Donor eligibility has now become a demanding and crucial factor in the blood transfusion supply chain, due, amongst others, to increasingly strict selection criteria. European medical practices rely on a safe and sufficient blood supply. Blood Establishments are responsible for that supply. To fulfil their duty, they need to maintain a sufficient number of eligible donors. Good Donor Management starts here and is defined as that set of actions that leads to a sufficient and reliable donor base selected from the general population. To achieve that objective, a specific manual aims to provide guidance for donor managers in Blood Establishments.

5.2. EU Guidelines and Directives in Transfusion Medicine

Regulatory requirements at the European Union level are given by Directives, which differentiate between requirements for plasma-derived medicinal products and blood and blood components. Directive 2001/83/EC applies to all medicinal products, defined as 'any substance or combination of substances presented for treating or preventing disease in human beings'. [29] By contrast, Directive 2002/98/EC and its current technical annexes - Directive 2004/33/EC, 2005/61/EC and 2005/62/EC - set the legal framework for blood and blood components. [5, 12, 13, 30] For those Member States that classify blood as a medicinal product as defined by the pharmaceutical legislation, requirements related to collection and testing of blood and plasma still apply[6]. Similar quality and safety requirements have been introduced for tissues and cells. Directive 2004/23/EC [31] and more recently Directives 2006/17/EC [32] and 2006/86/EC [33] have given minimal requirements for the donation, procurement and testing process of tissue and cells and for traceability, severe adverse reactions (SAR) and events (SAE) as well as coding, processing, preservation, storage and distribution of tissue and cells.

General standards: EU Directive 2002/98/EC [30] sets general standards for the quality and safety of human blood and blood components. The Directive is based on the earlier Directive 89/341/EC and Council Recommendation 98/463/EC on the suitability of blood and plasma donors and the screening of donated blood in the European Community.

Technical standards: More detailed norms on technical requirements have been laid down in Directive 2004/33/EC. [13]

Quality systems: Specifications relating to quality systems are found in Directive 2005/62/EC. [5] This Commission Directive 2005/62/EC sets out the technical requirements for blood establishments related to the implementation and maintenance of standards and specifications relating to a quality system. It covers general principles, personnel and organisation, premises, equipment and materials, documentation, blood collection, testing and processing, storage and distribution, contract management, non-compliance and self-inspection, audits and improvements.

As per the EU blood legislation [30] 'quality shall be recognised as being the responsibility of all persons involved in the processes of the blood establishment with management ensuring a systematic approach towards quality and the implementation and maintenance of a quality system. The quality system encompasses quality management, quality assurance, continuous quality improvement, personnel, premises and equipment, documentation, collection, testing and processing, storage, distribution, quality control, blood component recall, and external and internal auditing, contract management, non-compliance and self-inspection.

The quality system shall ensure that all critical processes are specified in appropriate instructions and are carried out in accordance with the standards and specifications set out in this Annex.

Management shall review the system at regular intervals to verify its effectiveness and introduce corrective measures if deemed necessary. All Blood Establishments and hospital blood banks shall be supported by a quality assurance function, whether internal or related, in fulfilling quality assurance. That function shall be involved in all quality-related matters and review and approve all appropriate quality related documents. All procedures, premises, and equipment that have an influence on the quality and safety of blood and blood components shall be validated prior to introduction and be re-validated at regular intervals determined as a result of these activities'.

Traceability: Details on traceability requirements and notification of serious adverse events (SAE) and reactions (SAR) are found in Directive 2005/61/EC [12].

---

[6] 'This Directive shall apply to the collection and testing of human blood and blood components, whatever their intended purpose, and to their processing, storage, and distribution when intended for transfusion'. Article 2, Para 1, Directive 2002/98/E.

5.3. Development of Tools Addressing the Implementation

With the technical and medical focus of the directives, common requirements are defined in order to guarantee the safety of blood throughout the EU member states. Following the publication of the directives by the EC, the requirements have been transposed to the national legal systems in each of the member states.

In order to further sustain the improvement of blood safety in Europe, the EC has given project funds to major topics of the 'vein-to-vein' chain:

- Donor management and self-sufficiency in blood supply based on the different cultural and structural variations in Europe
- Quality management focused to develop document systems using standard operating procedures
- Quality system requirements based on EU directives and commonly used standards in order to establish the process of self-inspection and regulatory inspections by competent authorities
- The optimal use of blood including the right amount of blood and quality criteria for the clinical transfusion process

The funded projects comprised several organisations in blood transfusion and intended to establish common standards, criteria and state-of-the art knowledge on those topics in order to give practical assistance for member states or institutions, that would need to improve their current transfusion system.

While the topics of quality system requirements, inspection and in part donor management are linked to directive requirements, the topic of optimal use of blood is not primarily addressed in the current blood legislation.

5.3.1. Donor Management and Self-sufficiency in the Blood Supply

The blood legislation gives detailed criteria for donor eligibility and the process of blood collection with respect to the information given to the donor and the traceability requirements, but there are no rules on how to find, motivate, retain or treat donors. The DOnor MAnagement IN Europe, or DOMAINE Project has been set up to provide the guidance needed in donor management.

Blood Establishments from 18 European countries, the Thalassaemia International Federation and a representative from the South-eastern Europe Health Network joined forces in DOMAINE.

In 2008 the EU DOMAINE Project began to survey current blood donor management practices in European Blood Establishments. The insights derived from this study have been used extensively to develop the current DOMAINE Donor Management Manual. [34] The general objective is to help to create within the EU a safe and sufficient blood supply, by comparing and recommending good donor management practice among the Member States. The process of donor management involves many factors that Blood Establishments should take into account in order to provide the right number and types of blood products needed for transfusion.

These aspects include the following.

- Development and usage of donor recruitment strategies
- Organisation of blood donor sessions
- Development and usage of retention strategies
- Blood donor data management
- Donor counselling and donor care

Summing up and describing these activities may be interesting, but will have little practical effect. Personnel, equipment, housing, ICT, quality systems and finances must also be included and considered.

The Donor Management Manual provides such an opportunity. Complementary to these achievements, training programmes have been developed in order to disseminate the information to Blood Establishments in all European countries.

5.3.2. Quality Management of Document Systems Using Standard Operating Procedures

The EU-Q-Blood-SOP Project listed under EQUAL-blood has formulated a set of SOPs to be used in blood banking.

The project developed a pan-European standard operating procedure (SOP) methodology European best practice within the area addressing the quality and safety of blood. It had the following core activities. [35]

- Assessing the existence of SOP manuals and guidelines currently used in the 16 blood services involved in the project in order to identify (i) international and national SOP manuals already in place, and (ii) the current inspection practice
- A manual to assist Blood Establishments to develop and implement their own SOPs
- Testing the new SOP methodology among the partner institutions
- Producing the manual in different languages and distributing it to the participating blood establishments.

The manual describes a methodology based on good practice that

(1) assists Blood Establishments to implement or expand their standard operating procedures (SOPs).
(2) contributes to the understanding and management of quality processes in blood services.
(3) assists Blood Establishments in preparing for the inspection of their services related to the implementation of quality relevant elements required by the EU directive 2002/98/EC. [30]

Using the example in figure 5, this could be done as follows:

5.3.3. Quality System Requirements Based on EU Directives and Commonly Used Standards in order to Establish the Process of Self-inspection and Regulatory Inspections by Competent Authorities

The European Blood Inspection Project (EuBIS) has developed and is implementing commonly accepted criteria and standards to ensure equivalent recognition of inspection of Blood Establishments among EU Member States.

Two manuals has been developed that define the following [36] –

- Define requirements for quality management systems of blood establishments based on the Directive 2005/62/EC. [5]
- Develop a manual covering pan European standards and criteria for the inspection of Blood Establishments based on GMP guidelines to assist national inspections in implementing the
  - common criteria and standards for the inspection of blood establishments
  - requirements for the implementation or expansion of quality management systems to be inspected
  - the development of inspection checklists which closely follow Directive 2002/98/EC and its technical annexes
  - evaluation criteria for inspections and a benchmark system for deviations and improvements

Table 2. Steps, actions and responsibilities testing request for blood components

Step	Action	Responsibility
1	Reception of request	technician
1a	Check if the request is complete and valid	
-	address of the customer	
-	type of test requested	
-	testing material and labelling	
1b	Register the sample information in your laboratory information system (LIMS)	technician
1c	In case all information is complete proceed to step 2, if the request/test material/sample identification is incomplete go to step 3	technician
2	Start to perform the analytical test	technician
3	No testing performed.	technician + physician
	Document the type of non conformance and return relevant information to the customer	

The EuBIS manual(s) are designed to be used as tools to advise

- Blood Establishments that wish to optimise their quality system and self-inspection process related to the requirements set by the EU blood directive
- Blood Establishments to prepare for regulatory inspections by competent authorities
- if wished by competent authority, to be used as a reference during the
- implementation process of the EU directive requirements

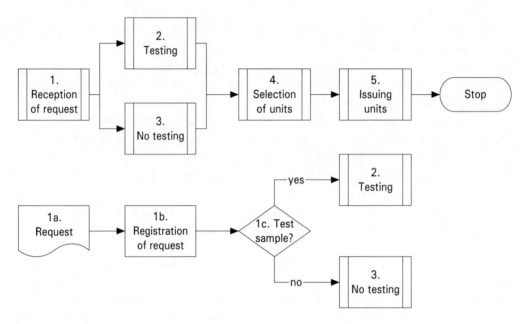

Figure 5. Example of a flow chart using international symbols to describe the testing request for blood component.

The EuBIS training guide [36] gives detailed information related to the blood directives including the cross-references to commonly used (required) standards as GMP, PIC/S and EDQM (CoE) Guide.

Chapter 3 of the EuBIS training guide is following the structure as presented in the annex of Directive 2005/62/EC [5] which gives legal requirements referring to quality management systems by the EC. The information in Chapter 3 is presented in the following form –

Column 1   Criterion number and primary reference to EU Directives
Column 2   Sub-process / control point (the manufacturing process step to which the audit criterion applies)
Column 3   Cross reference source
Column 4   Inspection criterion description
Column 5   Example evidence

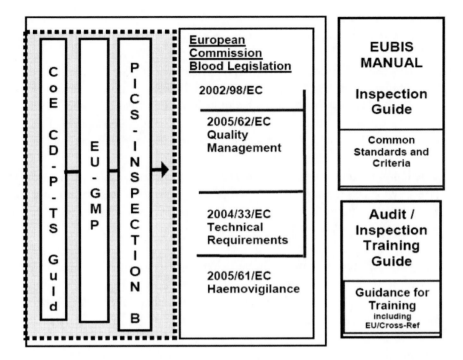

Figure 6. The EuBIS Project expert circle developing a manual for common European standards and criteria for the inspection of blood establishments (Inspection guide) for good practice following the EC blood legislation. The manual is supplemented by an audit / inspection – training guide on the relevant aspects to be addressed during the inspection process including cross-references for common European standards and criteria for quality management systems of blood establishments.

3 Inspection Guide

3.1 Licensing requirements

Blood Establishment Inspection Guide	EuBIS

Scope:	Licensing requirements

Criterion No. and Primary Ref. (EU Dir.)	Sub-process/ control point	Cross-Ref. source	Inspection criterion description	Example evidence
	Process(es) covered:	Licensing requirements		
LR 001 2002/98/EC Art. 5 – Licensing and authorisation Art. 11. Quality system for blood	Licensing requirements	GMP Annex 14 PIC/S Chap. 2 EDQM (CoE), Chap. 1	The Blood Establishment has submitted the information listed in Annex I (2002/98/EC) to the Competent Authority. The Competent Authority has verified that the blood establishment complies with the requirements of Directive 2002/98/EC and indicated which activities it may undertake and which conditions apply.	• Manufacturers license and whole sale distribution license as appropriate to the activity profile assigned by the Competent Authority • N.B. For those blood establishments that follow the requirements defined by 2001/83/EC, individual product licenses are required.

Figure 7. Inspection Cross reference guide for good practice following the EU blood legislation developed by the EuBIS experts. The cross-reference guide will assist Blood Establishments in implementing quality system requirements based on EU legislation.

The EuBIS training guide chapter 3 on inspection has 11 sections that walk the trainee through a number of QSEs as can be seen in figure 8.

5.3.4. Rational Use of Blood – the EU Optimal Blood Use Project

The EU Optimal Blood Use Project has developed a pan-European standard for optimal blood use [37]. It shares best practice on training in optimal use of blood components by developing and sharing a toolkit that can be used by a partnership of staff in blood establishments, hospital blood banks and hospitals' therapeutic departments, for the benefit of patients.

Also, it will provide a network of benchmarking on blood use in European hospitals.

This project will seek to identify good practice and start the development of a European quality management system for the therapeutic use of blood components, through the following steps [37] –

- Surveying the current situation in participating states in order to identify variations across Europe in blood usage, adverse effects, therapeutic practices and training
- Developing a toolkit in the form of a manual that will facilitate best practice implementation across Europe, raising awareness and training of health care staff about the use of blood components
- Developing a project website that will facilitate the sharing of best practice, the provision of a critically reviewed evidence base for optimal transfusion practice.

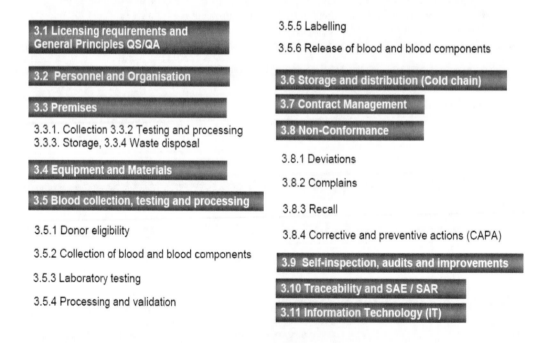

3.1 Licensing requirements and General Principles QS/QA

3.2 Personnel and Organisation

3.3 Premises
3.3.1. Collection 3.3.2 Testing and processing 3.3.3. Storage, 3.3.4 Waste disposal

3.4 Equipment and Materials

3.5 Blood collection, testing and processing

3.5.1 Donor eligibility

3.5.2 Collection of blood and blood components

3.5.3 Laboratory testing

3.5.4 Processing and validation

3.5.5 Labelling

3.5.6 Release of blood and blood components

3.6 Storage and distribution (Cold chain)

3.7 Contract Management

3.8 Non-Conformance

3.8.1 Deviations

3.8.2 Complains

3.8.3 Recall

3.8.4 Corrective and preventive actions (CAPA)

3.9 Self-inspection, audits and improvements

3.10 Traceability and SAE / SAR

3.11 Information Technology (IT)

Figure 8. Structure of content in the EuBIS training guide chapter 3.

6. Directions for the Future

Recent developments in quality management system paradigms have placed an increased emphasis on standardized documentation that allows continuous traceability and standardized procedures.

There has been a shift toward focusing on customer satisfaction and relationships, and this will likely continue to develop and mature. An example can be found in the ISQua approach to quality management for Blood Establishments and patient blood management programmes[7].

Within the EU much attention is being given to inter-country harmonization and standardized approaches in both the procurement (EUBis) and clinical transfusion practice (EUBUP), in addition to attempts through DOMAINE to harmonize donor management. However, the continued use of terminology that may be perceived as aggressive, terms like 'recruitment', 'donor camps' and the like, stemming from a period of enduring shortages and lack of public awareness, are still used. This may demonstrate poor understanding of the perceptions of the public.

In the age of social marketing, it is easy to imagine that blood collection establishments should be able to present a more collaborative and customer-friendly image where donors see themselves as critical partners in patient care rather than suppliers of raw biological materials (despite the attitudes of some regulatory bodies on this point). The key in the social marketing for blood donation is in motivation and the retention thereof. The culture and related attitude might change from the demanding and finger pointing '*I NEED YOU*' into a partnering through a supporting and offering – '*IF YOU NEED US, HERE WE ARE*'.

These developments are part of an ongoing process of refinement and review. In North America the current emphasis is on the promising though challenging development of comprehensive bio-vigilance and patient blood management, placing the patient in the centre of the transfusion medicine universe. However, the application of quality management systems to transfusion medicine can be limited by the growing gap between the advanced and developing parts of the world.

This gap may contribute to differences in cultures and the knowledge and skills available to the establishment. Increasing reliance on technology can create barriers to promoting a culture of quality that views human skills and intelligence as fundamental building blocks that are supported by the appropriate tools and systems.

With the 'touch screen and push button' culture that increasingly is replacing human awareness and understanding, the intellectual understanding of what a process and related procedures mean, or their purpose and intent of performance, and their place in an intelligent production chain from input into output, can all be lost. This phenomenon already has led to a decline in the basic understanding of physiologic and pathophysiologic processes of human blood and its elements to be used for clinical use. Building a culture of quality may therefore require building human capacity and should be viewed as a high priority. Quality is a multifaceted phenomenon, and the potential for a culture of quality is universally present, but deployment of quality management systems remains fully realized. In many instances, quality is not discovered, not observed, not identified, not applied and above all not entirely owned by the transfusion world to the extent needed to achieve real Total Quality Management.

---

[7] See also Chapter 9 – Patient Safety and Quality Management at the Clinical Interface

Annex 1. Isqua's International Principles for Healthcare Standards, 3rd Edition November 2007

Criteria	Revised Principles	Guidance
Principle 1	QUALITY IMPROVEMENT Standards are designed to encourage healthcare organisations to improve quality and performance within their own organisations and the wider healthcare system.	
1.1	The standards require healthcare organisations to define, as appropriate to their size and scope, their: • mission or purpose • values • ethics or code of behaviour and • strategic objectives.	
1.2	The standards define responsibilities for quality and performance improvement at different levels of the organisation.	Responsibilities may be defined for governance, management, clinicians, other staff and, where applicable, volunteers.
1.3	The standards define the responsibilities of a healthcare organisation for: • governance and • organisational management.	a) Governance responsibilities may relate to determining the organisation's direction, setting objectives and developing policy to guide the organisation in achieving its mission, and monitoring the achievement of those objectives and the implementation of policy. b) Organisational management responsibilities may relate to setting targets or goals for the future through planning and budgeting for the organisation's range of services, establishing processes for achieving those targets, allocating resources to accomplish those plans and ensuring that plans are achieved by organizing, staffing, controlling and problem-solving.
1.4	The standards require healthcare organisations to inform the public of: • the services they provide and • the quality and performance of the services.	
1.5	The standards require that policies, procedures or processes and plans for all key functions in the organisation are • documented • authorised • kept current and • implemented.	Authorisation may be demonstrated by the signature of a person with authority to approve policies and plans, or the recorded decision of a governing body.

Criteria	Revised Principles	Guidance
1.6	The standards require an approach to quality improvement that: • is systematic • is continuous • is organisation-wide • covers all aspects of performance • supports innovation • incorporates monitoring, including of all high risk processes and procedures, and evaluation.	
1.7	The standards require that key care and service processes and outcomes be measured through the use of: • performance indicators • patient/service user satisfaction surveys/assessments and • other performance measures.	Requirements could include: a) the use of these methods to measure functions such as human resources, infection control, risk management and patient/service user care and services; b) encouragement of the use of indicators expressed as ratios with defined numerators and denominators; c) use of other performance measures such as surveys, audits and feedback; d) the referencing of clinical performance indicators to evidence based medicine; e) encouragement for healthcare organisations to develop, implement or enrol in a quality indicators program.
1.8	The standards require the evaluation and analysis of data from performance measurement and its use to improve performance and services.	Data sources may include: a) indicators, patient/service user satisfaction assessments and other performance measures; b) complaints; and c) near misses, incidents and adverse events.
1.9	Law, regulations and health policy are recognised and integrated into the standards.	a) Common legal and regulatory requirements that may be referenced relate to employment, health and safety, building, environmental protection, reportable diseases, waste management, food and hygiene, health professional registration, health information, medicines and technical standards. b) Health policy may relate to new public health initiatives based on latest research or evidence that have been issued as guidelines but not incorporated into law.
Principle 2	PATIENT/SERVICE USER FOCUS Standards are designed with a focus on patients/service users and reflect the patient/service user continuum of care or service.	

Annex 1. (Continued)

Criteria	Revised Principles	Guidance
2.1	The standards cover the rights of patients/service users to: • dignity and respect • privacy • confidentiality and • safety and security.	Requirements could include organisations: a) documenting patient/service user rights and responsibilities; b) implementing training activities on them for staff.
2.2	The standards require a system for receiving, investigating and resolving patient/service user complaints and concerns in a fair and timely way.	
2.3	The standards require staff to involve patients/service users in their own care and services by: • respecting their preferences and choices; • informing them about their options for care and treatment; and • obtaining their informed consent.	Choices may include whether or not to be treated, the type of treatment, who they want involved in their care or service and end of life wishes. Preferences may relate to a) how they are addressed b) personal effects c) clothing and self care routines d) food, drink and meals e) activities, interests, privacy, visitors. Written consent is obtained for such activities as: a) participation in research or experimental procedures b) all operative and invasive procedures, anaesthesia and moderate/deep sedation and c) where there is a significant risk of adverse effects.
2.4	The standards require the cultural and spiritual sensitivities of patients/service users and their communities to be recognised.	This may include requirements to: a) provide access to spiritual care or advice that meets patients' /service users' needs; b) train staff on the cultural beliefs, needs and activities of different groups served; c) provide separate facilities and services for women and men where appropriate for the culture.
2.5	The standards cover access to services for patients/service users, including: • a range of services based on the needs of the community and the scope of the organisation • access for individuals with disabilities and special needs • coordinated admission or entry processes.	
2.6	The standards require that the assessments of patients/service users: • are comprehensive	Assessments may cover: a) patient/service user needs and risks appropriate to the type of service and patient/service user;

Criteria	Revised Principles	Guidance

	• involve relevant disciplines
	• are completed and documented in a timely manner.
		b) elements such as:
		   – medical
		   – physical
		   – mental, behavioural and emotional
		   – nutritional
		   – functional
		   – pain
		   – abuse and neglect.

2.7	The standards require that individual care/service plans are prepared and documented: • based on the assessment of patient/service user needs, including the results of diagnostic tests where relevant • involving the patients/service users and their families • including the goals or desired results of the treatment, care or service.	
2.8	The standards require that health professionals: • follow the care/service plans • monitor the progress of patients/service users in achieving the goals or desired results of treatment, care or service • reassess patients'/service users' needs when indicated • revise the care/service plan according to results.	
2.9	The standards require that referral, transfer of care, discharge or end of service is planned.	Requirements could include: a) planning commencing at first contact with the organisation and being ongoing; b) planning including patients/service users and their families; c) planning involving making links with referral agencies, other levels of health service and other organisations; d) if death is the expected outcome of the service, planning including the preparation of patients and their families for death, the management of pain and symptoms, linkage with support groups, counselling, and addressing spiritual and cultural needs.
Principle 3	ORGANISATIONAL PLANNING AND PERFORMANCE Standards assess the capacity and efficiency of healthcare organisations.	

Annex 1. (Continued)

Criteria	Revised Principles	Guidance
3.1	The standards require that organisations use a planning process to determine the level of staffing and skill mix required to meet the needs of the services provided.	Requirements could include: a) the plan considering the number of staff and independent practitioners needed, the levels of seniority and experience required, and the different disciplines and roles to match the needs of services to be provided; b) the planning process being documented and able to be evidenced.
3.2	The standards require that, for the positions they hold, staff, independent practitioners and volunteers where applicable, have relevant and current: • orientation and training • education • knowledge • skills and • experience.	
3.3	The standards require that those permitted by law and by the organisation to practice are credentialed and have their scope of practice defined.	Requirements could include: a) procedures for assessing or accepting healthcare professional training; b) credentials and scopes of practice being documented and regularly reviewed.
3.4	The standards require that staff, independent practitioners and volunteers where applicable: a) have their performance and competency evaluated on a regular basis b) receive relevant ongoing education and skill training and c) are provided with internal and external development opportunities.	Requirements could include competency assessments and performance evaluations being documented and shared with the staff member (or practitioner or volunteer) involved.
3.5	The standards require staff to follow current accepted standards, protocols and evidence based clinical practice guidelines.	
3.6	The standards require healthcare organisations to involve patients/service users, their families, staff and where possible the wider community in planning for the provision of services.	Requirements could include the documentation of the planning process and those involved in it.

Criteria	Revised Principles	Guidance
3.7	The standards require organisational planning to identify desired or expected service and organisational results and measure progress in achieving them.	Requirements could include: a) strategic and operational plans including longer term and short term goals and objectives for the organisation and its services; b) progress in achieving these goals and objectives through defined activities being measured and reported on a regular basis.
3.8	The standards require service planning to be based on the organisation's strategic direction and to consider environmental and financial factors.	
3.9	The standards require the planning of functions, activities and the development of departments and services to include provisions for coordination with each other and with relevant external services.	
3.10	The standards require that the efficient use of resources is regularly reviewed and is evaluated against organisational plans and budgets.	Reviews may include the utilisation of staff, equipment, supplies and space.
Principle 4	SAFETY Standards include measures to protect and improve the safety of patients/service users, staff and visitors to the organisation.	
4.1	The standards require a planned and structured approach to risk management that addresses all significant risks faced by the organisation and its services.	A risk management plan may include elements such as: a) policy b) context c) scope and objectives and criteria for assessing risk d) risk management responsibilities and functions e) staff training f) a list of identified risks – strategic, operational, financial and hazard g) a risk register or similar with an analysis of the risks and their level h) summary of risk treatment plans for major risks i) processes for communicating with stakeholders.
4.2	The standards require the risk management plan to be monitored and reviewed for effectiveness and results communicated within the organisation.	Requirements could include the organisation: a) undertaking routine surveillance of actual performance compared with required performance; b) investigating the current situation and specific issues periodically; c) using results from the monitoring and review processes to make improvements.

Annex 1. (Continued)

Criteria	Revised Principles	Guidance
4.3	The standards require healthcare organisations to have processes for reporting and investigating safety incidents, adverse events and near misses affecting patients/ service users, staff or visitors and for using findings to improve services.	The system may include: a) training for staff b) means for documenting and reporting incidents/events c) root cause analysis d) processes for informing patients/service users of adverse events
4.4	The standards require the organisation to protect the health and safety of staff.	The health and safety program for staff needs to be appropriate to the risks in the particular care sector and may include: a) protective clothing and equipment for staff b) workplace assessments c) workload monitoring and stress management d) staff vaccination e) prevention from needlestick or manual handling injuries f) protection from occupational hazards.
4.5	The standards require healthcare organisations to • train staff on the safe operation of equipment, including medical devices, and • ensure only trained and competent people handle specialised equipment.	
4.6	Standards require healthcare organisations to ensure that: • relevant safety law and regulations are met • the buildings, space, equipment and supplies necessary for the stated services are provided and • facilities and equipment are inspected, tested, maintained and updated or replaced in a planned and systematic way.	
4.7	The standards require healthcare organisations to undertake clinical risk assessments to safeguard patients/service users from unintended consequences of care/treatment.	Risk assessments could be required to include: a) medication management, covering issues such as patient/service user allergies and antibiotic resistance; b) equipment risks, e.g. fire/injury risks from use of lasers; c) risks resulting from long term conditions.
4.8	The standards require healthcare organisations to have a planned and systematic program for preventing and controlling infections which includes at least hand washing and cleaning requirements.	Other requirements may include, as appropriate to the care or services provided: a) structures and resources b) use of isolation and precaution techniques c) use of antibiotics

Criteria	Revised Principles	Guidance
		d) sterilisation activities e) monitoring f) collection, analysis and use of infection event data g) reporting e) staff education.
4.9	The standards provide guidance to assist organisations to manage issues of patient/service user safety relevant to the care sector, including any appropriate safety priority areas from the WHO Global Patient Safety initiative.	For acute services and others where applicable, this will include standards covering processes for: a) the safe management and use of blood and blood products b) right patient/right side/right site interventions c) safe practices before, during and after surgery, anaesthesia, moderate/deep sedation and invasive procedures d) safe medication management, including: - prescribing/ordering - transporting, storing and disposing - preventing, monitoring and documenting - responding promptly to adverse effects and medication errors.
4.10	The standards require patient/service user records to be current, complete, accurate and secure to assist the safety and continuity of care and treatment.	In the case of both electronic and hard copy records, requirements may include, as relevant to the service being provided: a) legible, dated, timely and signed entries b) alert notations c) progress notes, observations, consultation reports, diagnostic results d) all significant events such as alteration to patients'/service users' condition and responses to treatment and care e) any near misses, incidents or adverse events f) procedures for confidentiality, security and storage g) use of only recognised abbreviations h) procedures for retaining and destroying records.
Principle 5	STANDARDS DEVELOPMENT Standards are planned, formulated and evaluated through a defined and rigorous process.	
5.1	The need for new or revised standards and priorities are established by seeking the views of potential users, professional, purchaser, provider and patient/service user groups and governments and other stakeholders and using evaluation data from the use of previous standards.	

Annex 1. (Continued)

Criteria	Revised Principles	Guidance
5.2	Relationships with the standards of other organisations and professional and regulatory requirements are considered.	Links or overlap with other standards may be identified to aid implementation of the standards and avoid duplication where possible.
5.3	Standards are developed or revised in accordance with a plan that includes objectives, resources and timeframes.	
5.4	Standards are based on: • current available research, evidence and experience • internationally recognised guidelines • recommendations from WHO and national/international professional organisations and • input from technical experts and • legal requirements.	Standards based on those of other organisations/countries could be adapted to local culture and health service requirements.
5.5	Government, professional, purchaser, provider and service user interests have adequate opportunity for input into the standards development and revision process through direct representation and formal consultation.	Opportunities for other interested parties to participate may include publication of draft standards for comment, such as posting on the internet.
5.6	The scope and purpose of the standards are clear in terms of: • the type of healthcare organisation to which they apply; • whether they are designed for use by a whole organisation; • what range of services they cover; • the reason the standards are needed and used.	The purpose or reason for the standards may be: a) to set a minimal level of acceptable performance b) to facilitate quality improvement c) for accreditation or certification d) for licensing or e) for insurance eligibility.
5.7	There is a clear framework for the standards that makes them easy for organisations and assessors to use.	The framework may include: a) standards being grouped logically, e.g. by function or system; b) standards being labelled so that their content can be easily identified; c) the numbering system for the standards and their criteria or elements enabling them to be easily identified; d) A clear description of the standards framework in the documentation provided to users.
5.8	The wording of the standards is clear and unambiguous.	Clear wording may be achieved by: a) sentences having clear subjects and objects so it is clear what is required or who is responsible; b) words that may have more than one meaning or interpretation being clearly defined, e.g. good, well or sufficient; c) a formal review process to identify and clarify wording that is ambiguous or not clear;

Criteria	Revised Principles	Guidance
		d) material being available to assist users in the interpretation of the standards.
5.9	Standards are tested/piloted and evaluated by providers and assessors prior to approval to ensure they are understandable, measurable, relevant and achievable.	
5.10	New and revised standards are approved by the standards setting body or appropriate authority before general implementation in the sector.	
5.11	There is a process to determine the conditions under which the standards could be used by an independent assessment organisation, other than the body that developed the standards.	Requirements may include: a) the process being documented; b) expectations being defined and agreed, e.g. that the standards are used as intended and that the independent organisation provides feedback on the standards and the results of using them.
5.12	Information and education are provided to users and assessors of the new and revised standards to enable interpretation and implementation.	
5.13	Parameters, timeframes and any transitional arrangement for the implementation of revised standards are clearly identified and followed.	Requirements could include revisions of standards being publicised and distributed to users and assessors in sufficient time for them to develop an understanding of the standards before the date of implementation.
5.14	The views on standards and the satisfaction of users, assessors and stakeholder groups with them are obtained, documented and monitored and the analysed data is evaluated to assist with improving standards.	Processes could include: • feedback on the standards being sought from the organisation assessed and the assessors after assessments; • periodic surveys of stakeholders being used to obtain their feedback on the standards; • analysing feedback data on a regular basis, e.g. annually; • using the data in the standards revision process in a way that can be demonstrated.
Principle 6	STANDARDS MEASUREMENT Standards enable consistent and transparent rating and measurement of achievement.	
6.1	There is a transparent system for rating an organisation's performance on each standard, criterion or element.	
6.2	Guidelines or other information are provided to assist assessors to rate consistently and healthcare organisations to assess their own performance on the standards.	Guidance may be provided on how criteria or standards are weighted or how ratings are to be applied where there are identified risks or safety issues.
6.3	There is a defined methodology for measuring overall achievement of a set of standards in a consistent way.	Examples of how the methodology may define achievement include achievement on all compulsory standards, or all standards being achieved at a defined level, or no standards being rated at below a defined level.

Annex 1. (Continued)

Criteria	Revised Principles	Guidance
		b) The methodology may be used by organisations to assess their overall achievement of the standards as part of a self-assessment process. c) Overall performance on the standards may be used for the purposes of certification or accreditation, but these processes may use additional criteria that are not relevant here.
6.4	The satisfaction of healthcare organisations and assessors with the measurement and rating system is evaluated and results used to make improvements.	Processes could include: a) feedback on the rating system obtained after the assessment from the organisation assessed and the assessors, e.g. its usefulness and ease of use; b) analysis of feedback data on a regular basis, e.g. annually; c) using the data to improve the rating system in a way that can be demonstrated.

Annex 2. ISQua's International Principles for Healthcare Standards for Hospital Transfusion Services (CSIH Draft 2012)

HOSPITAL TRANSFUSION SERVICE
The organization protects and ensures the rights of its recipients.
Recipient's Informed Consent
Staff follow documented policies and procedures for recipient consent, including: a) obtaining consent for routine situations and emergency or high risk situations b) determining if a recipient is capable of providing consent and legally able to c) determining when someone other than the recipient can grant consent d) handling patients who are unsafe or refuse treatment and e) documenting consent decisions and who made them.
Appropriate information is provided to recipients and their families, in a way that they can understand: a) about the recipient's health status, including the clinical facts about their condition b) on any proposed tests or treatment c) on the risks and benefits of any proposed high risk treatment or procedure and d) on the alternatives available.

After information has been given and in line with legal requirements, recipient consent is obtained by signature or other indication:

a) at the first point of contact for tests or treatment
b) specifically and separately for high risk transfusion as defined by policy
c) documented in writing in the patient's record for such transfusion

Recipient records are current, accurate and complete.

There is evidence in the recipient record of the implementation of the plan of care, including:

a) observations and monitoring results
b) details and outcomes of transfusion
c) information given and consents received
d) any alterations in the patient's condition
e) responses to treatment and
f) any near misses, incidents or adverse events such as adverse transfusion reactions.

The organization addresses deviations, non-conformances and adverse events reporting to ensure compliances to the regulations.

Mechanisms are in place to recognize any adverse event related to transfusion of blood components. Additional steps include the evaluation and reporting of such events. The medical director is responsible for the development of procedures to address adverse event reporting.

The procedure is to include the steps for recognition, assessment and investigation to follow for the different types of adverse events related to transfusion:

a) Immediate Transfusion Reactions
b) Delayed Transfusion Reactions
c) Transmitted Diseases through Transfusion

The transfusion service is responsible to develop policies, processes and procedures to identify recipients involved in a look back and notify the recipient's doctor.

The organization ensures that the activities are performed in the best environment by qualified staff following best practices.

The transfusion service develops policies, processes and procedures for the collection of recipient samples, compatibility testing and distribution of units to the department for transfusion.

The transfusion service defines the information for collection of the samples with the request for the blood and blood components in the procedure. This includes:

a) the identification of the recipient with the blood sample matches at the time of collection
b) the request is signed by the authorized person and is complete, accurate and legible.
c) the sample is identified with two independent identifiers
d) the sample label is affixed to the tube prior to collection
e) the identification of the date and time and person who collected the sample is documented.

Annex 2. (Continued)

The procedure needs to include the retention period for the recipient's sample.
The transfusion service develops policies, processes and procedures for the serologic confirmation of the donor's ABO and Rh typing including autologous units.
The transfusion service develops policies, processes and procedures for pre-transfusion testing for allogeneic and autologous transfusion to include ABO and Rh testing. The procedure includes the selection of components especially when ABO and Rh compatible units are not available.
The transfusion service develops policies, processes and procedures for the methods to be followed for testing for unexpected antibodies to red blood cells and include the investigation when clinically significant antibodies are identified to ensure that the component selected meets the established policies.
The transfusion service develops policies, processes and procedures for performing serological cross match between the recipient's blood sample and the donor's red blood cells. This also applies to computer cross match.
The transfusion service is to develop policies, processes and procedures for testing requirements for transfusion of components to neonates.
The transfusion service is to develop policies, processes and procedures for the selection of blood and blood components in special situations such as: a) leukocyte-reduced components requests if not routinely available   b) Cytomegalovirus (CMV) selected units to reduce the risk of CMV transmission.   c) irradiation of components as requested   d) request for lack of Hemoglobin S in blood or red blood cells   e) compatibility testing indication for massive transfusion recipient
The transfusion service develops policies, processes and procedures for the final inspection and labeling of components prior to issue. The following applies: a) attachment of label to the component   b) final check of records at time of issue   c) the signature of the person picking up the component if applicable
The transfusion service develops policies, processes and procedures for the return of issued components and the reissue of these components.
The transfusion service develops policies, processes and procedures for the release of blood and blood components in the case of emergency release when components are not available based on the testing not being completed when a delay in transfusion could be detrimental to the patient.

Annex 3. Example of an Organogram for a Blood Establishment

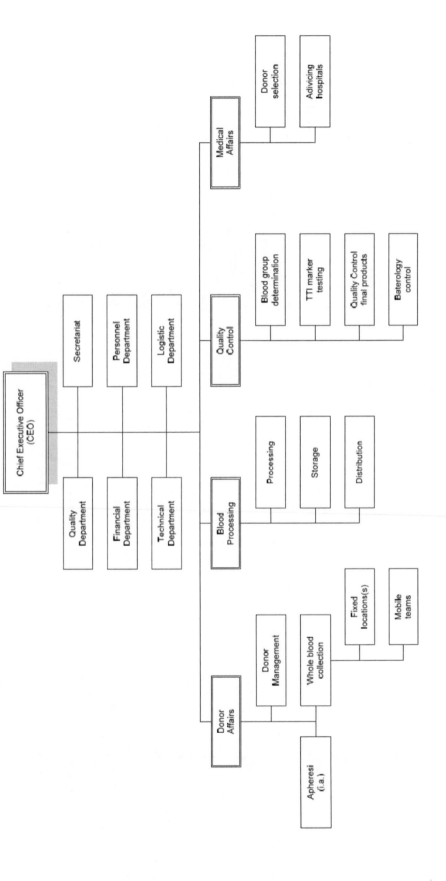

Annex 4. Example of a Stock Report Document

Daily report on stock of Red Cell Concentrates, Leukocyte depleted

Report Date: December 12, 2006

Blood Group	untested blood			tested blood			Balance		
	Units	previous stock	total	previous stock	tested	total	issued blood / issued	untested	Tested
A Pos.	100	10	110	500	105	605	102	5	503
A Neg.	20	2	22	88	22	110	18	0	92
B Pos.	50	5	55	243	53	296	45	2	251
B Neg.	5	0	5	21	5	26	3	0	23
0 Pos.	100	10	110	498	105	603	112	5	491
0 Neg.	75	8	83	369	81	450	75	2	375
AB Pos.	40	4	44	203	40	243	38	4	205
AB Neg.	5	0	5	24	5	29	3	0	26
Total	**395**	**39**	**434**	**1946**	**416**	**2362**	**396**	**18**	**1966**

Daily report on stock of Red Cell Concentrates, Leukocyte depleted

Report Date: December 13, 2006

Date:	untested blood		tested blood				issued	Balance	
	Units	previous stock	total	previous stock	tested	total	blood issued	untested	Tested
Team									
A Pos.	105	5	110	503	107	610	98	3	512
A Neg.	15	0	15	92	14	106	22	1	84
B Pos.	48	2	50	251	47	298	40	3	258
B Neg.	7	0	7	23	6	29	5	1	24
0 Pos.	92	5	97	491	93	584	108	4	476
0 Neg.	82	2	84	375	82	457	72	2	385
AB Pos.	43	4	47	205	45	250	35	2	215
AB Neg.	6	0	6	26	5	31	1	1	30
Total	**398**	**18**	**416**	**1966**	**399**	**2365**	**381**	**17**	**1984**

References

[1] United Nations. (1948) Universal Declaration of Human Rights. 22 March 2011 Retrieved 09 June 2012 from www.un.org/en/documents/udhr/index.shtml.

[2] International HACCP Alliance. Retrieved June 09 2012 from http://haccpalliance.org.

[3] *Food and Drug Law*, 3rd Edition 2007. Hutt PB, Merrill RA, Grossman LA. Foundation Press, New York, USA (pp 918 and 924).

[4] Commission Directive 91/356/EEC of 13 June 1991 laying down the principles and guidelines of good manufacturing practice for medicinal products for human use. Official Journal of the European Union, L*193, 17/7/1991, p30–33.*

[5] Commission Directive 2005/62/EC of 30 September 2005 implementing Directive 2002/98/ EC of the European Parliament and of the Council as regards Community standards and specifications relating to a quality system for blood establishments. Official Journal of the European Union, L256, 01/10/2005 p41-48.

[6] PIC/S GMP Guide for Blood Establishments PE 005-1, PIC/S secretariat, Geneva, CH, 2001 (actual version PE-005-3, Sept. 2007).

[7] Quality Management Systems – Requirements ISO 9001:2008. CEN European Committee for Standardization, Brussels, BE 2008.

[8] Environmental Management Systems Requirements ISO 14001:2004. CEN European Committee for Standardization, Brussels, BE 2004.

[9] AQAP and ISO. Retrieved from http://en.wikipedia.org/wiki/ISO_9000#Background.

[10] EFQM. Retrieved June 09 2012 from http://www.efqm.org/en/.

[11] ISQua. Retrieved June 09 2012 from http://www.isqua.org/about-isqua/about-isqua.htm.

[12] ASQ. Retrieved June 09 2012 from http://prdweb.asq.org/certification/control/index.

[13] Commission Directive 2004/33/EC of 22 March 2004 implementing Directive 2002/98/EC of the European Parliament and of the Council as regards certain technical requirements for blood and blood components. Official Journal of the European Union, L91, 2004, p25-39.

[14] AABB Technical Manual, current edition (ISBN 1-56395-155-X) AABB Press, Bethesda, MD, USA.

[15] Berthe L. *Quality Manual Preparation Workbook.* 2003 AABB Press, Bethesda, MD, USA.

[16] Commission Directive 2005/61/EC of 30 September 2005 implementing Directive 2002/98/ EC of the European Parliament and of the Council as regards traceability requirements and notification of serious adverse reactions and events. Official Journal of the European Union, L256, 1/10/2005, p.32-40.

[17] *Food and Drug Law*, 3rd Edition 2007. Hutt PB, Merrill RA, Grossman LA. Foundation Press, New York, USA (pp 918 and 924).

[18] Food and Drug Administration. Current Good Manufacturing Practice for Blood and Blood Components. 21 CFR § 606.

[19] Oberman H, ed. *Standards for Blood Banks and Transfusion Services,* 7th edition. AABB: Bethesda, MD, 1974.

[20] Oberman H, ed. *Standards for Blood Banks and Transfusion Services,* 8th edition. AABB: Bethesda, MD, 1976.

[21] Oberman H, ed. *Standards for Blood Banks and Transfusion Services,* 9th edition. AABB: Bethesda, MD, 1978.

[22] Clinical Laboratory Improvement Amendments of 1988. 42 CFR § 493.

[23] Widmann F, ed. *Standards for Blood Banks and Transfusion Services,* 14th edition. AABB: Bethesda, MD, 1991.

[24] Food and Drug Administration. Biological Products: Reporting of Errors and Accidents in Manufacturing (proposed rule), 62 Federal Register 496 (1997).

[25] Menitove J, ed. *Standards for Blood Banks and Transfusion Services,* 20th edition. AABB, Bethesda, MD, 1999.

[26] The WHO standard indicating levels of sufficient blood supply to hospitals for basic needs lies at 10 red blood cell units per 1,000 inhabitants. Source: World Health Organisation (2009) *Global blood safety and availability. Facts and figures from the 2007 Blood Safety Survey.* Retrieved June 09 2012 from http://www.who.int/mediace ntre/factsheets/fs279/en/index.html.

[27] Van der Poel CL, Janssen MP, Borkent-Raven B (2007). *Report on the collection, testing and use of blood and blood components in Europe in 2004.* Council of Europe, European Committee (Partial Agreement) on Blood Transfusion.

[28] Kort de W, Wagenmans E, Dongen van A, Slotboom Y, Hofstede G,Veldhuizen I. Blood collection and supply: just a matter of money? *Vox Sang,* 2010;98: e201-e208. doi:10.1111/j.1423-0410.2009.01297.x

[29] Directive 2001/83/EC on the Community code relating to medicinal products for human use. *Official Journal of the European Union,* L33, 8/02/2003, p 30-40.

[30] Directive 2002/98/EC of the European Parliament and of the Council of 27 January 2003 setting standards of quality and safety for the collection, testing, processing, storage and distribution of human blood and blood components and amending Commission Directive 2004/33/EC of 22 March 2004 implementing Directive 2002/98/EC of the European Parliament and of the Council as regards certain technical requirements for blood and blood components. *Official Journal of the European Union,* L91, 30/03/2004, p25-39.

[31] Directive 2004/23/EC of the European Parliament and of the Council of 31 March 2004 on setting standards of quality and safety for the donation, procurement, testing, processing, preservation, storage and distribution of human tissues and cells, *Official Journal of the European Union L 102, 7.4.2004, p. 48-58.*

[32] Commission Directive 2006/17/EC of 8 February 2006 implementing Directive 2004/23/EC of the European Parliament and of the Council as regards certain technical requirements for the donation, procurement and testing of human tissues and cells. Text with EEA relevance. *Official Journal of the European Union L 038, 09/02/2006, p. 40-52.*

[33] Commission Directive 2006/86/EC of 24 October 2006 implementing Directive 2004/23/EC of the European Parliament and of the Council as regards traceability requirements, notification of serious adverse reactions and events and certain technical requirements for the coding, processing, preservation, storage and distribution of human tissues and cells. *Official Journal of the European Union L 294, 25/10/2006, p. 32-50.*

[34] de Kort W, Veldhuizen I. *Donor Management Manual,* 2010.ISBN 978-90-815585-1-8 DOMAINE project Nijmegen, NL. Retrieved June 07 2012 from www.domaine-europe.eu/.

[35] Retrieved June 09 2012 from www.eu-q-blood-sop.de/pages/objectives.php.

[36] Retrieved June 09 2012 from www.eubis-europe.eu/objectives.php.

[37] Retrieved June 07 2012 from www.optimalblooduse.eu.

In: Quality Management in Transfusion Medicine
Editor: Cees Th. Smit Sibinga

ISBN: 978-1-62618-665-1
© 2013 Nova Science Publishers, Inc.

Chapter IV

Process Management in the Vein-to-Vein Chain

Jan Peter Jansen van Galen[1]*
and Cees Th. Smit Sibinga[2]

[1]Managing director Production Unit
Sanquin Blood Bank, Amsterdam, NL
[2]International Development of Transfusion Medicine,
ID Consulting for International Development of Transfusion Medicine (IDTM),
University of Groningen, Zuidhorn, NL

Abstract

This chapter outlines the principles of process management as applicable to the blood supply.

Following general principles, available tools for managing processes are described focused on statistical process control. A section is dedicated to the importance of the supplier-customer chain in relation to process management, followed by a detailed description of process management in the vein-to-vein transfusion chain – procurement and clinical consumption.

Keywords: Project management, Quality management, Monitoring and evaluation, Statistical process control, Vein-to-vein chain

Questions to be answered:
How can an organization keep up with the challenge and enhance the reliability of performance?
How can an organization ensure that every process delivers value every time?

---

* Tel: +31-6-2247.2821; E-mail: jpjvg@xs4all.nl.

1. Introduction

Project management has become recognized as an essential competence by those organizations, which need to effect change in order to prosper and survive. It has also been applied across a growing range of business activities including high technology projects, information technology and, more recently, complex business initiatives. The standardization of tools and techniques has led to the commodification of the blood supply. By contrast, the recognition of the difficulties of delivering multiple products (cellular and plasma derived) has led to increasingly sophisticated thinking in the areas of process management. [1, 2]

Despite these advances, there is still a high level of failure – even organizations that have robust processes often fail to deliver the benefits from processes and projects effectively. Although the investment in project and process delivery capabilities has never been higher, it is simply failing to keep pace with the scope, scale and complexity of the challenges that organizations have to take on to stay ahead. This is particularly true in low and medium HDI countries. [3]

Most initiatives to improve operational process delivery tend to focus on the obvious, tangible aspects and they fail to generate sustained improvement. It is not just that the skills and the expertise of the managers are limited; often the fault lies at the heart of the organization – it just does not have the corporate competences and quality culture for consistent success.

In addition to a sound foundation of well identified, analyzed and described processes, there are four other dimensions that are essential to deliver operations successfully and consistently:

- A set of key values and principles which catalyze the attitudes needed for successful delivery – *quality culture*;
- The right attitudes underpin a robust delivery chain – *clear process flow*;
- Processes create additional value when the inter-relationships (*supplier-producer-customer chain*) are managed in an integrated way;
- Organizations deliver consistently when a proper approach, attitudes and behaviour are embedded in their quality culture – *creation of ownership*.

1.1. Key Values and Principles that Drive the Right Attitude, the Quality Culture

It has long been recognized that attitudes and behaviours drive the effectiveness of management, but there has been no clear articulation of the '*values and principles*' that underpin a successful organization.

These key '*values and principles*' are to be used to determine how we recruit, develop, recognize and reward people, which enables to develop the attitudes and behaviours – the culture – in people, that are fundamental to success. These '*values and principles*' are the crucial catalysts for successful process management. [4] The key values and principles are:

- Preserving a strict and consistent vision and mission – the set goals;
- Ensuring total clarity – a basic quality principle;
- Confronting reality – the trigger for improvement;
- Behaving with integrity – the fit for purpose principle;
- Creating energy – commitment to the authorities and responsibilities provided.

Sub a. Preserving a strict and consistent vision and mission – the set goals

This requires the whole team to really understand the drivers of the business and the benefits required by the business strategy, the set goals. It is this understanding that enables the relentless focus on aligning decisions with the objectives, departmental and organizational. It allows ensuring that every action contributes to the delivery of benefits. People generally manage well downwards into a process, but are not always as efficient at managing upwards and outwards.

Additionally, the management often finds it difficult to communicate its needs, issues and priorities to the project teams. Developing people with this strict and consistent vision and mission is the key to bridging this gap and ensuring that everyone works together toward delivering the benefits fit for purpose.

Sub b. Ensuring total transparency – a fundamental quality principle

Vagueness and ambiguity of objectives and responsibilities are the root cause of many of the problems that exist in processes and production chains. It is crucial for people to understand what is expected of them and what they can expect of others.

Achievement of total transparency is the building block that enables people to perform effectively. This applies when communicating the goals and how they will be achieved (and who they will be achieved by) when agreeing all roles, authorities and responsibilities, and when promoting well-reasoned, firm and timely decisions – accountabilities. This is not an easy value to live up to. It requires a great deal of effort, particularly in the early planning stages of a process. It is one of the pillars of quality culture.

It then calls for people to consider the target audience (internal and external), what the message is and what actions are necessary to ensure that they fully understand what is required every time they communicate. It necessitates continuing self-appraisal, validation and evaluation that clarity is being achieved.

Sub c. Confronting reality – the mirror phenomenon and trigger for improvement

It is human nature to look on the bright side and avoid looking for trouble – it usually manages to find us without help! The result is that we often face unpleasant surprises. Successful managers cannot afford unpleasant surprises; they need to actively confront reality and be open to deviations and non-conformances. This means engaging the politics and powers within the organization, understanding personal goals and aligning them with the process. Being pragmatic about what can be delivered and the way it can be done, key to proper time management. It also means having a passion for actively looking for threats to success and ensuring that these devils are dealt with promptly – the principle of improvement based on regular SWOT (Strengths, Weaknesses, Opportunities and Threats) analysis. We need the courage to challenge what we observe and find, to ensure that it represents the real situation. It is no good complaining that others have obscured reality; process managers must assure it for themselves.

Sub d. Behaving with integrity – the fit for purpose principle

Processes rely on team working and teams are built on trust, mutual respect and confidence. Also, stakeholders need to be able to trust the team because, while processes are repetitive, the external customer has to live with the outcomes for years. This is fundamental to the principle of '*fitness for purpose*' and '*customer orientation*'. Without integrity, trust disappears, teams do not function effectively and time is wasted because opinions are not respected. Often more time is spent protecting positions than in delivering the expected outcomes. Managers have to create an environment of trust and confidence, where people work as a team, contributing to the good operations of the process. They have to take personal ownership for consistently meeting expectations and deal with problems in an open, honest and timely manner (non-conforming policy and strategy). Above all they have to maintain respect for the individuals, culture and market forces that drive the organization.

Sub e. Creating energy to make things happen – commitment to the assigned authorities and responsibilities

Energy is perhaps the greatest differentiator. Good managers do not sit back and monitor history; they actively go out and manage the future – the Deming cycle of improvement. They create energy and enthusiasm toward achieving their objectives – and departmental managers need to be good leaders. They have to be able to drive the processes forward, finding creative solutions and working in partnership to release the power of the individual and the team. They have to be able to motivate people and recognize the importance of acknowledging and rewarding achievement. It is their determination and persistence that makes things happen. This does not mean rushing about like a headless chicken; it is about the focused and sincere application of influence and determination to find the means to deliver – *not finding out why things can not be done, but how things could happen.* These 5 values and principles drive success integrally on the vein-to-vein process chain. All involved should aspire to demonstrate commitment to them in all that we do – develop ownership. Good managers create the energy in themselves and in their teams to make things happen.

2. The Process Flow

The foundation of successful process management is a toolkit of well analyzed and described processes. However, success requires more than just a good toolkit of processes; they need to be linked together to form an integral and robust purchase, production and delivery chain. [5] Even this is not enough unless people with the right set of values, principles and behaviours underpin this operational chain. '*Doing the right process*' sounds simple, but a common cause for processes failing is that the wrong process was started at the wrong time, the process initiation having been inadequate to drive out the real scope required. An effective process initiation ensures that the rationale for the process is properly defined, sound and achievable; input, production and output from supplier to customer. Often the link between the capability delivered by the process and the realization of benefits is overlooked and/or considered too difficult to describe. Unfortunately, this is a recipe for disaster and chaos. The key is in the available 'capabilities' which will allow benefits or outcomes to be delivered fit for purpose. When the 'capabilities' are clearly defined, timescales and costs will contribute to what the organization really needs. The management has to understand what the organization really needs and be able to articulate and document how these benefits will be created from the outputs – *if it cannot be stated, it cannot be delivered.* The other side of the equation is just as important – it must be feasible to deliver to the time, cost and quality defined in the mission statement. Developing a robust mission requires energy, to get the best information available and drive out all the risks and obstructing issues. So, good main and working process design ensures achievability and defines the functional requirement –

- what the totality must deliver; *the work breakdown*
- how many processes and procedures are required and what each must do; *the operational and technical architectures*
- how the processes and procedures fit and work together; *the work flow.*
- It also defines the assurance process; *how to prove that the processes and procedures will fit and work together like a chain.*

Top-down planning is crucial as is proper flow charting the serial events. It is essential to see the whole picture and not get lost among the individual processes and procedures. If the main and working processes are done well, there can be high confidence that, if the design is built, the benefits will be achieved. A comprehensive and properly defined management plan is essential. The management plan consists of a clear statement of the process objectives, how the process will be managed and the plan for delivery. Its development represents an opportunity to get the team and other stakeholders involved and committed. Unless they buy into the plan (*develop feeling of ownership*), it is unlikely that they will understand what is expected of them and what they can expect of others, the supplier-customer relationship. Developing the plan is the manager's opportunity to get clarity and commitment. It forces resolution; what can not be written down, is not thought through, and represents an issue or risk to the process.

2.1. Securing the Infrastructure that Provides the Ability to Deliver

Resources provide the fuel for delivery –

- getting the right quality (competence) and quantity of people,
- supported by the right technology (operational tools),
- with an effective infrastructure (managerial and operational),

These represent one of the most critical tasks facing the manager. The right quantity and quality of people who are able to operate effectively from day one, are required. Communicating what the processes really need, in terms of competencies, quantity and time, is a fundamental starting point. It then takes real determination to obtain these resources at the right time, whether internally or externally.

Most of us rely on access to the right communication technology such as e-mail, intranets, CAD, and other technologies, but the problem comes when we put together a team that crosses departments or other organizations – such as in the Donor Department or the Distribution Department – and the technology does not work. It is necessary to define how the team is going to work and to then provide the technology required to allow it to happen and not the other way around. Fortunately, this is getting easier with today's information and communication technology, but it is still up to the manager to ensure that the technology works for the team.

Another important aspect is an effective infrastructure. In reality, the ability of people to perform effectively is still heavily dependent on good infrastructure. While co-location is not always practical, it remains one of the most powerful levers available to build the team and influence attitudes and behaviours. An infrastructure that works well would not just happen; it needs to be carefully thought through, planned and properly implemented.

2.2. Processes Provide the Vital Foundation for Good Control

Management processes provide the foundation to '*do it right*'. The core or working processes are typically well understood and documented and will support sound planning and effective control.

However, for the more complex operations, specialist processes, such as system engineering and ICT, may be needed to enable effective management. It is crucial that the set of management processes selected are appropriate to the challenges created by a specific process. Sound planning is key to communicating the current status and work to be done. It is essential to clear understanding and communication of the work to be done and its current status.

This starts with the top-down planning for the process design. An effective planning process will continuously reconcile these top-down plans and milestones with the detailed bottom-up plans that are developed as the main processes evolve. This 'big-picture thinking' is needed to look for the best structures and identify and manage the implications of key interactions.

Effective control is required to manage disruptions. However, there is a tendency to think that all that is needed for good process management is to '*turn the handle*' on these processes. Nothing could be further from the truth. Effective process management requires that the information provided by the controls is acted upon (Quality Assurance or QA) – because having the information (Quality Control or QC) is only a starting point. What really differentiates the successful process manager is the way the information is used and that is all about the attitudes and behaviours of the manager – the quality culture.

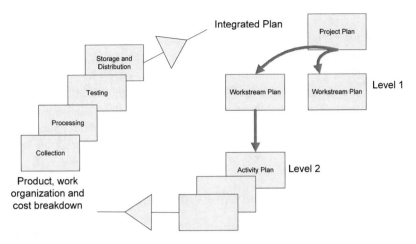

Figure 1. The planning hierarchy leading to an integrated process plan in blood procurement.

While system engineering has grown out of the need to manage technological processes of increasing sophistication, it has a wider application. It is particularly suited to larger complex processes, or those that operate within complex environments, such as large regional or national blood establishments.

It embodies the lessons learned from successes and failures over the last 60 years. A good working definition for system engineering is:

"System engineering is the set of activities which control the overall design, implementation, and integration of a complex set of interacting components or systems in order to meet the needs of all users and other stakeholders".

System engineering makes it possible to control the most complex technical solutions and to ensure that the solution will actually deliver what is required. It will typically –

- reduce overall delivery time and cost of products and services - *cost-effectiveness*
- reduce, and promote earlier discovery of rework and discard - *efficiency*
- create resilience to change and improvement - *development*
- increase the probability of delivering the real user needs – *fitness for purpose*.

In summary, it is a vital tool in the right circumstances.

2.3. No Process is Isolated – Interfaces are Crucial

The organization moves on, and so must the processes. The manager has to understand how the organization – in terms of its strategy, priorities and resource constraints – is changing in relation to its external environment, such as competitors, regulators, suppliers and customers. It is important to consider how these changes will affect what the organization wants from the processes and how the processes should respond, because preserving a strict and consistent mission is crucial. Few processes can deliver in isolation; usually there are interfaces and dependencies with other parts of the organization. The process may need access to an asset or a resource for which there are competing demands, e.g. blood collection with the demand for processing and the simultaneous demand for testing. This makes it essential for managers to identify and manage the interfaces with other processes or departments and maintain effective relationships with '*business-as-usual*'.

The process manager needs an effective network of relationships. He can not afford to leave the external environment unmanaged as it impacts a typical process or project in so many diverse ways. This requires energy and integrity from the manager to develop relationships (e.g. professional, operational, scientific) and keep abreast of developments.

2.4. Aligning the Organization and its Processes

Most processes have to operate within the culture and working practices of the organization; they need the co-operation and support of the main supportive and steering functions to succeed. This needs to be considered in terms of sponsorship and politics, processes, systems and people. Every process needs effective leadership from within the organization. Without it, stakeholders will build unrealistic expectations and play to their own political agendas; doors that need to be open for the process to succeed will remain closed. Effective leadership unlocks these doors. Even with effective leadership, the manager still has to be relentless in engaging the organization to ensure that aspirations of stakeholders are effectively managed. It is also vital for the manager to gain trust and confidence of stakeholders. Time spent by the leader and manager, to clarify their respective roles and to develop trust in each other's ability to deliver, will be repaid many times in the success of the processes and the satisfaction of the customers, internal and external.

Processes need to provide information for exchange with the rest of the organization and rely on some of its key systems and supportive processes such as procurement and payroll. It makes sense to align systems and processes as much as possible to avoid conflict and disruption. Processes need the best people and, in order to get them, it must be clear that taking on a process role can be a career enhancing experience.

The effective manager will establish and address the development needs of the team and ensure that their efforts are recognized and appropriately rewarded. Time spent on promoting the image of the process within the wider organization will pay dividends. After all the strength of the entire chain is determined by the weakest link. Above all: communicate, communicate, communicate. The really successful managers spend at least as much energy communicating with the other stakeholders, telling them what the process is doing, establishing how it will affect them, and enquiring what the stakeholders are doing that will in turn affect the process, as in managing the process itself.

2.5. Added Value of Complex Inter-relationships When Managed in an Integrated Way

Almost every organization is faced with a multiplicity of drivers of change, both internal and external. Managing parallel initiatives is an important core corporate competence. Conventional management approaches are often inadequate for dealing with the scale and complexity of change required. This is particularly true in developing countries. Programme management enables robust realization of benefits that rely on outputs from multiple initiatives, especially where:

- There are shared objectives across a number of processes, such as where the outputs of a number of processes have to be combined to deliver the ultimate benefits required (e.g. collection, component production and QC)
- There is complexity of inter-relations, such as where there are strong dependencies between processes that require close co-ordination to harmonize design and preserve integrity at the interfaces (e.g. storage/distribution and collection)
- There is a need for efficient utilization of shared resources, such as where resources from a common pool are in demand across multiple processes and departments (e.g. human resources, finances, technical services)
- It can help implementation efficiency, for example where integrated planning will significantly reduce disruption to current operations (e.g. supply logistics, donor availability and access).

A programme approach aims to harness synergies and produce a wider set of benefits than the sum of its individual processes. A primary objective is to realize a defined set of benefits (customer satisfaction) – not a set of outputs. If the set of processes within the programme is not going to deliver the planned benefits, then the processes have to be changed.

A variety of methodologies exist to cater for programmes of different types, generally reflecting the dominant technical content such as re-location, organizational design, systems development, Enterprise Resource Planning (ERP) and Result Oriented Management (ROM) implementation, etc.

The common mistake is to assume that programmes are just like large projects and therefore have the same set of success factors.

There are five critical success factors that are fundamental to effectively managing programmes for processes and delivering the organization benefits from them –

- set clear directions and a high-level road map;
- gain commitment of key stakeholders;
- organize to balance conflicting influences;
- drive to realize the organizational benefits;
- integrate and assure for a coherent solution.

Effective integration means harnessing synergies and simplifying interactions. Assurance, on the other hand, is concerned with providing confidence that the programme will deliver a workable solution that will deliver the benefits intended – the right people doing the right things in the right way and at the right time to achieve the right result.

Both potentially impact the programme organization, as well as its governance, management and control processes, and are required on a number of levels within the programme:

- Scope – ensuring clarity of scope between processes within the programme and externally with related initiatives (e.g. cryopreservation of collected stem cells);
- Design – ensuring the design of any process component fits within the overall programme design and within the wider operational and technical architecture (e.g. validation, maintenance and repair);
- Delivery – managing internal cross-process dependencies, external dependencies (with other programmes, internal departments and third parties) to ensure that delivery of change is coherent and synchronized (e.g. development of cellular engineering for cellular therapies);
- Resources – ensuring optimal use of limited skills and facilities given multiple competing demands of individual processes and procedures (e.g. primary and secondary processing of blood);
- Organizational impact – ensuring the impact of each process on individual departments is clearly understood so that implementation may be managed efficiently and excessive demands are avoided (e.g. human resource management, education programmes).
- Disruption – ensuring that exceptions, issues, risks and changes, which may affect more than one process, are managed in the wider context (e.g. error and non-conformance policy)
- Communication – integrating communications into the infrastructure of a programme will increase its effectiveness, improve the likelihood of its acceptance among staff and also help those charged with delivery to focus on the key issues (e.g. ICT and MIS).

The manager assures that his programme will deliver to its full potential – not just the sum of its individual parts. A good, well designed and operated programme always delivers more.

2.6. Organizations Deliver Consistently when Operational Approach, Attitudes and Behaviours are Embedded in the Culture

Project-based working is an increasing feature of professional life, often representing a third or more of an organization's work.

Increasingly organizations transform themselves into projects-focused establishments, driven by three major influences –

1. They must be highly responsive to customer demands (demand driven);
2. Time to 'market' is absolutely critical if opportunities are to be fully exploited; The need to deliver blood components more quickly and reliably puts enormous pressure on blood establishments irrespective of environmental and climate/season conditions;
3. The ability to recognize and respond to change distinguishes the 'first class' establishment from the merely adequate. Health care changes rapidly and often unpredictably as new technologies and approaches are exploited and new players bring new concepts. Flexibility is vital.

Project-based working is now widely accepted as vital to the future of transfusion medicine (vein to vein) and much effort has gone into improving the capability and performance of the managers involved, both top and middle management [6] However, those who adopt it do not always achieve the high performance they seek. Clearly, individual performance alone is not enough.

It has been observed that many blood establishments and hospital blood banks are failing to achieve high performance from their programmes and processes because they have not appreciated the distinction between the effectiveness of a good individual and the far more effective power of that person working within a supportive culture of teamwork. All aspects of the organization must focus on the performance goals, where processes, structure, people and systems are the four key elements. As project-based working increases, this 'streamlining' becomes ever more significant to performance.

Understanding and acting upon the success factors that underpin this 'streamlining' really do make a difference in the ability of the organization to deliver programmes and projects reliably and consistently.

These success factors cover the four key areas of an organization:

- Structure,
- Supporting processes,
- Information and measurement systems,
- People.

In an effective corporate culture, these factors mesh together to influence performance and deliver results. Changing the culture of an organization is challenging, because culture is intangible and no single action will change it. Successful change is only achieved by the coordinated and integrated effect of changes across all four areas. Many attempts to establish a corporate culture fail because managers do not recognize that each of these parameters has the capacity to influence or defeat the whole change process. Consistent success is achieved only when all aspects of the organization are focused on the integral performance goals.

2.7. Project-based Roles and Clarity in Responsibilities

In many organizations, project and process management is a 'parallel activity'. People are assigned to it without clear understanding of the relative authorities, responsibilities and inter-relationships that exist between process and line functions – it is simply an add-on to their routine job. Successful process delivery requires that these organizational boundaries are defined and agreed at all levels. Organizations that consistently deliver projects and their associated benefits are likely to have a flat, process-led and role-based structure.

A *process-led structure* is one where the focus is on accountability for outcomes rather than functional inputs and skills. This results in a high level of personal autonomy – for managers this means real accountability for delivering their processes.

A *role-based organization*, with many people having multiple roles, creates significant fluidity (a marked contrast to most conventional organizations), and enables migration through roles to act as a mechanism to develop management competence. If processes are to be consistently successful throughout the organization, then *'the way we do things'* must also be consistent and excellent. This means that there must be a delivery process for the work that is clearly understood and well communicated to all those involved. To the extent necessary, standard tools and techniques should be installed so as to allow flexibility of resource between processes and consistency of reporting at all management levels (communication). A robust outcome or work delivery process will be focused on the technical development lifecycle with process and supportive management disciplines stitched around it. These disciplines will be designed to actively support process working. All parts of the organization will share a common understanding of objectives, processes and tools.

Resource management is a key factor in optimizing the deployment of people in processes and developing people's skills and competencies. [6] This is the nearest equivalent in a projects-based organization to operations management in a traditional procurement setting. The indicators that an organization chooses to measure and monitor have a great influence on behaviour.

Many organizations have not yet recognized that the drivers of performance in processes are not the same as those in a conventional situation. The key to good control over processes is quick data turnaround (monitoring) and forward-looking reporting (evaluation), so that people are focused on continually thinking about how best to complete the outstanding work – creating a culture of determination to deliver based on ownership. Project focused measures and controls, such as –

- action-orientated predictive reporting,
- well defined baselines and milestones,
- market-orientated budgeting,

will provide a powerful dashboard of information with which to 'drive' projects forward.

Most organizations monitor the time and cost of their projects and processes once they have started; some also have efficiency indicators such as project management expense and benchmark data (internal and external).

Project selection also has an enormous impact upon operational performance since this ensures that the organization puts its resources in the optimum portfolio of investments.

This plays a role, not only when projects are initially selected for investment (e.g. introduction of pathogen reduction), but also in enabling rapid decision-making once the project is up and running, including closing down a project that is no longer delivering what is wanted by the organization to properly manage the related processes. In this way, successful project-based organizations promote a robust portfolio management discipline that continuously addresses the question of which projects best satisfy the strategic objectives and what processes need to be in place.

Perhaps because of the transient nature of projects, staff are seldom recognized and nurtured in quite the same way as a high-powered technical specialist or a senior management high-flyer. Yet, the value and consequences to the organization from successful projects are immense. People involved in projects get a real insight into the workings of their organization and what it takes to implement change effectively. Project working has the potential to provide real development opportunities. The 'people or human resource' dimension of a successful project-based organization has to embed the attitudes and behaviours driven from the value set described, the quality culture. There are two critical enablers to achieving this. The first is a reward system that directly reflects the success of projects, and the contribution of the individual to that success. The second is recognized career paths that provide development opportunities to those who have proved their ability to deliver.

These incentives will help to motivate, retain and develop the individuals whose ability to deliver is critical to the success of an organization.

3. How to Implement

The introduction of a corporate quality culture will almost certainly demand a revision to values and behaviours. This means that new people may rise to prominence because they are naturally inclined to the new approach and, not surprisingly, some existing senior people may be very resistant to the concepts. Winning people over is a key to change. Experience suggests that it is possible to get performance benefits from corporate quality culture quite quickly, and sustained performance improvement within one to two years. The levers for securing benefits and their potential impact are well defined; the skill lies in knowing when and how to pull the levers.

Introducing a corporate quality culture is a significant change program in itself, but one that has been shown to deliver significant improvement in performance in many organizations. The key to success is a robust change process that makes a robust case for change to the operations, that makes it real to those involved, that makes it happen – moving all the levers to make change happen, and that makes it sustain – continuing to embed the changes until they really are owned and become part of the culture.

The chain of processes as they routinely appear for instance in a blood establishment or a hospital blood bank could be seen as a series of interrelated and repetitive projects, each with their own specific objective and outcome. Hence, process management could also be seen as a continued project management. Additionally it includes automatically the management of change of processes to improve performance and quality of output and hence customer satisfaction.

Processes are composed of smaller elements – procedures, identified through proper process description. To visualize the chain of processes and procedures as well as the sequential order of steps within a process or procedure, analysis and consequent mapping could help to understand better and therefore provide a useful tool for process and change management.

3.1. Flowcharting

Flowcharts or process or procedure maps are strong tools in the management of processes, process descriptions and SOP writing. In the past when a flowchart had to be made manually, it was often omitted because of the amount of time needed to draft one with the risk that it had to be done again in case of a change.

There are good software programmes like Microsoft Visio™ [7], that are useful to help making flowcharts easy and quickly. Changes are easily applied without having to re-do the whole chart. Flowcharts have always made use of symbols as shown in figure 4.2. Usually one page is sufficient to make a flowchart, but sometimes the process contains so many steps, that one page is not enough or the flowchart is so complex that the process must be split and flowcharted over more pages. In such case the *reference symbol* (last one mentioned) can be used to refer to the page where (that part of) the flowchart continues.

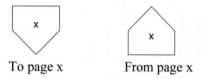

To page x   From page x

On the page where the flowchart continues the same symbol (upside down) can be used to refer to the page with the previous part of the flowchart.

Each flowchart has a start point and an end point.

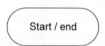

The *start / end symbol* must be used at least twice in every flowchart. It can be used more often in case there are more end points of the process. Either the first and last step are mentioned or the symbols contain the title and the result of the process described.

Commonly used international flow chart symbols -

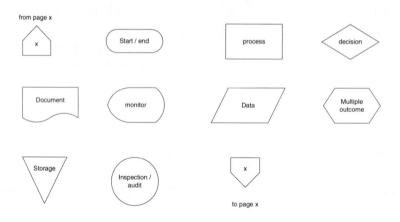

Figure 2. The most commonly used international flow chart symbols.

The *process symbol* is the most often used. Brief information is given about the action that must be taken at this point in the process. It always has an input and an output.

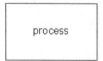

The *decision symbol* - the diamond - is used to identify Critical Control Points (CCPs). There is always an input from the previous step and a choice must be made how to proceed: either to go back in the process, to stop the process or to proceed.

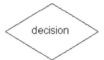

The *document symbol* can be used either to find or to retrieve documented data or to document data manually.

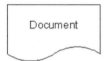

The *monitor symbol* is used in the same way as the document symbol to retrieve information or to enter and store data into the computer. In both cases data have to be documented (either manually or automated). It is a Critical Control Point and should therefore be followed by the decision symbol with the question whether the documentation procedure is completed or not.

The *data symbol* can be used for all kind of data that are handled either manually or automated.

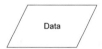

The *multiple outcome symbol* is used when in a process several activities that have to be performed simultaneously, are the outcome of a previous step.

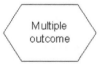

For example when the blood and sample collection have been performed at the same time –

- the samples are sent to the laboratory for both blood group determination and TTI marker testing, where

- the whole blood is sent to the blood processing department for the production of the various components.

The *storage symbol* is used when the process is temporarily interrupted. This can be the storage of a consumable or blood component that will be used or issued later, or bringing data to someone else who will handle these data subsequently.

The *inspection symbol* can be used either to indicate that

- a specific inspection must be performed by the operator himself, or
- by a third party (colleague), or
- an internal audit, peer audit or mandatory inspection must be performed.

There are many more symbols that can be used but usually are not very often used. These depend on the programme that is used like *iGrafX Process*™, *SigmaFlow*™ or *Traxion*™. There are two different ways how to present a flowchart:

- The common used line charts, or
- Lane charts.

The *Line Chart* is a straight forward flow that starts at the top of the sheet and ends at the bottom. For an example of a simple flowchart see figure 4.3. It must be clear who is doing or performing the various steps.

At this stage, nobody is worried about the details of what happens inside each of these boxes. The goal is to capture each of the steps, identify their basic function, and connect them in a manner that represents the process.

They provide an immediate overview of the sequence of events and steps from start to end, from input to output, from supplier to customer. Once a process map is drawn, the next step is to define explicitly each of the map objects. This must be done accurately and quantitatively; the accuracy of the process or project model depends on it. If a process modelling tool is used, the tool will include attributes at each element in the process.

shopping

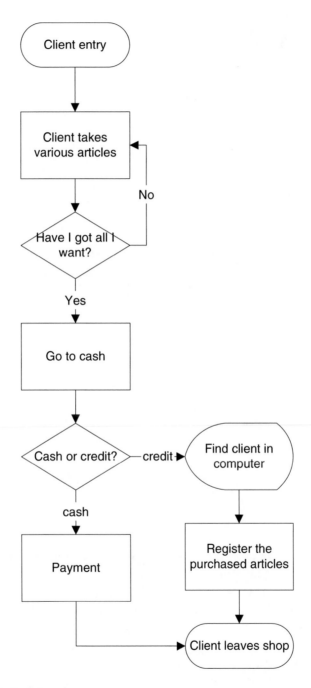

Figure 3. A simple flowchart of shopping.

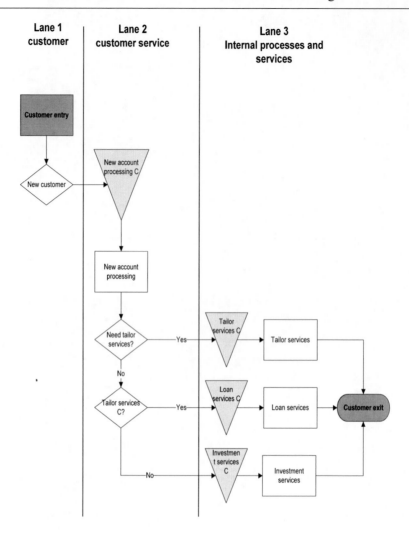

Figure 4. Swim lane flow chart of shopping. The customer is in lane 1, the customer service (shop personnel) is in lane 2 and the internal processes are in lane 3.

The attributes are numerous. The categories of process element definitions include:

- Operation cycle time of the process element, including its average time to complete, the variation in time called the standard deviation (SD), and perhaps a distribution curve to represent all the possible completion times as well.
- Resources used in the process element, including human, capital, and natural resources.
  The better tools will permit identification of resources by name and type and then later track their utilization during simulation. Value added by the process step or element in the units of measure that mean the most to the organization. At a minimum, it must be possible to define whether the process step is value-adding (VA) or non-value-adding (NVA). Cost of the resources consumed. These include the costs of personnel, facilities, direct material (consumables), and even include indirect costs.

If it is not clear whether there are clearly distinct functions or departments involved in the process than a *lane* or '*swim lane*' flow might be more practical (see figure 4.4). In this example three parties are involved: the customer, customer service and banking service.

Swim Lanes represent a more recently developed visualization technique for process modelling.

The *line flow* is always within one Department or operational entity performed and at the end there could be an interface connecting to the next process.

The swim lane flow is particularly used when more than one interface is involved and especially if these interfaces are 'borders' or connections between Departments. Here interface management (supplier-customer principle) is important to ensure that the end of the process is indeed 'fit for purpose' as a start for the next process in the connected Department or Departments.

For the manager of a process or project it is important to

1. *set the baseline* – before you will be able to measure the effects of process management, you must first characterize the current conditions.

By using the same process modelling technique of flowcharting for the running processes and procedures as well as for the future (changed or adjusted) processes and procedures, you will have the basis for measuring the effectiveness of the management of your process optimization efforts.

2. *see the process* – there are three conventional views of a process
- What you think is going on;
- What is really going on;
- What should be going on.

Obviously these three are distinctly different.

The only way to achieve a realistic view of the processes to be managed is the second view – mapping what is really going on.

Only then you will be able to move on to the third view – what should be going on, allowing proper measuring and achieving maximal control and effectiveness of process management.

3. *stimulate closed-loop behaviour* – to continue the cycle of improvement the model chosen should be a dynamic, living entity where at any point in time model and reality are synergistic.

Modelling the current operations of processes and procedures from the beginning, stimulates closed-loop behaviour of your personnel avoiding deviations that interfere with the aspired consistency of performance and output.

3.2. Statistical Process Control (SPC)

Process control through proper and consistent monitoring and evaluation (MandE) is necessary to measure the quality of a product or service.

The first question arising is *"What is quality?"*

For a long time quality was individually defined by the company making products or delivering services. Terms like "Top Quality", "A-Quality", or "High Quality" were used.

Since more and more companies and organization have developed their quality systems and quality management also the meaning of the term "quality" has further developed. Today it is understood and comprehended as the level of customer satisfaction, the ultimate fitness for purpose or use.

The second question is *"What is a process?"*

A process is the transformation of a set of inputs, like materials, actions, methods and operations, into desired outputs, like products or services. Outputs shall be delivered to the customer, both internal and external customers.

The third question is *"What is control?"*

Before the industrial revolution each product was controlled personally by the craftsman who had made it. From the moment products were made on a little larger scale 100% control was necessary. When, however, the scales of production increased it became too expensive to check 100% of the products. This was the moment Statistical Process Control or SPC was introduced. This is only possible if equipment, processes, procedures etc. are standardized, validated and documented. Statistical Process Control (SPC) must be embedded in the quality system and owned as an integral part of the quality culture. [8-10] Validated equipment, processes, procedures etc. must be controlled regularly to ensure they meet continuously the requirements. A given percentage of each batch must be sampled for quality control. For blood establishments it is internationally accepted to practise a routine sample frequency of a minimum of 1% of all products or 4 per month, whichever is the largest [11]. The results of these tests are statistically analyzed. For this purpose basic statistical tools are sufficient though needed to allow proper and reliable monitoring and evaluation of a process or procedure. Testing does cost money. However, not testing does cost more money due to costs for re-work, repair or loss of unsatisfied customers and transmitted infections.

3.2.1. Definitions

Some of the most commonly used terms are –

Mean   the sum of all sample values divided by the number of samples:

$$X_{mean} = 1/n(\sum X_{(1-n)}),$$

where X is the sample value and n the number of samples.

Median   the middle observation
Mode   the most frequent observation

The mode, median and mean are not necessarily the same. Only in the exceptional symmetric distribution they become the same (see Figure 5)

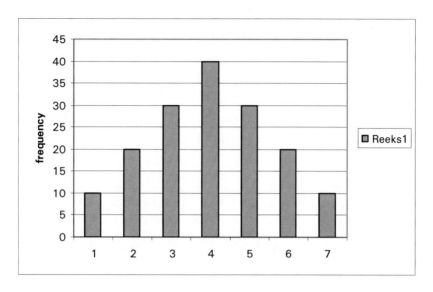

Figure 5. Bar chart of frequencies.

Deviation   the positive or negative difference between the value and the mean.

$(X_i - X_{mean})$

Variance   the averaged of the squared deviation
$(X_i - X_{mean})^2/n$

Standard Deviation   the square root of the variance

$\sigma = \sqrt{(X_i - X_{mean})^2/n}$ or $\sigma = ((X_i - X_{mean})^2/n)^{1/2}$

The meaning of the standard deviation (SD) can be explained with the Gaussian curve or normal distribution (Figure 6).

When the standard deviation is calculated it is known which % of the data are reliable.

Maximum value   the highest value among a series of data; interesting in relation to standard deviation

Minimum value   the lowest value among a series of data; interesting in relation to standard deviation

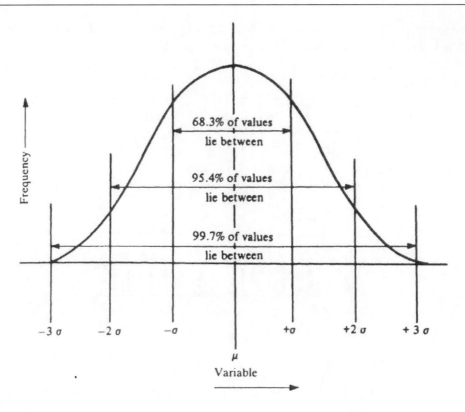

Figure 6. Gaussian curve showing plus or minus one, two or three Standard Deviations.

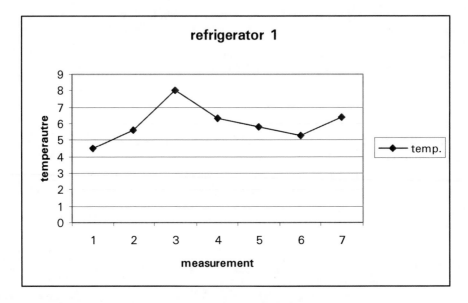

Figure 7. Line plot of temperature recordings of a refrigerator.

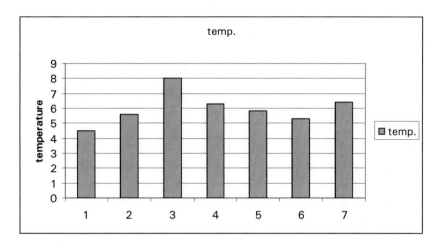

Figure 8. Column or bar plot of recorded temperatures of a refrigerator (see figure 7).

3.2.2. Visualization of Data

Data can be visualized or plotted in a variety of ways using e.g. MicroSoft Excel™ [12]:

Line plots:

This is often done, even if it is actually not allowed. It is allowed if there is a relation (development) in the time between the data, e.g. the twice daily measured temperature of a refrigerator. An example of a line plot is given in Figure 7.

Column plot:

This should be the most commonly used plot as usually there is no relation between data e.g. the weight of individual bags of whole blood or the measured temperatures of various refrigerators. An example of a column plot is given in Figure 8.

Pie chart:

Pie charts provide a lot of information in a relatively small area. Pie chart applications are limited to the presentation of proportions since the whole pie is normally filled, but usually are rather illustrative. An example of a pie chart is given in Figure 9.

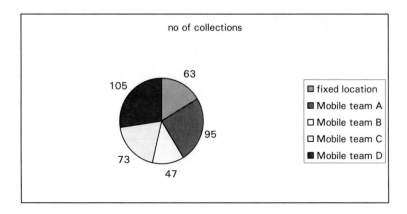

Figure 9. Pie chart of collection numbers: fixed location and four mobile teams (A-D).

Shewhart chart:

This is a good tool for trend analysis and provides an early warning if the trend is approaching the warning level or action level.

The Shewhart chart is the plot of a few lines and the data of the measurement:

- the mean + 3 x σ
- the mean + 2 x σ
- the mean + 1 x σ
- the mean
- the mean - 1 x σ
- the mean - 2 x σ
- the mean - 3 x σ

σ = standard deviation

Actions must be taken if:

1 value is larger than 3 x σ or lower than -3 x σ (action level)
2 consecutive values are between 2 and 3 x σ (warning level)
4 consecutive values are between 1 and 2 x σ, or
10 consecutive values at the same side between the mean and 1 x σ.
An example of a Shewhart chart is given Figure 10:

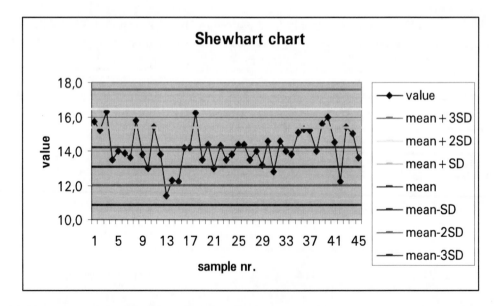

Figure 10. Shewart chart of sample values indicating a mean and one, two or three Stadard Deviations.

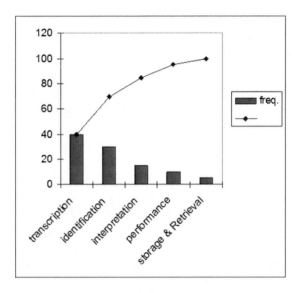

Figure 11. Pareto plot. In this example transcription and identification should be improved to solve almost 80% of the total non-conformities.

Pareto analysis:

When solving 20% of the causes of non-conformities 80% of the problems will be solved. This is based on the theory of the Italian economist Pareto who stated that 20% of the population had 80% of the wealth. The types of non-conformities, rework, repair, process capacity are plotted in a column plot against the frequencies plus a line with the cumulated frequencies. This shows how many types of non-conformities, rework, repair, process capability must be solved to solve 80% of the total problems. An example of a Pareto plot is given in Figure 11.

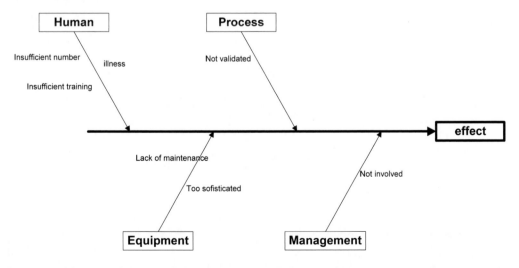

Figure 12. Ishikawa or fish bone chart showing causes (human, equipment, process and management) and effect.

Cause-Effect analysis:

For almost all non-conformities the effect is clear, but the question is what is the cause. The Cause-Effect analysis, also called *Ishikawa* or *fish bone diagram* is a good tool to find a cause. The diagram shows at the end of the central spine the effect and the cause categories at the end of the ribs. These categories are usually – Human, Equipment, Management, Processes etc. On the ribs all kind of causes in the particular category can be written. An example is shown in Figure 12.

3.2.3. Sample Taking

For a reliable Statistical Process Control it is important to know who is taking the samples, how the samples are taken and how many and how frequent samples are taken. There are no general rules for the frequency of taking samples. It is very much a function of the blood component being made and the process used – routine bulk production versus specialized procedures such as pooling or washing of blood components. It is recommended that samples are taken quite often at the beginning of a process capability assessment and process control – the introduction of a new preparation process. When it has been confirmed that the process is in control, the frequency of sampling may be reduced. [8] The selection of products to be sampled must be objective. Staff involved in the manufacturing should not be the first choice to sample; this should be done independently and non-biased by staff from the testing laboratory. Samples must be taken in such way that they are representative for the component and the related preparation process. [11]

Components should be well mixed immediately prior to sampling. Sampling often follows a 'worse case' approach, where sampled are taken from close to or even just expired components. Random sampling has the advantage of minimising bias, but 'fixed' sampling has the virtue of operational convenience. In blood establishments where large volumes are processed, control testing should be increased above the statistically determined minimum (usually 1.0 – 1.5%) to a level of approximately 1 – 10% of the annual production to address process variations.

Table 2. Quality control tests for blood components

Whole Blood	Volume
	Haematocrit
Red Cell Concentrate	Volume
	Haemoglobin
	Haematocrit
	Leucocyte count
	Platelet count
Plasma	Volume
	Total protein
	F VIII
	Leucocyte count
	Platelet count
	Reddishness (red cells/haemolysis)
Buffy Coat	Volume
	Haematocrit
	Leucocyte count
	Platelet count
Platelet concentrates, single unit or made from a pool of 4 or 5 buffy coats	Volume
	Platelet count
	pH at end of shelf life
	Swirling

A practical method of choosing components to be sampled is the following – out of each 100 collections of whole blood randomly 1 - 5 donation is chosen for quality control. The following tests can be performed on the donation and routine components made out of that donation (Table 2). It is important to realize what can be achieved with statistics. However, if not properly used it can give the wrong impression or result in unreliable or even false conclusions. If one axis of a graph is much more stretched than the other it can give the wrong impression. If in a graph there is no justification for the extrapolation of a line, it may result in a false conclusion if the line is extrapolated. An example is shown in Figure 13.

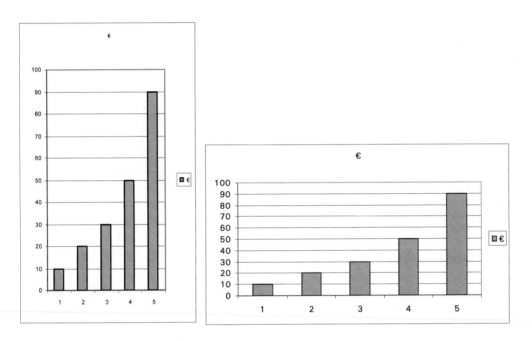

Figure 13. Two ways of plotting (column or bar) the same data.

4. Supplier-Producer-Customer Chain

Processes are the managerial and operational entities that allow an orderly functioning of any organization. Processes can be studied at several levels of complexity, where each identified process may be composed of a series of procedures or Key Elements (KE).

The interfaces between the procedures within a process or between processes are named Critical Control Points (CCP). CCPs indicate a transfer of outcome or result from one point to another and therefore need documentation to prove fitness for purpose.

An outcome or result is supplied as a starting material or input to the next step in the chain – so there is a continuum of supplier-customer interactions [13]. The production process can be complex as in for example a pharmaceutical industry and simple as in a regular bakery or carpenter workshop.

4.1. Primary, Supportive and Steering Processes

In an organisation three types of processes are distinguished:

- primary processes or primary activities.

This is the so called 'core business' of an organisation.

- supportive processes.

All support outside the primary process, for example human resource management, finance and administration, facility management, procurement, the legal department, but also the company restaurant

- steering processes (in literature also known as management processes).

All activities intended to steer the company's primary and supportive processes: formulation of year plans, checking results, coaching and leading personnel. Finally, long term strategy formulation is a process in this segment.

This is considered one of the working areas or tasks of top management.

4.2. Process Elements

When studied at a basic level, each process consists of chain(s) of activities. Moreover each process is built up of five elements: *results* (input), *activities, people, resources, scope and constraints* and *results* (output).

A good approach is in result oriented management (ROM) [14] which is based on the eleven key management principles –

1.	Division of Labour and Specialization
2.	Authority and Responsibility
3.	Unity of Command (one captain on the ship)
4.	Unity of Direction (common goal)
5.	Discipline
6.	Organization vs Individual Interest
7.	Pay and Reward (performance/outcome)
8.	Chain of Command (reporting relationships) and Team Spirit (top, middle and lower levels)
9.	Materials: should be in their proper place
10.	Equity and Fairness: equal and fair treatment of all employees (HRM)
11.	Initiative: managers should encourage

Results (input):

Here we mean the input from a preceding process or step into the following process or step. In case of a purchasing process, raw materials are bought from manufacturers or vendors. After testing and approval (also a process) raw materials are the input for the ultimate primary production process.

Activities:

Each process is a continuous chain of activities or procedures. These can be simple activities as in the example of a bakery. In more complex situations activities can be clustered into sub-processes.

Each step must have a relation with

- the final product or service,
- value added, and be essential to the production.

Non value adding activities should be eliminated (lean principle).

People:

People perform a part of the activities within a process. A proper division of tasks, authorities and responsibilities is essential for an effective process. A balance should always be established between prescribed process steps and professional skills and competence – the right people at the right place.

Resources:

In this category we find equipment, information, documents, etc. Contrary to raw materials, these resources are not 'consumed' or converted during the process. However, they are essential for the operation of a process.

Scope and constraints:

With scope and constraints we mean elements from 'outside' that 'steer' the process. For example constraints with respect to number of available personnel or timely delivery of raw materials or consumables, but also facilities, working conditions and power supply.

Results (output):

The *'raison d'être'* of each process is its output, in fact the ultimate product, service or result for a customer. Working with the concept of 'processes' is similar to steering on results or ROM. Each result can be measured in number and quality, consequently a performance indicator can be established for each process based on pre-set standards or specifications.

Whatever serves as an input or an output needs to meet set criteria of acceptance. In other words, needs to be 'fit for purpose or use'. The receiver of an input or output actually has the position of customer, while those who provide an input or output function serve as a supplier. So, the supplier-producer-customer chain actually represents a continuum or circle. Between supply of input and reception of output is the production of the ultimate output, the product or service.

In the following paragraphs the primary processes of a blood establishment will be discussed.

4.3. Processing (A Blood Establishment As Example)

The total process of a blood establishment is quite complex and several departments are involved. Usually interfaces within a department are not very difficult to manage. Problems arise with interdepartmental interfaces. This means that it is important to analyse these interdepartmental interfaces (see lane chart page 28 and figure 4.5).

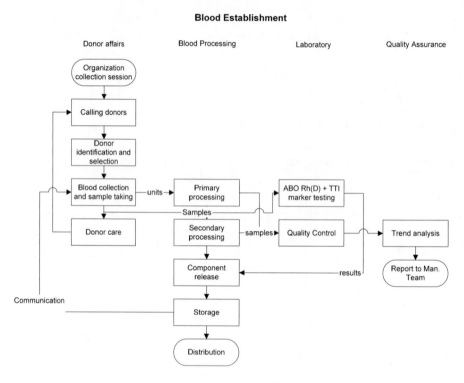

Figure 14. Flow chart of the procurement of blood (lane chart).

4.3.1. Donor Care is Important for Donor Retention

There should be a regular - more than daily - communication between the Distribution Department and the Blood Collection Department about the total number of units to be collected and the type of blood bag to be used (e.g. double or triple, depending on platelet production and/or production of cryoprecipitate). Units of whole blood should be delivered to the processing department as to optimise the condition for blood processing procedures. All collected units should arrive without delay at the processing department.

All samples for the mandatory quality control - blood group determination and TTI marker testing, must be correctly labelled and arrive without delay at the laboratory. The results should be available in a timely manner to the Processing Department to enable timely release and final labelling of the blood components. Delays in handling cause unnecessary quarantine storage and reduce the actual shelf life for issue and clinical use. Samples from blood and blood components (usually 1%) should be taken, labelled and sent to the Laboratory for in-process quality control (compliance with set specifications or technical standards).

The results of these tests should be sent to the Quality Assurance Department for SPC and trend analysis.

In the simplified workflow of a Blood Establishment the Processing Department is situated between the Blood Collection Department and the Storage and Distribution Department. This trias (see Figure 15) is usually indicated as the procurement process and supported by the Laboratory Quality Control functions. Each of these three represents a main or core process and can be divided in the various work processes and detailed procedures for which not only basic description at managerial level (process descriptions) are needed, but attached the operational documents describing the operational flow of the procedures (SOPs) but also the standardized operational handling of equipment (EOP). Obviously this equally importantly relates to the Quality Control as a main process.

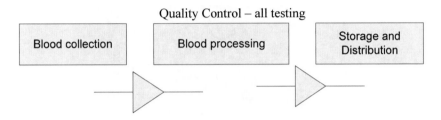

Figure 15. Trias of core processes controlled by QC.

4.3.2. Source Material Collection

Blood components, like pharmaceuticals, are produced in a *process focussed production* environment. Process equipment is used in the conversion or production process.

A batch of product or in case of a blood establishment a blood component e.g. a bag of erythrocytes concentrate, is the planning unit. A finished product inventory policy must be determined. Two possibilities exist:

1. Production to stock, or
2. Production to order.

In case of a blood establishment 'production to stock' (demand driven) is the general approach, although in many a less developed situation we can see the daily practice of 'production to order' (supply driven). Source material collection starts with a long term supply forecast (products to be delivered in future months or years). Historical data of requests and deliveries of blood components to hospitals are extrapolated to determine a forecast for a certain coming period. Trend analysis should be included to predict the 'production or sales volume' for a certain year. Seasonal variations should be part of the forecasts at month level or even week level. Based on forecasts with a time-horizon of e.g. one year, the necessary number of donors, blood collection bags, test-tubes and personnel is planned. This planning level is used to establish the number of production personnel, donor attendants or laboratory technicians. For example the number of collection bags to be used is the basis for contracting a supplier. The same applies for the number of TTI marker tests in a screening laboratory and the necessary supply of test kits.

Using short term planning procedures personnel and materials are planned at a week level. Numbers of donors to be called for a donation are based on the stock situation in the blood establishment. When stocks are below or above the required level, the number of donors that are invited to visit the blood collection centre or mobile team session will be upgraded or downgraded, this to prevent out of stock situations (shortages) or unnecessary expiration of unused finished product (excess). So the input is closely related to the output and a balance between expected output (demand) and needed input (supply) needs to be achieved based on a documented continuous monitoring and evaluation of the actual dynamics of demand (hospitals) and supply.(blood establishment) in a well documented system of stock or inventory management.

Blood is collected with the intension to produce components as requested (demand) in the hospitals for specific supportive haemotherapy – appropriate and rational use or component therapy.

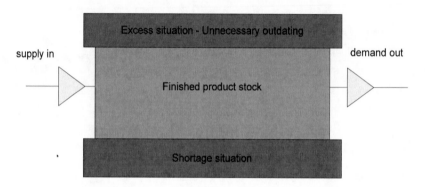

Figure 16. Stock management dynamics.

The market for source material selection and collection is the community. The management of the process of source material collection needs an analysis of needs and availabilities. In the blood supply the market situation has a number of different aspects as compared to regular industrial markets:

1. Blood is regarded to be a national resource;
2. Blood is a living tissue to be used for transplantation;
3. Collected blood is perishable and has a limited shelf life;
4. Blood is not a merchandise to be bought or sold commercially;
5. Blood is in principle abundantly available;
6. Access is limited;
7. There is a special relation needed between the 'holder' of the source material and the 'collector' based on ethical principles;
8. Not all 'holders' are *a priori* eligible for collection;
9. The 'holder' should become part of a system for regular collection (retention);
10. Quality of the source material blood is highly depending on personal behaviour and life style.

For the source material collection process market research is needed, based on continuous evaluation of consumption needs of customers. Additionally, the processing of source material will unavoidably lead to production losses.

Statistical monitoring and evaluation of the entire chain will provide proper information to management the process of collection.

Potential blood donors need to be identified from 'low risk' groups in the society. Potential blood donors need to be informed and motivated about the need for sharing some of what they 'hold' with those in need – so, be brought to awareness of contributing to a social act of solidarity in the community. Once identified and informed, there needs to be a policy and strategy to continuously treasure the growing relation – donor retention.

Potential blood donors then become a source to be mobilized when needs are indicated. For this reason a set of basic information has to be provided to the community.

As an example, EU has composed such set of basic information (see annex 4.1). [15]

For the management of mobilization, selection and collection simple algorithms should be developed and applied to avoid both over and under collection, leading to shortages or unnecessary outdating.

These algorithms have to be based on current information:

- Where to mobilize potential donors;
- How to mobilize potential donors; call-up strategies, blood groups;
- What is the minimum and maximum to be mobilized; cost-effectiveness, needs;
- Are there seasonal effects to be observed; harvest times, holidays, raining season, etc.;
- Are there climate restriction; Tropic, moderate, cold
- Are there religious circumstances to be observed; Ramadan, Christmas;
- Relation staff numbers to numbers of potential donors to be handled;
- Logistics of session organization; mobile team, fixed sites, walk in;
- Logistics of transport to and from;
- Logistics of consumable supplies;
- Team composition; competencies - authorities, responsibilities and accountabilities;
- Communication.

The main target is to have sufficient input for the processing of blood to allow an adequate stock of finished product to continuously satisfy the needs of the consumers – the patients in the hospitals. So, the main process of source material collection actually breaks down into a number of work processes and related procedures which need a carefully designed plan, based on accurate information and with set targets, monitoring and evaluation.

4.3.3. Processing of Blood: Manufacturing Blood Components

On a routine base blood components are produced from whole blood donations – component policy. The basic need is red cells and platelets, and occasionally plasma. This means the selection of the appropriate collection bag system. There are currently two approaches –

- a regular conventional double or triple bag system to allow platelet production in the conventional platelet rich plasma method, or
- a specific 'bottom and top' system to allow buffy coat recovery for platelet production.

The conventional anticoagulant and preservative fluids used are two-fold
CPD = Citrate Phosphate Dextrose during collection and primary
      processing;
SAG-M = Saline, Adenine, Glucose and Mannitol is added to the
      recovered red cells and used as a preservative for red cells.

The SAG-M is an additive solution for preserving and stabilizing the red cells following processing and is standard in 'bottom and top' bag systems, but could be used also in conventional multiple blood bag systems. In the example of a 'bottom and top' system, approximately 450 ml of whole blood is processed routinely into the three basic components - red blood cell concentrates, plasma and buffy coats.

When the source material – whole blood – has been inspected and accepted (fit for purpose) and documented, the process starts with centrifugation. Subsequently a separation step results in three different components. The production of platelet concentrates actually is a secondary processing step out of the primarily produced buffy coats or in the conventional approach out of platelet rich plasma (PRP). Similarly, the plasma could be secondarily processed into cryoprecipitate and cryoprecipitate-poor or supernatant plasma (CPP). Additional secondary processing steps may take place on specific demand of the hospital such as –

- irradiation of red cell concentrates or platelets,
- washing of red cell concentrates,
- concentration steps,
- pooling (platelets, cryoprecipitate), or
- splitting into small volumes for paediatric use (paedipacks)

Processing steps of a unit of whole blood collected in a ' bottom and top' multiple (triple or quadruple) blood bag system leading to the production of three final components – red cells in additive solution (SAGM), plasma and a buffy coat for platelet production.

The processing logistics will depend on the calculated needs in the hospitals. So, the demand will trigger the supply and the decisions what type of collection system to be handled and in what quantities. The need for red cells is the driving force in the production process, where the need for platelets usually can be met by processing 20 % of the buffy coats. The management of the manufacturing process needs an equally careful planning as applies to the source material collection process.

The main process depends at its output side on the needs and requests of the customers, the patients in the hospitals and for its input side on the supply of the source material from the donor department. As processing and the integrated in process QC as well as the mandatory ABO/Rhesus and TTI marker testing do need time to be accomplished, planning should be properly timed and phased. Week-ends and public holidays are known well in advance and should be used to plan accordingly. Manufacturing of blood components requests an operational planning because of the differences of characteristics in behaviour and operational treatment of the various key blood components, the overall preservation conditions of blood as a tissue and the logistics of supply, capacity of separation equipment (centrifuges) and storage capacity.

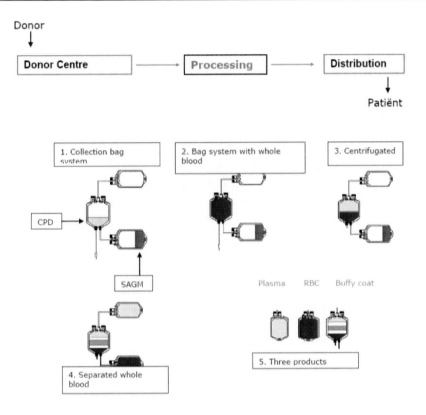

Figure 17. The processing steps using a 'bottom and top' additive solution collection system are shown clockwise – 1: the empty set; 2: the 'top and bottom' collection bag filled with whole blood; 3: following centrifugation – plasma at the top, buffy coat in the middle and the red cells in the bottom part of the collection bag; 4: plasma is separated in the empty satellite bag, red cells are drained in the SAG-M bag and the buffy coat remains in the collection bag.

4.3.4. The Process of Quality Control (QC)

The quality control or QC is necessary to ensure product conformity with set specifications. QC has two key elements – the mandatory ABO/Rhesus and TTI marker testing, and the in-process control for product specifications. Safety and clinical efficacy of blood components starts at the time of donor selection and blood collection in a Donor Centre or Mobile Team collection site (donor information, questionnaire, informed consent, medical tests). This process represents the source material selection and collection, necessary as a key input of the source material 'whole blood' fit for the purpose of blood component production. So, information, motivation and selection of donors and proper collection of whole blood are essential to quality of the starting or source material. The community is the market from where the source material has to be selected and collected.

Specifications begin with specifications for whole blood and continue into the production process with specifications for each intermediate and finished product. There are two basic processes defined as Quality Control –

- *mandatory quality control*, to be done on each unit of whole blood collected: TTI markers (HIV, HBV, HIV and Syphilis) and immunohaematology markers (ABO and Rhesus D);

- *in-process quality control* to monitor and evaluate the production of finished blood components for compliance with set product specifications. This in-process QC is done following a pharmaceutical sample size principle (1 to 1.5% of total annual production).

It is obvious that for each of the QC tests (procedures) protocols or SOPs have to be written together with result documents to capture the outcomes of the various QC tests done. Additionally, based on the described strategies of a blood establishment, the methodologies have to be defined and validated before starting the testing procedures.

So, in preparation to each process and related procedures, a plan needs to be developed to allow proper introduction of the elements of the entire chain in routine operations.

The *routine mandatory QC* is done on each collection following a fixed protocol –

- reception, inspection and documentation of the collected samples,
- division of the samples over the ABO/Rhesus and the TTI marker part of the laboratory,
- preparation of the test methods; reagents, equipment and documentation,
- documentation and evaluation of outcomes.

The *in-process QC* follows a different scheme and is usually planned for a specific day, e.g. Monday or Sunday morning following a week-end, where the Donor Department has started to collect and the routine testing of the last batches of the previous week have been handled and completed. A sampling protocol and plan is needed to allow proper process control of the various manufacturing procedures and steps. An example of in-process QC tests based on set criteria, is the list in use within the EU (see annex 4.2). [16]

In-process QC should follow a fixed protocol –

- sampling of the source material, intermediate 'products' and finished 'products' based on statistical sample size (1-1.5%),
- inspection and documentation of samples (ID and integrity,
- preparation of the test methods; reagents, equipment and documentation,
- documentation and evaluation of outcomes.

With incidentally produced components each component has to be tested for compliance with the set specifications. Appropriate bacteriological control of the collection and manufacturing process must be performed to guarantee the validity of aseptic handling.

4.3.5. Specifications and Labelling Process

After each processing step, a labelling step is required. The essence of labelling is in traceability at each step of the procurement chain – collection, processing, storage and distribution. Labels are outcome or result level 4 documents.

They represent the outcome of a process and indicate what is in a container. There are various label systems available. However, in transfusion medicine the most commonly used system is the ISBT-128 labelling system (Figure 18).

Each product has its own specific label. The final label is produced or printed at the moment of matching the laboratory tests with the historic data and affixed on bag surface of the produced component.

Collection data: Unique unit identification number Blood Centre Identification Collection date	Quality information: ABO blood group Rhesus D factor TTI markers Alloantibodies
Product information Component code Component name Anticoagulant/preservative Component information Storage conditions	Expiry date Special information (if applicable) Rhesus phenotyping Other blood groups

Figure 18. Basic ISBT 128 code label with its four quadrants for Collection data, Quality information, Product information and Expiry date/special information.

All information is bar-coded and eye readable. The label has four quadrants each dedicated to a specific set of information.

Left upper - *Collection data:* unique unit ID number, blood establishment ID, collection date.
Right upper - *Quality information:* ABO and Rhesus D blood group, TTI markers and alloantibodies.
Left lower - *Product information:* ISBT-128 blood component code, component name, anticoagulant/preservative used, component information (referral to brochure), storage conditions.
Right lower - *Expiry date and Special information:* Rhesus phenotype, other blood groups (Kell, Duffy, Kidd, etc).

The total size of the label covers completely the blood bag manufacturer's label except the lower row containing blood component code and batch number of the blood bag (system).

The labelling process builds up over the production process, from collection through intermediate product into final component with the complete label. Control steps of the labelling process must take place after each labelling procedure. The principle followed is a double check, which may be done by two independent people or through the computer

Following the final labelling as an outcome of the critical quarantine release process, the produced component is ready for storage and ultimate issue to the customer (hospital).

4.3.6. Traceability

Labelling should comply with the relevant national legislation and international agreements. An international example of required information within the EU is given in annex 4.3. [17] The EU requires that Member States shall take all necessary measures in order to ensure that the system used for the labelling of blood and blood components collected, tested, processed, stored, released and / or distributed on their territory complies with the identification system referred to in art. 14, paragraph 1 and the labelling requirements listed in Annex III. Paragraph 1 states the following –

DIRECTIVE 2002/98/EC OF THE EUROPEAN PARLIAMENT AND THE COUNCIL

Of 27 January 2003
Setting standards of quality and safety for the collection, testing, processing, storage and distribution of human blood and blood components and amending Directive 2001/83/EC

Article 14
Traceability

Member States shall take all necessary measures in order to ensure that blood and blood components collected, tested, processed, stored, released and / or distributed on their territory can be traced from donor to recipient and vice versa.

To this end, Member States shall ensure that blood establishments implement a system for identification of each single blood donation and each single blood unit and components thereof enabling full traceability to the donor as well as to the transfusion and the recipient thereof. The system must unmistakably identify each unique donation and type of blood component. This system shall be established in accordance with the requirements referred to in Article 29(a).

With regard to blood and blood components imported from third countries, Member States shall ensure that the donor identification system to be implemented by blood establishments permits an equivalent level of traceability.

This implies a traceability or labelling plan with a sequential build up of the label from collection to released final product.

4.3.7. Storage and Distribution

Storage conditions for blood components should be designed to preserve viability and function during the storage period, until final use - transfusion into a patient. For the different blood components different storage conditions apply. As an example the conditions as required by the EU are listed in annex 4.4. [18] The management of the storage and distribution process relates to

- the calculation of adequate storage capacity including extra capacity in case of break down of a refrigerator freezer;
- regular performance control of the storage and distribution part of the cold chain;
- separate storage capacity for whole blood and components in quarantine, finished products and rejected (bio-hazardous) or returned products;
- continuous inventory monitoring and evaluation;
- accurate and documented request and issue procedures and related documentation;

- supply of hospitals with an appropriate working stock of red cells and plasma, sufficient to cover consumption during a regular week and week-end period.

For a proper management of this process of blood stock management regular statistical evaluation of request patterns from hospitals is needed, including trend analysis. The storage of issued blood components in hospitals relates to the managerial responsibilities of the supplier – appropriate information on how to store and control the storage conditions.

As a principle, the manufacturer remains liable for the components produced, and therefore should take the necessary precautionary measures to avoid unnecessary deterioration of product as well as to avoid unjustified or wrong use. This means the building of a working relation with consumers, and a formal agreement or contract on –

- how to order,
- how to store, and
- how to handle blood and blood components in the hospital,
- conditions for return of stock, and
- accounting for the final destination of each unit issued and received (traceability principle).

Such agreement or contract requires a regular revision.

4.4. What if Outcomes Deviate from Set Standards?

Each process or procedure ends with a result or outcome. The result or outcome serves as the input or starting point of the next step – procedure or process. The interface represents a Critical Control Point (CCP), the delivery of a result or outcome (supplier) to the next step (customer). Critical Control Points are essential documentation points. They are monitored against the set standards or specifications and the results are evaluated statistically – benchmarking through SPC. [8, 9]

The conclusion might be a trend that has to be corrected or a deviation of the specifications. This might be caused by a system error or by a human error. Also in other stages of the process deviation from set standards might be observed. It is of critical importance how to deal with these non-conformances and deviations. The basic approach should be educational and not punitive. The main objective is improvement through correction and prevention of re-occurrence.

If an employee would be punished for having made an error, no or under reporting of nonconformities might happen in the future.

Error management includes the terms error, deviation, non-conformance, accident and incident. However, there are differences in importance between a deviation, a non-conformance, an error, an accident and an incident[1].

---

[1] See Chapter 7 – Event Management - a Total Organization Commitment to Quality and Safety and the Tools and Techniques Available to Achieve this Foal.

Deviation	Intentional (authorized) or unintentional departing from the originally specified requirements of a product prior to completion
Non-conformance	Non-fulfilment of a requirement
Error	A mistake possibly resulting in non-compliance or non-conformance, or an unintentional or unplanned deviation attributable to a mistake by an individual
Accident	- An unexpected occurrence in a process causing damage
Incident	An unexpected occurrence in a process not causing damage due to timely detection, corrective and preventive action

Deviations, non-conformities and errors usually are detected before the product or service has been delivered to customers.

They may, however, pass several inter-departmental interfaces before being detected (Murphy's law).

When detected before a product or service is provided to the outside world, the consequences will not affect the confidence of customers or society. When a deviation, non-conformance or error is not detected and passes the interface with the outside world, consequences may lead to serious loss of confidence and trust in the operations of the organization. [19] The management of errors is described in Chapter 7.

A useful classification might be the one suggested by Dr. Howard F. Taswell from the Mayo Clinics Blood Bank, Rochester, MN [20] –

- Identification
- Performance
- Transcription
- Interpretation
- Storage and Retrieval.

Errors may occur incidentally or systematically.

Whatever the pattern, there always should be introduced a root cause analysis to be able to correct and prevent re-occurrence of the same error.

5. Process Management in the Vein to Vein Transfusion Chain

The vein-to-vein transfusion chain is depicted on the painting below (Figure 20)[2]. The painting shows a hospital technician literally pumping blood – under supervision of a doctor - from a donor (the nurse on the right in the painting) to a patient (the pale lady on the left).

This painting shows a simple process. In words, a process can be described as a number of sequential activities that are aimed to satisfy a need of a customer.

---

[2] Painting of an early blood transfusion (The Hague, the Netherlands: A.C. van der Lee, 1933)

In case of the old painting the pale lady is, for medical reasons, in need of a blood transfusion. The process is bringing donor and receiver/patient together in a ward, connecting the donor and the patient with a system to pump blood from a donor directly into the circulation of the patient. In process terms:

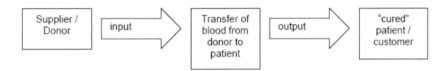

Figure 19. Supplier – producer – customer chain.

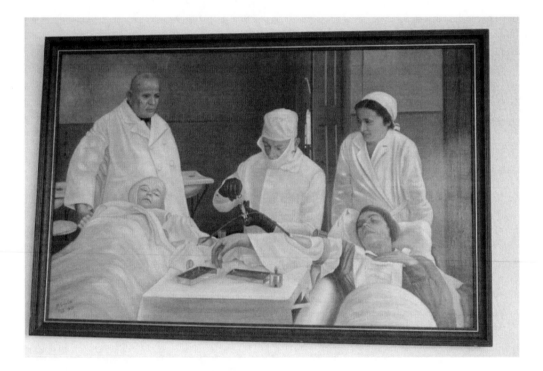

Figure 20. Painting of an early blood transfusion.

5.1. Processes, What Is It About?

In general there is no product or service without a process and inversely there is no process without a product or service. Processes are the managerial and operational entities that allow an orderly functioning of any organization.

All processes, regardless their complexity share common elements: supplier, input, activities, output and (internal or external) customers. Assume the preparation of meals, ingredients, the input for the process, are supplied by a food store or market. This input is the starting point for the process. Subsequently in a number of process steps the ingredients are cleaned, washed, prepared, cooked, the output of this process is the meal served to the customer/client. Hopefully the meal is in conformance with customer expectations (e.g. price, taste and quality). Value for the customer leads to customer satisfaction, but also in this case to an income for the owner of the restaurant preparing meals.

5.2. Historical Background of Thinking in Terms of Processes

In 1911 Frederick Winslow Taylor (1856-1915) published *"The Principles of Scientific Management"*. [21] His approach is the first example of studying process steps, by observing and measuring each individual task in a process in order to increase productivity and quality. Subsequently Henri Ford (1863-1947) translated processes into mass production lines based on standardization and simple (however often monotonous tasks for his employees) tasks for his employees. Numerous other process oriented approaches have been established in the 20th century SPC (statistical process control), lean manufacturing, TQM (Total Quality Management), ISO, JIT (Just-In-Time), PDCA (Plan Do Check Act, by Duran and Deming) and more recently Six Sigma and Lean Six Sigma.

As far as applicable for transfusion medicine these concepts will be used and explained in the following pages. The bottom line of all these process oriented concepts is delivering good quality end results in terms of products and services. End results based on *effective, efficient* and *flexible* processes.

5.3. Definition of Key Concepts

Before going into more detail, we will review a number of keywords and definitions that will appear in this chapter.

Process: activity or a number of activities, that use an input, add value to the input and result in an output to a customer (internal or external). Processes need to be described in a logical way indicating the steps from input to output and the resources needed (e.g. human resources).

Procedure: Specific activity that forms the basic unit of a process or a specified way to carry out an activity or a process. Written instructions (SOPs, EOPs) are used to describe all activities.

Production process: a process involving equipment or software resulting in a product for a customer. Mostly only the conversion is part of this process, not distribution and shipping processes. Sometimes the concept "primary process" is used to the describe the core business of a company, so producing steel is the "primary process" of a steel company, producing pharmaceuticals is the primary process of a pharmaceutical company and producing blood components is the primary process of a blood establishment.

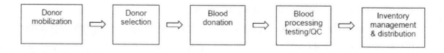

Figure 21. Processes in a blood establishment.

Operations: all conversion or production processes that are carried out by organizational units (departments) of any organization leading to specified goods and services intended to satisfy customer needs in markets.

Business processes: processes that support the main/primary process e.g. order taking and processing, human resource management processes (contracting, training, personnel), bookkeeping processes, product or service design processes.

Control systems: the interfaces between procedures in a process step or between processes lead to critical control points (CCP's). The systematic use of control systems leads to intermediate products that are fit for use in the next production step.

Organization: a company, hospital, division, production unit, department, etc

Function: a number of people in a classical organization with a similar educational background and the same task e.g. marketing and sales dept., purchasing, quality assurance, medical department, etc. A function can have several departments that fulfill different tasks.

Department: a number of employees reporting to a manager.

Most companies daily run several production processes (primary processes) and hundreds of business processes split up over many departments. Taking the human resources department as an example, more than 10 sub processes can be observed: hiring and firing, management development, record keeping, employee relations, salary and benefit programs, assessment programs …

5.4. Processes in Blood Establishments and Hospitals

As an example, the blood transfusion process in a clinical setting will be presented. In general, blood establishment maintains a contract with the hospitals to which services and blood components are supplied.

The contract defines the mutual legal relationship and the mutual responsibilities and accountabilities, including the financial agreement for cost recovery.

The final part of the blood procurement and supply chain ends in the blood components stock mostly located in the facilities of the clinical laboratory of a hospital, under the responsibility of, for example, clinical chemist or pathologist. In (logistic) process terms:

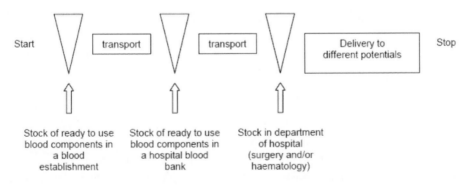

Figure 22. Transport logistics from blood establishment to patient/recipient.

Of course a blood component ordering process has to be performed to guarantee sufficient blood stocks in a hospital. Orders are based on historical data and trend analysis with respect to the clinical use or epidemiology of blood transfusion.

Minimal stock levels, estimations with respect to planned patients and emergencies supply of the blood establishment have to be incorporated in the order calculations.

Blood order or request forms are the input for supply of blood components to the hospital. The processing of a hospital order or request in a blood establishment is depicted below:

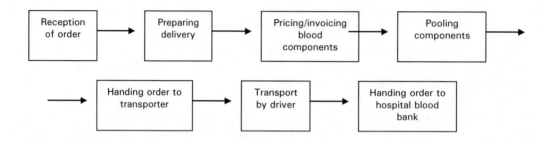

Figure 23. Processing customer order for blood or blood components.

The hospital blood component stocks are intended to be used for patients with a clinical need for blood products.

The clinical transfusion process [3][2, 23] follows the principle: *transfusion of the right unit of blood to the right patient at the right moment and according to appropriate guidelines*, e.g. anaemia that cannot be treated in another way. Below the abbreviation RBC-unit will be used (RBC: Red Blood cell Concentrate).

This process covers a number of 4 important operational steps or processes: Ordering and sampling, selection and pre transfusion compatibility testing, delivery of a blood component to the clinical area, administering the blood component and monitoring the transfused patient. This requires a number of steps[4].

5.5. Process of Bedside Administration of Blood Products

The bedside administration of blood components has a number of process steps (see flowchart) and is normally well described in procedures that must be followed. [22, 23]

The process starts with a clear objective, for example rising patients Hb-level in order to improve oxygen supply to tissues.

A clear indication must be present to prescribe and administer red blood cells, e.g., the bedside administration of RBC *starts* with the reception of the blood component from the clinical laboratory or blood bank in the hospital. It *ends* with a clear report.

The process of bedside administration of an RBC-unit has a number of critical control points (CCP) that need to be well documented.

---

[3] Manual www.optimalblooduse.eu
[4] See Chapter 9 – Patient Safety and Quality Management at the Clinical Interface

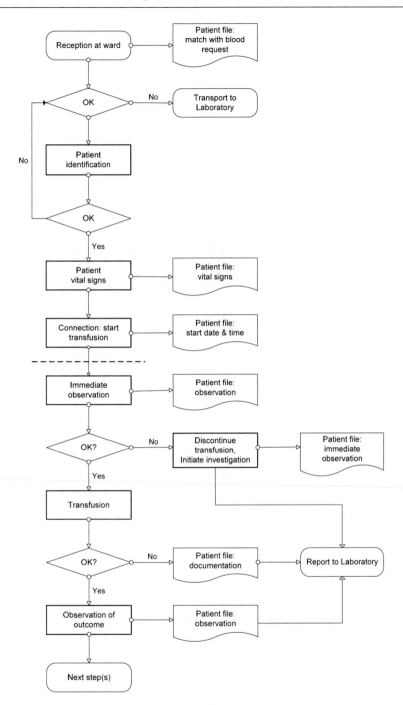

Figure 24. The bedside administration of blood components.

These CCP's include: a visual quality check on the RBC-unit to be administered (integrity of the bag, absence of blood clots, expiry date), patient identity and blood group compatibility. Other important CCP's: vital signs before the transfusion starts, during the first 15 minutes of the transfusion at low infusion rate (be aware of potential transfusion reactions) and after the transfusion. Finally a clear report of the whole process is prepared covering at least the following elements: ID and type of blood component administered, start time and end of the transfusion, vital signs, (pre) medication, volume administered, transfusion reactions (if any) and clinical outcome. This report is part of the (electronic) patient file.

Ignoring or neglecting agreed upon process steps and critical control points may lead to serious hazard to the patient. Bedside errors include using unsuitable administration sets, unhygienic conditions and substandard facilities. This type of errors may lead to bacterial contamination and bacteraemia. Early bedside complications are haemolytic reactions, allergic and pyrogenic reactions, air embolism, citrate toxicity, volume overload.

Transfusion of the wrong blood component to the wrong patient may be fatal to the patient and to the trust in the entire blood supply system in a hospital.

6. Final Recommendations

The management of any organization is based on five intimately related elements – organization and structure, including the necessary infrastructure, human resource and legal framework; standards for both quality of practices and the technical operations; documentation, managerial and operational; education (teaching and training) of all involved and finally assessment (monitoring and evaluation) focused on improvement.

6.1. Organisation and Structure

Organisation and structure in a blood establishment or hospital blood bank are essential building blocks to define tasks and roles in the different processes in the organisation.

A lot of literature exists with respect to different types of (professional) organizations and structures, and in particular Henry Mintzberg being a 'guru' in this field has described the design of effective organizations. [5] In blood banking a wide range of organisational structures can exist, sometimes different from country to country, linked with historical developments and based on the technology level available. In this chapter no specific recommendation has been made for an optimal organization.

All organizational structures share a number of essential elements. Of course there should be sufficient qualified personnel to carry out all tasks which are the responsibility of the organization. Individual authorities, responsibilities and accountabilities should be well defined and described in clear job descriptions. This 'Good Organizational Principle' (GOP) applies for all functions present in the organisation (see also chapter 3). GMP requirements are part of the legal system in e.g. the US, Australia and EU, and consequently a legal obligation.

More important the frame work of functions should be clearly understood by every level or layer in the organisation. Staff should always have appropriate access to their line management and should be properly supervised in accordance with the (critical) tasks being performed in the blood supply or clinical haemotherapy process. When inspected by the Competent Authority the organization should be able to present a clear organisation charts (general and Departmental), clear job descriptions, proofs of qualification and competency of all personnel, on-the-job training records, list of existing posts end their occupancy. [24, 25]

6.2. Standards

Standards represent the minimum acceptable level of performance of an organization and serve as the reference for improvement through progress. There are two levels of standards, those that describe the minimum criteria for quality that allow customer satisfaction, safety, efficacy and sustainability of the operations and the expected outcomes, and those that related to the minimum technical requirements or specifications of the outputs, whether products or services. Less is not acceptable, more is encouraged

6.3. Documentation

Documentation is the core element. Process management systems are usually described in documents available for personnel in the organization. These documents can be provided in different levels.

The *organization process management manual* (level 1) is a fundamental document and provides a clear mission statement, summary of management policies and strategies, a.o. the organizations objectives and vision. Top management is responsible to communicate these aspect to all stakeholders within the organization, but also to external stakeholders such as donors, customers, suppliers, authorities, etc.

The *procedures manual* (a level 2 document) describes the internal structure/organization and responsibilities. The *work instructions,* SOPs (Standard Operating Procedures) and related EOPs (Equipment Operating Procedures), and the JDs (Job Descriptions) describe in detail the methods for performing activities. These are level 3 operational and instructive documents that end in the outcome documents or records as an evidence of what was done. In blood transfusion activities all processes must be adequately documented. To be able to perform in a standardized way, personnel/operators follow the procedures as documented. All significant changes are validated and authorised. Staff education (teaching and training) records ensure that personnel is aware of changes in work processes or specific tasks starting at the day the changes have become effective.

Finally document archiving should follow state of the art standards to allow adequate traceability and retrievability.

6.4. Education (Teaching and Training)

Personnel involved in the collection, testing, processing, storage, distribution, prescription and clinical use of blood products should be appropriately qualified for their jobs. This applies to medical doctors, nursing staff, laboratory technicians, assistants, etc. Personnel should be provided with timely, relevant and regularly updated teaching and training. Written proof of proper education and written evidence of on the job (re)training must be available within the organisation.

Education is an ongoing fuelling of people to remain competent for the tasks assigned.

6. 5. Assessment

Assessments of all processes and related procedures, and key-competencies of all personnel can be done on an annual basis in organization wide programmes. Regular internal assessments and evaluation at employee level of the results on objectives, is the start of an improvement cycle – the Deming cycle known as the Plan – Do – Check - Act (PDCA) cycle, is considered a valuable mechanism for this purpose.

Annexes

Annex 1

Information Requirements
(as referred to in Article 2 and 3)
PART A
Information to be provided to prospective donors of blood or blood components

1. Accurate educational materials, which are understandable for members of the general public, about the essential nature of blood, the blood donation procedure, the components derived from whole blood and apheresis donations, and the important benefits to patients.
2. For both allogenic and autologous donations, the reasons for requiring an examination, health and medical history, and the testing of donations and all the significance of 'informed consent'.

For allogenic donations, self-deferral, and temporary and permanent deferral, and the reasons why individuals are not to donate blood or blood components if there could be a risk for the recipient.

For autologous donations, the possibility of deferral and the reasons why the donation procedure would not take place in the presence of a health risk to the individuals whether as donor or recipient of the autologous blood or blood components

1. Information on the protection of personal data: no unauthorized disclosure of the identity of the donor, of information concerning the donor's health, and of the results of the tests performed.
2. The reasons why individuals are not to make donations which may be detrimental to their health.
3. Specific information on the nature of the procedures involved either in the allogenic or autologous donation process and their respective associated risks. For autologous donations, the possibility that the autologous blood and blood components may not suffice for the indented transfusion requirements.
4. Information on the option of donors to change their mind about donating prior to proceeding further, o the possibility of withdrawing or self-deferring at any time during the donation process, without any undue embarrassment or discomfort.

5. The reasons why it is important that donors inform the blood establishment of any subsequent event that may render any prior donation unsuitable for transfusion.

6. Information on the responsibility of the blood establishment to inform the donor, through an appropriate mechanism, if test results show abnormality of significance to the donor's health.

7. Information why unused autologous blood and blood components will be discarded and not transferred to other patients.

8. Information that test results detecting markers for viruses, such as HIV, HBV, HCV or other relevant blood transmissible microbiologic agents, will result in donor deferral and destruction of the collected unit.

9. Information on the opportunity for donors to ask questions at any time.

Annex 2

Commission Directive 2004/33/Ec
Annex V –
Quality and Safety Requirements for Blood and Blood Components

2.1. Blood and blood components must comply with the following technical quality measurements and meet the acceptable results.

2.2. Appropriate bacteriological control of the collection and manufacturing process must be performed.

2.3. Member States must take all necessary measures to ensure that all imports of blood and blood components from third countries, including those used as starting material/raw material for the manufacture of medicinal products derived from human blood or human plasma, shall meet equivalent standards of quality and safety to the ones laid down in this Directive.

2.4. [For autologous donation, the measures marked with an asterisk (*) are recommendations only]

Component	Quality measurements Required The required frequency of sampling for all measurements shall be determined using statistical process control	Acceptable results for quality measurements
Red cells	Volume	Valid for storage characteristics to maintain product within specifications for haemoglobin and haemolysis
	Haemoglobin (*)	Not less than 45 g per unit
	Haemolysis	Less than 0,8% of red cell mass at the end of the shelf life
Red cells, buffy coat removed	Volume	Valid for storage characteristics to maintain product within specifications for haemoglobin and haemolysis
	Haemoglobin (*)	Not less than 43 g per unit
	Haemolysis	Less than 0,8% of red cell mass at the end of the shelf life

(Continued)

Component	Quality measurements Required The required frequency of sampling for all measurements shall be determined using statistical process control	Acceptable results for quality measurements
Red cells, leukocyte-depleted	Volume	Valid for storage characteristics to maintain product within specifications for haemoglobin and haemolysis
	Haemoglobin (*)	Not less than 40 g per unit
	Leukocyte content	Less than 1×10^6 per unit
	Haemolysis	Less than 0,8% of red cell mass at the end of the shelf life
Red cells in additive solution	Volume	Valid for storage characteristics to maintain product within specifications for haemoglobin and haemolysis
	Haemoglobin (*)	Not less than 45 g per unit
	Haemolysis	Less than 0,8% of red cell mass at the end of the shelf life
Red cells, buffy coat removed, in additive solution	Volume	Valid for storage characteristics to maintain product within specifications for haemoglobin and haemolysis
	Haemoglobin (*)	Not less than 43 g per unit
	Haemolysis	Less than 0,8% of red cell mass at the end of the shelf life
Red cells, leukocyte-depleted, in additive solution	Volume	Valid for storage characteristics to maintain product within specifications for haemoglobin and haemolysis
	Haemoglobin (*)	Not less than 40 g per unit
	Leukocyte content	Less than 1×10^6 per unit
	Haemolysis	Less than 0,8% of red cell mass at the end of the shelf life
Red cells, apheresis	Volume	Valid for storage characteristics to maintain product within specifications for haemoglobin and haemolysis
	Haemoglobin (*)	Not less than 40 g per unit
	Haemolysis	Less than 0,8% of red cell mass at the end of the shelf life
Whole blood	Volume	Valid for storage characteristics to maintain product within specifications for haemoglobin and haemolysis 450 ml +/- 50 ml For paediatric autologous whole blood collections – not to exceed 10,5 ml per kg body weight.
	Haemoglobin (*)	Not less than 45 g per unit
	Haemolysis	Less than 0,8% of red cell mass at the end of the shelf life
Platelets, apheresis	Volume	Valid for storage characteristics to maintain product within specifications for pH
	Platelet content	Variations in platelet content per single donation are permitted within limits that comply with validated preparations and preservation conditions

Component	Quality measurements Required The required frequency of sampling for all measurements shall be determined using statistical process control	Acceptable results for quality measurements
	pH	6,4 – 7,4 corrected for 22 °C, at the end of the shelf life
Platelets, apheresis, leukocyte-depleted	Volume	Valid for storage characteristics to maintain product within specifications for pH
	Platelet content	Variations in platelet content per single donation are permitted within limits that comply with validated preparations and preservation conditions
	Leukocyte content	Less than 1 x 10^6 per unit
	pH	6,4 – 7,4 corrected for 22 °C, at the end of the shelf life
Platelets, recovered, pooled	Volume	Valid for storage characteristics to maintain product within specifications for pH
	Platelet content	Variations in platelet content per single donation are permitted within limits that comply with validated preparations and preservation conditions
	Leukocyte content	Less than 0,2 x 10^9 per single unit (platelet-rich plasma method) Less than 0,05 10^9 per single unit (buffy coat method)
	pH	6,4 – 7,4 corrected for 22 °C, at the end of the shelf life
Platelets, recovered, pooled, leukocyte-depleted	Volume	Valid for storage characteristics to maintain product within specifications for pH
	Platelet content	Variations in platelet content per single donation are permitted within limits that comply with validated preparations and preservation conditions
	Leukocyte content	Less than 1 x 10^6 per pool
	pH	6,4 – 7,4 corrected for 22 °C, at the end of the shelf life
Platelets, recovered, single unit	Volume	Valid for storage characteristics to maintain product within specifications for pH
	Platelet content	Variations in platelet content per single donation are permitted within limits that comply with validated preparations and preservation conditions
	Leukocyte content	Less than 0,2 x 10^9 per single unit (platelet-rich plasma method) Less than 0,05 10^9 per single unit (buffy coat method)
	pH	6,4 – 7,4 corrected for 22 °C, at the end of the shelf life
Platelets, recovered, single unit, leukocyte-depleted	Volume	Valid for storage characteristics to maintain product within specifications for pH

(Continued)

Component	Quality measurements Required The required frequency of sampling for all measurements shall be determined using statistical process control	Acceptable results for quality measurements
	Platelet content	Variations in platelet content per single donation are permitted within limits that comply with validated preparations and preservation conditions
	Leukocyte content	Less than 1×10^6 per pool
	pH	$6,4 - 7,4$ corrected for 22 °C, at the end of the shelf life
Plasma, fresh-Frozen	Volume	Stated volume +/- 10 %
	Factor VIIIc (*)	Average (after freezing and thawing): 70 % or more of the value of the freshly collected plasma unit
	Total protein	Not less than 50 g/l
	Residual cellular content	Red cells les than $6,0 \times 10^9$/l Leukocytes: less than $0,1 \times 10^9$/l Platelets: less than 50×10^9/l
Plasma, fresh-frozen cryoprecipitate-depleted	Volume	Stated volume: +/- 10 %
	Residual cellular content	Red cells les than $6,0 \times 10^9$/l Leukocytes: less than $0,1 \times 10^9$/l Platelets: less than 50×10^9/l
Cryoprecipitate	Fibrinogen content (*)	Greater than or equal to 140 mg per unit
	Factor VIIIc (*)	Greater than or equal to 70 international units per unit
Granulocytes, apheresis	Volume	Less than 500 ml
	Granulocyte content	Greater than 1×10^{10} granulocytes per unit

Annex 3

Directive 2002/98/Ec of the European Parliament and the Council
Annex Iii – Labelling Requirements

The label on the component must contain the following information

- the official name of the component
- the volume or weight or number of cells in the component (as appropriate)
- the unique numeric or alphanumeric donation identification
- the name of producing blood establishment
- the ABO Group (not required for plasma intended only for fractionation)
- the Rh D group, either Rh D positive or Rh D negative (not required for plasma intended only for fractionation)
- the date or time of expiry (as appropriate)
- the temperature of storage
- the name, composition and volume of anticoagulant and / or additive solution (if any).

Annex 4

Commission Directive 2004/33/Ec
Annex Iv – Storage, Transport and Distribution Conditions for Blood and Blood
Components
(As Referred To In Article 5)

1. STORAGE
1.1. Liquid storage

Component	Temperature of storage	Maximum storage time
Red cell preparations and whole blood (if used for transfusion as whole blood)	+ 2 to + 6 °C	28 to 49 days according to the process used for collection, processing and storage
Component	Temperature of storage	Maximum storage time
Platelet preparations	+20 to +24 °C	5 days; may be stored 7 days in conjunction with detection or reduction of bacterial contamination
Granulocytes	+20 to +24 °C	24 hours

1.2. Cryopreservation

Component	Storage conditions and duration
Red blood cells	Up to 30 years according to processes used for collection, processing and storage
Platelets	Up to 24 months according to processes used for collection, processing and storage
Plasma and cryoprecepitate	Up to 36 months according to processes used for collection, processing and storage
Cryopreserved red cells and platelets must be formulated in a suitable medium after thawing. The allowable storage period after thawing to depend on the method used.	

2. Transport and Distribution

Transport and distribution of blood and blood components at all stages of the transport chain must be under conditions that maintain the integrity of the product.

References

[1]   Proctor R. *Managerial accounting for business decisions*. Second edition. Harlow UK. Pearson Education Ltd. 2006

[2]   Bossidy L and Charan R. *Execution – The discipline of getting things done*. First edition New York, NY USA. Crown Business. 2002

[3]   Smit Sibinga CTh and Pitman JP. Transmission of HIV Through Blood – How To Bridge the Knowledge Gap. In: Nancy Dumais editor. *HIV and AIDS - Updates on Biology, Immunology, Epidemiology and Treatment Strategies*, InTech, Riyeka, Croatia. 2011 Chapter 23, pp 583-618. Available from: http://www.intechopen.com /articles/show/title/transmission-of-hiv-through-blood-how-to-bridge-the-knowledge-gap

[4]   The Art and Science of Program Delivery. London UK. PA Knowledge Ltd 2002.

[5]   Minzberg H. *Structure in Five, Designing effective organizations*. Second edition Upper Saddle River, NJ, USA Prentice Hall Inc. 1993, Chapter 2.

[6]   van der Zwaan AH. *Organizing Work Processes. Engineering work and managing workers*. Second edition Assen NL. Koninklijke van Gorcum 2002.

[7]   Microsoft Visio™ 2010, Microsoft Office™. Available from http://office.microsoft. com /en-us/visio/

[8]   Oakland JS. *Statistical Process Control*. Fourth edition Oxford UK. Butterworth-Heinemann, 1999.

[9]   Walters LM and Carpenter Bradley JK, eds. *Simple Six Sigma for Blood Banking, Transfusion and Cellular Therapies*. AABB Press, Bethesda, MD, USA. 2007. ISBN 978-1-56395-249-4.

[10]   Gygi C, DeCarlo N, Williams B eds. *Six Sigma for Dummies*. Wiley Publishing Inc. Hoboken, NJ, USA, 2005. ISBN 0-7645-6798-5.

[11]   Guide to the Preparation, Use and Quality Assurance of Blood Components. Annex to Recommendation No. R(95)15, Committee of Ministers of the Council of Europe. Latest edition, Strasbourg, F Council of Europe Publishing. Chapter 6 – Statistical Process Control.

[12]   Remenyi D, Onofrei G, English J. *An Introduction to Statistics using Microsoft Excel*. First edition Reading UK. Academic Publishing Ltd. 2009.

[13]   Slack N, Chambers S, Johston R, Betts A *Operations and Process Management*. Second edition FT Prentice Hall, Pearson Education Ltd UK 2009, Chapter 7.

[14]   Shah RM. *Result Oriented Management*. First Edition Jaico Books on Business Management, India, 1976.

[15]   Commission Directive 2004/33/EC of 22 March 2004 implementing Directive 2002/98/EC of the European Parliament and of the Council as regards certain technical requirements for blood and blood components. *Official Journal of the European Union*, L91, 30/03/2004, Annex II part A, p29.

[16]   Commission Directive 2004/33/EC of 22 March 2004 implementing Directive 2002/98/EC of the European Parliament and of the Council as regards cer4tain technical requirements for blood and blood components. *Official Journal Of the European Union*, L91, 30/03/2004, Annex V, p.36-39.

[17]   Directive 2002/98/EC of the European Parliament and of the Council of 27 January 2003 setting standards of quality and safety for the collection, testing, processing, storage and distribution of human blood and blood components and amending Directive 2001/83/EC. *Official Journal of the European Union*, L33, 8/02/2003, Annex III, p.33.

[18]   Commission Directive 2004/33/EC of 22 March 2004 implementing Directive 2002/98/EC of the European Parliament and of the Council as regards certain technical requirements for blood and blood components. *Official Journal of the European Union*, L91, 30/03/2004, Annex Iv, p.35.

[19] Smit Sibinga CTh. Haemovigilance: An approach to risk management and control. In: Smit Sibinga CTh and Alter HJ eds. *Risk Management in Blood Transfusion: The Virtue of Reality.* Kluwer Academic Publ. Dordrecht, Boston, London 1999. pp 181-189.

[20] Taswell HF, Sonnenberg CL Error analysis: Types of errors in the blood bank. In: Smit Sibinga CTh, Das PC, Taswell HF eds *Quality Assurance in Blood Banking and its Clinical Impact,* Martinus Nijhoff Publ. Boston, The Hague, Dordrecht, Lancaster. 1984, pp 227-237.

[21] Taylor F W. *The Principles of Scientific Management Processes.* First edition New York, NY, USA and London, UK. Harper and Brothers, 1911.

[22] McClelland DBL, Pine E, Franklin IM, eds. *Manual of Optimal Blood Use.* EU Optimal Blood Use Project. Scottish National Blood Transfusion Service, Edinburgh, Scotland, 2010. Available from www.optimalblooduse.eu.

[23] Kajja I. *The Current Hospital Practices and Procedures in Uganda.* PhD thesis University of Groningen, NL. 2010 (ISBN 978-90-367-4619-9) Chapter 1.

[24] Seifried E and Seidl C, eds. *Common European Standards and Criteria for the Inspection of Blood Establishments.* EuBIS project. Frankfurt, D. 2010 Available from www.eubis-europe.eu.

[25] AABB Standards for Blood Banks and Transfusion Services. AABB Press, Bethesda, MD, USA, current edition.

In: Quality Management in Transfusion Medicine
Editor: Cees Th. Smit Sibinga

ISBN: 978-1-62618-665-1
© 2013 Nova Science Publishers, Inc.

Chapter V

Value and Role of Information and Communication Technology (ICT) and Management Information System (MIS) in Transfusion Medicine

Johan A. van der Does[*1] *and Thomas W. de Boer*[†2]
¹Consultant in Transfusion Medicine, The Hague, NL
²University of Groningen, Groningen,The Netherlands

Abstract

This chapter is about Quality Management Systems (QMS) and how to support them with adequate ICT systems like a Management Information System (MIS). First attention is paid to the relevant elements of a QMS and the Primary Process in blood establishments. As different types of organizations need a different approach, we introduce three types of organizations: the small blood establishment, the medium blood establishment and the nationwide organization of blood transfusion. Next attention is paid to typical problems in QMS and ICT and to the ICT-support of the management and operations. Finally the assurance and the maintenance of the quality of the ICT-systems itself is described. Throughout it is assumed that ICT is a service to and a support for the employees. It helps them in performing their tasks and their responsibilities.

Keywords: ICTsupport, Information Systems Design, Functional modelling, User Requirement Specification (URS), Service delivery, Validation

---

* Former Director of Red Cross Blood Bank, The Hague, The Netherlands, Former project leader Information Systems Sanquin, The Netherlands, Johan van Oldenbearneveltlaan 56, 2582 NV the Hague, NL. Tel: +31- 70 3554985, E-mail: ja.vander.does@worldonline.nl
† Former Assistant Professor of Information Science, University of Groningen, The Netherlands, Van Swinderenstraat 6, 9714HD Groningen, NL, Tel: +31- 6 41582426, E-mail: t.w.de.boer@gmail.com

1. Introduction

In the organization and operation of a blood establishment it is very important that high quality standards are maintained by an organization wide Quality Management System (QMS). Nowadays this can only be achieved by extensively using information and communication technology (ICT). Although mostly in the form of operational support systems and information systems, one sees that also data warehouses and (semi-)intelligent systems are used. This brings forth the question of how to organize this complex supporting ICT architecture. In our view the start of it all is in the structuring of the organization. The description of the processes, procedures, standards, responsibilities et cetera, that comprise the well-structured organization is the only basis on which an appropriate design of the needed ICT-systems is possible. In this way the systems are adapted to the organization. If this is not the case, the organization will run the risk of being adapted to the ICT-systems available. Of course an organization will always be adapted to a certain degree. Especially when there are systems available that have a proven quality. But care should be taken that organizational and user requirements come first. In this chapter we investigate the characteristics of QMSs and how information and communication technology (ICT) can be used to support it.

2. Elements of Quality Management Systems (QMS)

When we think of maintaining high quality standards, it is clear that it is necessary to have a structure, processes and procedures et cetera that build a quality system. Figure 1 shows the main elements in such a system.

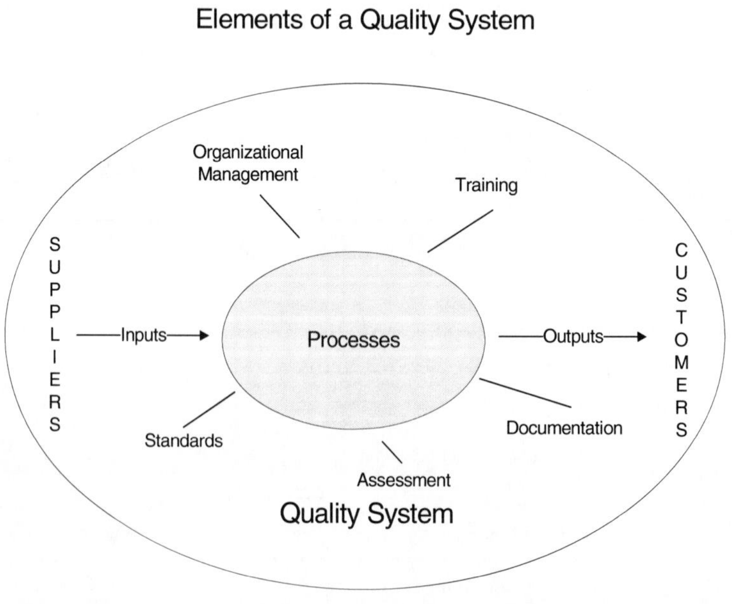

Figure 1. Elements of a Quality System.

An organization transforms the input from employees and suppliers into an output that is delivered to customers. This transformation process is the Primary Process. We will elaborate on that in the next section. In figure 1 we see five Quality Elements (QEs). These are the essential elements that must be properly set to guarantee a sound Quality Management.

1. Organization

   A well-structured organization and ICT support are the *conditio sine qua non* for Quality Management. Unless the organization is well defined and processes, procedures and tasks are described in detail and clear to every member, a good Quality System is impossible. Each product has to comply with all the quality criteria for each of the activities in the production process in each of the Main Business Processes (MBP). All these data have to be checked at release and at shipment after ordering, and this is impossible to perform by hand. ICT is therefore indispensable.

2. Standards

   Standards define and describe the processes and procedures, i.e. the way people should act, and set the targets to which results can be compared. Standards become a Plan in the Deming cycle when they are accepted and employees are committed to them.

3. Documentation

   The organization, the processes and procedures, tasks and activities must be documented to show that work is done according to standards, to train the employees and for reference.

4. Education (Teaching and Training)

   Employees should be familiar with the standards and be able to perform accordingly. Training is the only way to reach competence and attain that goal.

5. Assessment – Monitoring and Evaluation

   Any Quality Management System needs continuous monitoring. Without monitoring and fast feedback based on proper evaluation, the QMS will become ineffective.

Next to these quality system elements there are several prerequisites.

2.1. Detailed Knowledge

To maintain a high level Quality System it is necessary to go into details. Especially concerning the primary process, it is necessary to know in detail what the process is about, what is going on, who is responsible for what. This means that there must be a detailed description of the primary process and the roles and functions in it. More importantly, there must be agreement on the description and commitment to act accordingly.

2.2. Check, Check and Recheck

Monitoring is not just a matter of controlling the flow. It is a continuous check of the results of every part of the primary (and supporting) processes. That is why the cycle Plan-

Do-Check-Act is so important in Quality Management. The cycle was worked out by Deming [1] and the actual standard is described in detail in ISO 9001:2008.

In short the four stages are:

- Plan: establish the objectives and processes necessary to deliver results in accordance with customer requirements and the organization's policies.
- Do: implement the process.
- Check: monitor and measure processes and products against policies and requirements for the products, report the results and compare to standards by evaluation.
- Act: take actions to continually improve process performance.

3. ICT-Support

Because of the complexity and extensiveness of the processes, a QMS cannot do without a support by ICT systems. For a proper support, every system should be developed in a well defined project. In the project plan for the development of an information system the standards that will be used in operation should be described, next to the functionality and other user requirements, the tasks and the responsibilities. Care should be taken that the system is adapted to the organization and not *vice versa*. We will come back to these topics in the second half of this chapter.

4. The Primary Process

Transfusion Medicine comprises the clinical and laboratory processes in hospitals, and the procurement of blood products in blood establishments. In general, the Primary Process of a blood establishment is the production and delivery of blood components to customers. This process is demand driven, as it is not thinkable that someone will give blood when nobody needs it. This is depicted in figure 2.

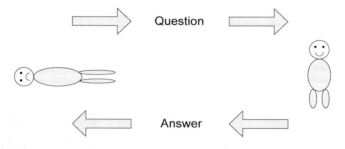

Figure 2. Demand driven blood donation.

Although there will be differences between individual organizations, it is possible to give a general description of the Primary Process. The blood components are extracted from blood, supplied by donors. In this Primary Process we distinguish six sub-processes that will be denoted by the term Main Business Process (MBP).

1. *Stock keeping, ordering and delivery* –
   Management of different components, as agreed with the hospitals. Taking care of incoming orders, transport of ordered components, transfer to an agreed point (mostly transfusion laboratory).

2. *Release of components from quarantine* –
   Physically labelling a unit as 'fit for use', guaranteeing that all parameters in donation, production and quality control are met. Units can then be transferred to the final stock. Units not complying are put back in quarantine (data not complete yet) or in isolation (possibly harmful for patients).

3. *Laboratory tests (Quality Control or QC)* –
   Performance of all the mandatory tests, on all donations. Quality Control and Quality Assurance of all the tests done.

4. *Preparing standard blood components* –
   Component preparation, with specifications as agreed with the hospitals.

5. *Donations* –
   Examination of donors, to prevent complications with the donors and in the patients; taking a unit of blood and making the donation a pleasurable experience.

6. *Donor management* –
   Creating awareness in society on the need for voluntary donors, informing prospective donors, motivating, accepting and retaining donors, maintaining donor administration, planning donor sessions.

The sequence of the sub-processes are depicted in figure 3. We call this chart the Logistic Model. It gives an overview of the Primary Process and also distinguishes the separate sub-processes.

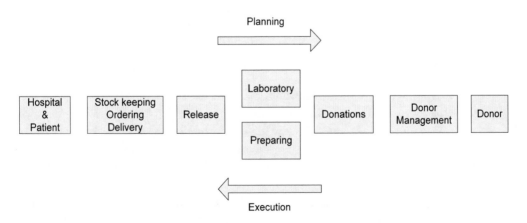

Figure 3. The general Primary Process.

It should be clear that each MBP is a process on its own with its own suppliers and customers and a Primary (sub)Process that is governed by a Quality Subsystem. Almost always each MBP is the responsibility of one head of a department, and he or she is responsible for both the execution and the planning of the daily operations as well as on the next abstraction level, the control. E.g., the laboratory receives from its (internal) supplier (donor department) blood samples that must be tested. The results of the tests are reported to the (internal) customers. This process is governed by a QMS that prescribes procedures for testing and standards for comparison.

5. Supporting Information Systems

Each of the processes will be supported by an information system. The design of these information systems is a long and tedious process. At the start of it there should be agreement about the organization and the Primary Process. Partly the agreement can be reached by agreeing on the Logistic Model as depicted in Figure 2. However, that is not enough. There should also be a clear vision and agreement on the necessary content of the information system and the authorities and responsibilities of the users. Therefore it is necessary to develop a so-called Static Structure Model (SSM) of the organization of the Primary Process.

The Static Structure Model is derived from the Class Diagram that is used in the Unified Modelling Language UML. [2] A Static Structure Model (see figure 4) describes which entities play a role in the organization. To begin with, there are two main organizations: the hospital and the blood establishment. In figure 4 they are represented by two large rectangles. In the rectangle of the hospital there are four small rectangles. They represent the entities that are relevant in the hospital. Of course, there are much more entities, but in a Static Structure Model we only represent the entities that are relevant for the topic at hand. So in this case we represent four entities: patients, transfusions, blood components and stock. Each rectangle in the model represents a set of entities in reality. In the model we call this set a class. The class contains one or more individual objects. E.g., the class Patients represents all the individual patients in the hospital. Classes are connected by lines that indicate a relation between them. Finally, classes are not only grouped by organization (hospital, blood establishment), but also grouped by the primary process in which they play a role. In figure 4 the several Main Business Processes (MBP) are indicated by dotted rectangles with their names attached. This connects the Logistic Model with the Static Structure Model. For several reasons the Static Structure Model is important.

1. It gives an overview of the relevant objects in the system. For each object a list of data that we want to know about that object should be defined. E.g., what do we want to know about a donor object? Name, date of birth, gender, address, blood type, dates of donation, availability due to special conditions, this list can become very long and diverse. The resulting data list is the basis for the data content of the information system to be.
2. It clearly defines authorities and responsibilities. It shows the different MBPs and the objects that are contained in it. For each MBP someone will be responsible; not only for the process but also for the objects that are involved. Within each sub-process a set of functions, tasks and procedures to perform the MBP will be defined.

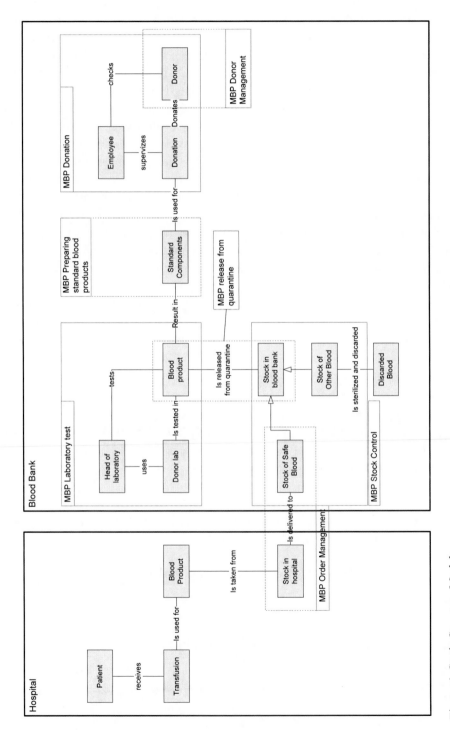

Figure 4. Static Structure Model.

Concluding, the Main Business Processes (MBP) have to be described in detail. Then these MBPs have to be translated into information, to become part of the information system. Also the responsibilities and authorities of all staff members and other employees are to be defined. To become clear to all participants, this process may take several months to one or two years,. Especially it is important to have everyone's agreement on the points where responsibilities for tasks, products or information is transferred from one department to another department, or from one staff member to another staff member.

As an example let us take a look at the process 'final release'. One essential process in each blood establishment is the process 'final release', where all data pertaining to one blood component are checked and where, only if all data are present and within the defined values or specifications, some visible sign will be attached to that component to indicate that it complies with all requirements. It will be clear for all concerned that data are to be gathered from donor management, donations, component production and QC laboratory, and that all data have to be within clearly defined limits, to be able to declare a blood component 'fit for use'. That bag with a blood component will then be physically transferred from the 'quarantine' stock to the 'safe, standard' stock. This process is owned by the Quality Manager, and mostly performed by the employees in the component production department . If not all data are within the set limits, two possibilities remain: the bags stay in quarantine stock, when data are (still) missing, or they are declared unfit for clinical use, and are transferred to the 'isolation stock', to be dealt with later. These units are physically transferred to refrigerators and freezers, that are clearly marked as 'Isolation', and are locked, with only authorized experienced employees having access to determine what has to happen with the units. In most cases they will be destroyed.

6. Three Types of Organizations

Because the opportunities for QMSs differ very much between organizations, we introduce three types of organizations. A local blood establishment, with for instance 10.000 donations per year, a larger blood establishment or a regional system of blood establishments, with for instance 50.000 units drawn, and a national system, comprising of 10 or more blood establishments, and more than 100.000 donations per year.

Table 1. Three types of organizations

Situation	Units drawn / year approximately	Quality development	Responsibility for the development of the ICT system	Hardware	Software
small blood establishment	10.000	Start	Each department separately	Separate PCs	Office (Word, Excel) or home developed system
bigger or system of blood establishments	50.000	On going	Each department with ICT dep.	PCs separate and in networks	
			Management Team / ICT dep.	Servers, backup systems	Quality certified specific blood bank software (of the shelf)
National system	100.000	cGMP	ICT dep.; service management	Servers, backup systems,	

In all countries of the world society demands better health care from governments, and this translates to the need for quality development in the blood supply. All blood establishments will move to formal quality systems, aiming (and eventually achieving) the level of cGMP, current Good Manufacturing Practices. [3] We will describe the small blood establishment as starting with a QMS, the bigger blood establishments as having an ongoing quality development, and the national system as functioning on the level of cGMP. Much of what will be said holds true for both the departments in the Primary Process (donor management, donations, component production, QC laboratory, release, stock, ordering and delivery), as well as for the departments in the supporting functions (book keeping, human resource management, quality assurance, technical services, etc.). In this chapter we will focus on the Primary Process.

Table 1 shows an overview of the characteristics of the three types.

6.1. The Situation in the Small Blood Establishment

In the situation of a (small) blood establishment, starting with a quality system, some computers will be available, mostly for office use, and often in the laboratory. Most administrative work is done by hand, on paper lists or in paper books.

The easiest way to start using computers is probably to automate each of the defined Main Business Processes separately. The advantages are that the amount of work to be done can be overseen, and each Head of a Department, often responsible for one well defined Main Business Process, can be the 'project owner' for his or her processes to be automated.

For each MBP a project group has to be formed, often consisting of (at least) the Head, the Quality Manager, one experienced employee of the department, and a person who will be responsible for the technical side: the computers, disks, service delivery and also the management of the software.

In reality, this does not happen: Heads of departments, in this phase of information system development will keep everything within their department, and the technical and service (to the users) side is often neglected. The data in this phase of development of each information system will be in separate files on the hard disks of PC's. These PC's will in general not be connected into one system. Possibly there are external hard disk units as backups. The Operating System will mostly be Microsoft Windows, the software will mostly be Microsoft Office (especially Word and Excel).

6.2. The Situation in the Medium Sized Blood Establishment

Often small blood establishments work together with a local ICT firm. That firm knows the business processes and, because of the small scale of the systems, is a nice and sufficient partner. This changes when we look at a medium size blood establishment or an organization consisting of several blood establishments. In this case the separate ICT systems in the organization or between organizations have to be connected. That means that the programmes, and databases, used in the small, individual blood establishments will, more or less, act as one system. That is often difficult to achieve. Even more problems arise when it turns out to be necessary to add more functions to the existing systems. Main problems lie in the fact that the systems are home grown, there is hardly any documentation, so only a few people understand how the systems work and can be connected. Also personal preferences tend to play a bigger role than is acceptable. Even in this situation senior management of the blood establishment(s) can decide to continue with the further development of the home grown programme. But this way is doomed to fail, it will cost much time and even more energy, and will never be able to give an information system that will comply with any quality standards. It is to be left as soon as this phase of development is recognized.

We think that in the case of a medium size blood establishment or an organization of several blood establishments it is time for bold, and important choices.

It should be recognized that the planning, development and introduction of an ICT system at this level is a major project, and should be dealt with accordingly.

This project can only be started when the top management, the Director, the Board of Trustees, the Management Team, all are convinced that this is necessary. In this phase the Ministry of Health or the state inspectorate should also be contacted. Topics to be considered are:

1. Strategy: what kind of blood establishment (system) do we want to be in 5 – 10 years time, what standards do we want to adhere to (or have to adhere to), what quality system do we develop, etc.
2. Do we want the ICT system to have functionality on four levels, support on the control level, the operational level, the strategy level and the policy level?
3. How do we get enough knowledge of professional ICT systems available to be able to develop requirements for the system, not only for the dedicated blood establishment primary process applications, but also for quality documentation, the financial system, Human Resource Management, etc.

The phase from recognising the need for developing a professional ICT system to the moment of charging an employee (current or specifically attracted) to start writing a project plan can easily take half a year or even a year. All senior staff and supervisory bodies have to be convinced that now this is a priority, and that by choosing this one, other necessary projects will have to wait.

6.3. The Situation in a National System

Here the same choices have to be made as in the previous section. However, the governments of all countries will prefer to have a system that is up to international standards. This is also advised by the World Health Organisation (WHO). However, the efforts needed will be many times greater because of the complexity of the organization and the resulting systems. Nevertheless, the advantages are clear enough. But the costs will be high:

1. It is expensive to design, develop and implement an information system at this level, both in money as well as in employee time.
2. Filling the data tables of the programme takes much time from senior staff members and other employees. This will be very difficult to explain to both the management and the governing board and Ministry of Health.

3. Middle and top management find it difficult to accept that there is a lot of home work to be done before anything useful can be seen from the system.
4. The formal service delivery system has to be up to standards too. Often no one has any knowledge or understanding of service delivery and hardware and software management. Change control and management are essential from the start.
5. Hardware is expensive, and has to be bought, installed and maintained according to standards, which are beforehand agreed upon.

It is important for top management to set up a project, with the explicit aim to make a real project plan, and to express the commitment of the top for this very time and energy consuming work. For the first, initial, project plan often an external consultant is necessary to support the development of that plan.

7. Applying ICT

Applying ICT means in the first place to match the organization, the processes and the people with the information systems to be. In this case the focus will be on functions, processes and procedures, and tasks in the organization and the matching functionality of the ICT-systems. So first we should have a clear view on the organization. Morgan [4] has shown that there are many possible views. Here we will narrow our view of the essentials of an organization to what is depicted in Figure 5. Figure 5 contains a functional overview of an organization. It consists of three perspectives, the Business Objective, the Functional and the Process perspective.

7.1. The Business Objective Perspective

The Business Objective perspective is about the goals of an organization. In this case we are interested in the Quality Management goals. Quality Management sets the goals and they are translated into Standards. The Standards are translated into measurable performance indicators and into a specification of who is responsible for attaining them.

7.2. The Function Perspective

In the Function perspective the functions in the organization are central. Each function has responsibilities that are described in the documentation, it has authorities to perform activities and it needs capabilities to perform. A function is connected to a position that is fulfilled by a human being. In fact this means that the human being has authorities, responsibilities, and needs capabilities. However, one should keep in mind that this is because the human being and the function are connected. Finally, we take into account that capability needs training.

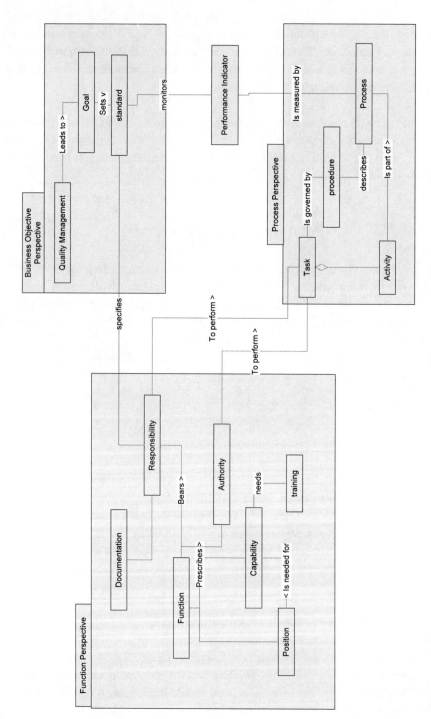

Figure 5. Functions, tasks and procedures.

7.3. The Process Perspective

In the Process perspective we look at the operations in the organization. There are tasks to be performed, based on responsibility and authority. A task is an order (a 'command') to do something. These tasks are governed by processes and procedures that describe what is to be done and how it is to be done. Tasks and procedures lead to activities that build up processes. The processes are monitored and results are compared with the performance indicators that are set by the standards. The functional overview gives all the ingredients that we want to know and that are needed to describe the organization in full detail. This description is a sound basis for the design of the supporting information systems. To give support, there must be a close connection between the functions in the organization and the functionality of the system.

8. On the Functionality of ICT Systems

The QMS manages the quality at three levels:

- The quality of the products
- The quality of the production process
- The quality of the organization.

This matches with the levels in the functionality of ICT systems. [5] The functionality of ICT systems is the way they are used in organizations. The functionality can be very diverse as each organization has its own requirements. But in general we can distinguish four levels of functionality that are common to all organizations.

1. Operations:
   The most basic level of functionality is the support of the daily operations. The time scope is one or two days. This functionality is almost always provided by databases that are used in the primary process. The systems are closely related to parts of the primary process. A typical characteristic of these systems is that their content is continuously updated and resembles the actual state of the production process and the organization. As they are connected to the primary process, we may call these systems primary systems.

2. Control:
   A second level of functionality is based on the primary system. It is the functionality that gives the ability to control the production process. The time scope at this level is the week. You may think of production lists and overviews of good and of fault products per hour per machine. It is tempting to call these systems secondary systems, but that may give the false impression that these systems are separate from the primary systems. That is in general not the case. The functionality is mainly offered by the primary ICT-systems. But it is different from the support of the daily operations, as the level of information is different. Let us give an example – Supporting the production process in a blood establishment implies a database with

the data of donors. These data are among others used to invite a donor to come and donate on a certain day. When the donor arrives, the data are checked and changed when necessary. This is primary support of the daily operations by the database. On an hourly or daily basis the same database produces the number of donations and other statistics. After analyzing these statistics, a manager could decide to increase e.g., the number of employees in the morning. This is support on a different level (control) and so we think of it as another level of functionality.

3. Organization:

Typical both operation and control functionalities are fairly static. Once the wanted support and reports are defined, the system will be unchanged for a relatively long period. This is different with the third level of functionality. In this case the data from the primary systems are collected and stored in a different type of database, often called a data warehouse. This data warehouse contains historic data from the primary process and is extended with data from other sources as appropriate. The data warehouse is used for analysis. From the historical data in the warehouse it is possible to detect weaknesses in the primary process and to find ways for improvements. Typical questions could be: "is the number of fault products evenly spread across the days of the week?" or "what could be the cause of differences in the number of donations per hour?" The time scope is from one month to a year.

4. Strategy:

At the strategy level one thinks about the way the organization has a responsibility to the community to perform a task. This leads to questions in general ("are we doing the right thing") and specific questions ("are we doing the thing right"). Here is where the historical data in the information systems come in. Historical data are mostly put in a so-called data warehouse. It can be thought of as a place where all the data about the performance of the organization is stored, that can be used for analysis. This opens opportunities to answer questions like: "How well/badly did we perform and what were the causes?". This will lead to improvements in e.g., procedures. The time scope at this level is more than a year.

When using ICT systems in an organization, it is necessary to develop systems that provide all four functionalities. Especially quality management needs the first three of them, and for planning purposes, senior staff needs the strategy view and possibilities. Although in principle all four levels should be supported, there will be differences in priorities depending on the organization. In general we can say that the smaller the organization, the more the focus will be on supporting operations. A general indication of the importance of ICT support in the different management levels for different organizations is given in table 2.

Table 2. Organization size and levels of functionality

Organisation size	Operation	Control	Organization	Strategy
Small	+	?	-	-
Medium	+	+	?	-
Big	+	+	+	+

9. Management Information Systems

Throughout the sixty years that computers have been applied in organizations, there has been the notion of Management Information Systems (MIS). That is, all these years the importance of information for the management has been recognized and ICT systems have been used to produce the needed information in time. But at the same time the content of the notion 'information' has developed. So there is a large range of all kinds of information delivered by 'information' systems to the management. To be able to specify the wanted information, a manager should have a clear view on what is possible and what is useful.

The basic notion in the story of management information is the datum (plural: data). In plain English we may call a datum a fact. A fact usually tells something about an object. Most often a fact (or datum) tells us the value that goes with an attribute of an object. For instance, a person (object) may have a length (attribute) of 1.90 meter (value). In principle every fact can be described as an Object-Attribute-Value combination. Data are used to fill databases. Data in databases are mainly used to support the daily operations in the primary processes. So when designing a data base, it is best to focus on the needs for data in the daily operations.

The second notion is the notion of information. Data (or facts) are representations of the state of nature. However, information is more than that. It is the selection of data that a manager needs to make a decision. So not all data are information in a given situation. On the other hand, information consists of data. But raw data are not always applicable as information. Very often the raw data need to be transformed into a form in which a manger can use them. Statistics like a mean, or diagrams are examples of transformed data. Information is widely used. It is used in daily operations and there raw data will suffice. But at a slightly higher level, e.g., at the level of control, organization and strategy of the processes, raw data always must be transformed in one or another way. So in designing an Information System, employees at every level must specify the data that they need as information and the way the information should be presented. Also factors like periodicity (how often does one need the information) are important.

The third notion is knowledge. Knowledge is not something that is found in ICT systems, although the science of Artificial Intelligence developed so-called Knowledge Systems. The Knowledge that is meant here is the insight developed by reflecting on decisions made in the past. To give an example, the management of a blood establishment will periodically evaluate the production of blood components. They will investigate what efforts were made and how much the costs were. Analysis based on these data will develop insight in what decisions lead to optimal results, what decisions did work out less well and which ones were just wrong. This insight is knowledge. Management should develop their knowledge continuously. The data needed to develop knowledge are more than just the production data from the primary processes. In addition to these internal data, developing insight needs also external data. Typical questions to ask are: "*What is the influence of external factors like the weather on the behaviour of donors?*" To answer such question, one needs next to the data about the donors and donations, also data about the weather. These data are collected in huge databases called 'data warehouses'. Analysis on data from data warehouses can be straight forward like in the case mentioned above. But also advanced analysis is possible. That is the domain of Business Intelligence. Business Intelligence is among others, the search for meaningful patterns in data. What correlations can we detect? What causal relations can be induced?

In conclusion, management information comes in many ways. At every level in an organization information is needed. Sometimes it is a simple raw fact, sometimes information is the result of an advanced analysis of a large set of historical data. It is the responsibility of the user of the system to specify the information he or she needs and the knowledge he or she wants to induce from it.

10. Project for the Design and Development of ICT-Systems

In a project for the design and development of an ICT-system, specialists from very different domains work together. This can easily lead to problems as specialists tend not to understand each other. That is why ICT projects are complex and tend to surpass budgets and time limits. In the case of an ICT project it is, more than with other projects, necessary to take care of the project organization and its management and control. To begin with, there are prerequisites that must not be neglected.

1. A clear project organization structure, with a defined Board (one or more persons), a well defined project team, or senior staff, with documented authorities and responsibilities.
2. Documented business processes. Ideally this documentation is maintained according to a good quality documentation system that results in controlled and authorized documents as part of a formal quality system. Special attention should be paid to the documentation of the user requirements.
3. Acceptance of the need for a high percentage of total time for most or all middle and top management for the project. An average ICT project easily lasts 1 to 2 years. During that period care must be taken not to start another major project, as this may change the organization and consequently the requirements for the ICT-system and add to the work load of the middle and top management.
4. The big impact, in man power (time) and also money, has to be accepted by all stakeholders. Commitment is needed from all participants: Ministry of Health, hospitals, Supervising Board, Executive Board, employees. Anyone who is involved.
5. An ICT-system needs continuous monitoring and servicing. At an early point in time of the whole project, the organization of the service delivery should be taken care of. This means that it has to be advised, discussed, decided, started and carefully built. As the service is thought of as something that is needed in the far future, both the senior staff within the blood establishment organization, as well as the stakeholders outside the blood establishment, will tend to minimize the importance of this part of the total project. That is a mistake.
6. Even if it is the first time for the blood establishment organization, there is a need for a strict defined project, with a formal project plan, formal acceptance, formal authorities, et cetera.

11. Planning and Execution of an ICT Project

An ICT project is a project in its own right. As for any project there are general characteristics.

1. A project is a temporary combination of people, equipment and materials, to produce a defined end-product. This end-product is a means to obtain a goal. It should be clearly specified, so that partial projects can be defined and the activities, materials and time needed can be defined.

2. The director of the blood establishment or national blood transfusion service will most probably be the deciding authority, and will order to prepare the project plan, will decide to accept it (or not) and to execute the project. The sponsors are the persons or organizations that provide the money, often outside the blood supply organisation, for instance the Ministry of Health or an international organisation.

3. Figure 6 gives an overview of a project. The figure clearly distinguishes between the whole project and developing the project plan and the execution of it. In fact it includes several phases:
    *   the partial projects to make a project plan
    *   the acceptance (or not) of the plan
    *   the execution of it
    (at the end) the formal acceptance. In the phase to create the project plan, the commitment and ownership of all concerned has to be developed. If middle or top staff will not commit themselves and own the project, sometimes they then have to be given other positions, or even dismissed.

4. A project is a way to regulate a complex set of activities, and will give the participants an idea of what is expected from them. It can be situated between normal routine work and improvising. A project has the advantage of explicitly describing the 5w2h – why, what, who, when, where, and which means are necessary (how and how much). The disadvantage is the relatively large (management and administrative) overhead. A well-defined and documented project complies with high quality standards.

5. The ICT project plan is a proposal to the director, who can decide on it, then accepting the means necessary in *inter alia*: Internal man power, external man power (hired specialists), costs for hardware, work stations, networks, software, and for the service delivery organisation. The project plan, when accepted, has now become a contract. It is the backbone of the project; all documentation should be related to the paragraphs of the project plan.

6. The project plan is also a means of communicating the project to all stake holders, within the organisation and outside of it. The plan will have a separate chapter on communication, as the project absorbs much of the capacity of middle and top management and all employees have expectations, which have to be either fulfilled, or changed by good information. Resistance has to be prevented, and, when present, solved as much as possible. During the execution of the project information may become available that enables improvement of the project. That should be formally handled – a change in the project plan should be proposed, discussed, and decided

upon. This complies with the formal change control and management, an essential part of any quality management system.

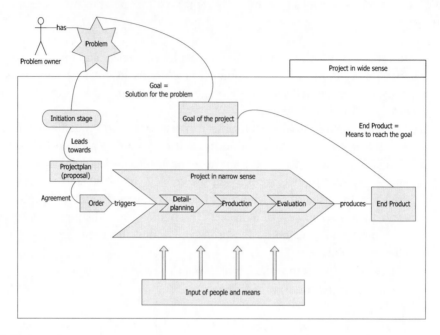

Figure 6. Project scheme.

12. Service Management

Service management is the management of a service to ensure that it meets the critical outcomes the customer values which the blood establishment wants to provide.

When one works with a stand-alone Personal Computer, one knows the frustration when the computer and software do not perform as expected. When a blood establishment or service has a centralised computer system, the expectations should be formalised in a service level agreement (SLA) between each Head of a department and the ICT department.

Incidents in the automated system will occur, but the Head of the ICT department must ensure that service delivery is resumed as quickly as possible, that the problems are dealt with, and that preventive measures are taken.

Service management should be planned, and has to support the strategies, organization, control level and operational goals of the blood establishment. The planning, operation, evaluation, improvement, and changes in the service delivery will be performed according to the Plan – Do – Check – Act principles (Deming).

A set of best practices for service management is the Information Technology Infrastructure Library (ITIL). This library consists of 5 books: service strategy, service design, service transition, service operation and continual service improvement.

Service management is about fulfilling customer expectations. It is essential to know the expectations for now and for the future. Expectations from employees regard their work. All business processes have to be documented, and for each the ICT services needed should be defined. This can imply office software, blood bank information systems, quality management software, statistical packages, etc. All these software applications together are called 'the software'.

The same applies for the hardware. There will be many computers, servers, scanners and automated equipment, that read, store, change and delete data. Software, hardware and data all have to be managed, with the objective that all employees have an optimal support in their work.

Managing a blood bank information system will involve many servers, housed in data centres, possibly in different parts of a country or province. The users (blood establishment employees) will be working in many places, from large laboratories, and several blood component storages to small donor centres, operating only a few days per month. When all users of the information system are housed in one building, and the Information Technology (IT) department is in the same building, often all employees know each other, and can communicate easily, often at the coffee machine area. Then problems can be discussed, and hopefully solved. But at larger centres, or with multiple geographical work places, this is impossible. Then a formal Service Management has to be instituted. One advantage of that is a uniform way of documentation, which can be used in audits, and for security reasons. A starting point then is the Configuration Management Data Base (CMDB), with as its basis the identity data base and the asset management data base: people and machines, including communications and software. The service desk is the primary contact for all questions involving information systems and its functioning, with the objective of solving problems as quickly as possible, and to get the information system functioning again. When incidents/problems are related to other parts of the service management, the service desk will maintain the communication with the clients, the employees in the blood establishment. Those other parts of service management can be Configuration and Change Management, Desktop and Service Management, System Management, Software Support, Network Management, Data Base Management and IT Security.

The International Society of Blood Transfusion has adopted Guidelines for Information Security in Transfusion Medicine. [6]

For each of these parts, personnel is needed, and especially in large blood establishments and national blood transfusion services, the director and management team will not easily fund a new and expensive IT organisation. It is nevertheless very important to have a good IT staff to minimise risks of service failure. The expectations of the customer have to be satisfied, and Key Performance Indicators (KPIs) have to be agreed on as part of the Service Level Agreements (SLAs) with the departments of the blood establishment. The KPI are the results of careful assessment of the services and are part of the monitoring and evaluation – the Check and Act of the Deming cycle Plan – Do – Check – Act.

13. Validation and Acceptation

The main Blood Bank Information System is one of the critical tools in the organisation and blood procurement operation of the blood establishment activities – donor management, donations, component preparation, laboratory, release of components, stock and delivery. It is the blood establishment's responsibility to prove that the programme that is selected, introduced, documented, tested and brought into operation will perform according to pre-set criteria and will fulfil the defined requirements.

It has to comply with the rules of cGMP (Good Manufacturing Practices), European Union requirements, FDA regulations or other, national regulations.

The start of introducing an information system is always documenting what the system should do – the User Requirements Specifications (URS). This is the responsibility of each of the Heads of the different Main Business Processes, together with the IT department or project staff. It is a list of all functions that the programme will have to support.

As validation is last major activity before allowing the programme to be implemented in routine operation, this will have to be done some time after the writing of the URS (1 – 2 year). The URS will have to be a controlled document, that is continuously kept up to date. This requires much effort of all concerned.

The ISBT has published the 'ISBT Guidelines for Validation of Automated Systems in Blood Establishments' [7], in which the objectives of validation are described as follows: to demonstrate control, to ensure compliance, to generate knowledge and to establish future requirements e.g., training, maintenance and calibration.

In these guidelines, all aspects of introducing, testing and validating a blood establishment information system are discussed. The total costs of such a project are major, not only in money, but certainly also in man power, and especially configuring the programme, writing the test cases and evaluating the results of the tests will all burden the senior staff for at least 1 to 2 years. In those years, no other major projects can be undertaken.

Conclusion

ICT is a support to employees in their tasks and responsibilities. It will often start in one or more departments separately, but then it will never be possible to develop one organization wide ICT system, that will comply with the needed quality requirements (cGMP). To develop an ICT system at GMP level will always involve buying the right of use of an off-the-shelf programme. Introducing such a programme can best be done in a formal project, which needs the support (and time and energy) of each member of the senior and middle management staff. The logistic model and the static structure model need to be developed, discussed, and accepted. Parallel to the development of the information system to support the primary process, all other information requirements should also be defined and the system to deliver these services to the employees organized: service delivery. The quality of the entire ICT system should be demonstrated before starting to use it in routine production by proving that it conforms to the User Requirements Specifications, which should be a controlled document, with formal change control and management. This is called validation.

References

[1]   Deming WE. *The New Economics For Industry, Government & Education.* Cambridge: Massachusetts Institute of Technology Center for Advanced Engineering Study, 1993, pp. 134 – 136

[2] Chaffey D and White G. *Business Information Management: improving performance using Information Systems,* Prentice Hall, Hemel Hempstead, UK, 2011, ISBN 0-273-71179-2

[3] Chaffey D and Wood S. *Business Information Management: Improving Performance using Information Systems*, Pearson, Pearson, Upper Saddle River, NJ, USA. ISBN 9780273686552

[4] EudraLex - The Rules Governing Medicinal Products in the European Union, 2010 Vol. 4. Good Manufacturing Practice (GMP) for Medicinal Products for Human and Veterinary Use, To be accessed through *http://ec.europa.eu/health/documents/eudralex /vol-4/index_en.htm*

[5] Morgan G. *Images of Organization*, 1986 Sage Publications, London, UK

[6] ISBT Guide for Information Security in Transfusion Medicine, *Vox Sang*, 2006;91 (Suppl. 1).

[7] ISBT Guidelines for Validation of Automated Systems in Blood Establishments, *Vox Sang*, 2010;98 (Suppl. 1).

In: Quality Management in Transfusion Medicine
Editor: Cees Th. Smit Sibinga

ISBN: 978-1-62618-665-1
© 2013 Nova Science Publishers, Inc.

Chapter VI

Haemovigilance: Big Brother or Kindly Light?

Lorna M. Williamson[*1] *and D. Michael Strong*[†2]
[1]NHS Blood and Transplant, England, UK
[2]Department of Orthopaedics and Sports Medicine,
University of Washington School of Medicine, Seattle, WA, US

Abstract

Total quality management in blood collection and transfusion requires monitoring risks from 'vein-to-vein' i.e. from blood collector and manufacturer to transfusion at the bedside and back. Haemovigilance is a set of surveillance procedures covering the entire transfusion chain from the donation of blood and its components to the follow-up of recipients of transfusions. Haemovigilance was initiated in Japan in 1993 and by France in 1994 and has been adopted since in countries throughout the world. Some of these systems reside within and are mandated by a national ministry of health, while others are primarily organized through professional societies or the country's blood collection system. The main objective should be sharing of data to all concerned. .

A good haemovigilance system should include data collection (including both numerators and denominators), analysis by experts, production of recommendations to improve practice, communication back to the front line, and education. Clear definitions are essential, and it is critical that experts examine each reported case carefully. Well-established systems, such as SHOT in the UK, have demonstrated, in various ways, how haemovigilance data can improve outcomes for patients. A good example is the reduction in Transfusion Related Acute Lung Injury (TRALI) due to implementation of male only plasma. The ability to monitor outcomes of interventions, such as this, is critical in improving safety. Likewise, donor systems can assist in reducing errors and accidents in the donation process. Haemovigilance should be an integral part of the system wherever

* Lorna M Williamson, MD, Medical and Research Director, NHS Blood and Transplant, Oak House, Reeds CrescentWatford WD24 4QN, England, UK, Tel: +44-7711 447117 (8) 7117, email: lorna.williamson@nhsbt.nhs.uk
† D. Michael Strong, PhD, MT(ASCP), BCLD, Department of Orthopaedics and Sports Medicine, University of Washington School of Medicine, Seattle, WA, US, Tel: +1-206-683-9045, E-mail: dmichaelstrong@mac.com

transfusion medicine is practised, and should also be expanded to include biovigilance for other substances of human origin such as cells, tissues and organs.

Keywords: Haemovigilance, Adverse event reporting, Errors

1. Introduction

Improving quality is a never-ending goal and putting new quality systems in place is not easy because providers, professional societies and even governments may tend to be resistant to change and mistrust of new systems is a major hurdle. Advancement of quality in transfusion medicine faces unique challenges from country to country stemming from cultural differences, government structures and resource availability and health issues that have different priorities for different countries. Improving quality systems has become more and more of an international effort in transfusion medicine due to many factors including increased communications, transport of blood components across national boundaries in wartime, recognition of differences in terminology, labeling and emerging infectious disease agents requiring more intense surveillance efforts.

Total quality management in blood collection and transfusion requires monitoring risks from 'vein-to-vein' and from blood collector and processor to transfusion at the bedside and back. Although risk is inherent in substances of human origin (SOHO), one key to reducing risk is to actively investigate adverse events and reactions and learn from these experiences. In most cases, this requires the development of a culture of quality and multidisciplinary participation in reporting and problem solving. It also depends on creating a culture where reporting is encouraged and praised, and where staff are not afraid to report errors in case they are disciplined or lose their job. Much of transfusion risk reduction has focused on infectious disease transmissions resulting in establishment of haemovigilance reporting systems. These systems have been established around the world and have made major contributions to improvements in safety, not only in reducing infectious disease risks, but also in identifying and reducing non-infectious disease risks such as mis-identifying the patient and so transfusing blood intended for someone else.

2. History of Haemovigilance

Haemovigilance was initiated in Japan in 1993 and by France in 1994 and has been adopted since in countries throughout the world. These efforts eventually have resulted in the establishment of the European Haemovigilance Network (EHN), partially in response to the European Blood Directive 2002/98/EC. [1] The definition of haemovigilance has been established by the EHN as follows:

> Haemovigilance is a set of surveillance procedures covering the entire transfusion chain (from the donation of blood and its components to the follow-up of recipients of transfusions), intended to collect and assess information on unexpected or undesirable effects resulting from the therapeutic use of labile blood products, and to prevent the occurrence or recurrence of such incidents. [2]

Haemovigilance systems grew out of a series of events that led to questions regarding the safety of the blood supply. The Acquired Immunodeficiency Disease syndrome (AIDS) epidemic led to many HIV transmissions from blood transfusion in a number of countries in the 1980's. This led to public debates, commissions of inquiry, prosecutions and convictions stemming from how the issue had been handled. It also provided additional stimulus to assess the safety of transfusion services through ongoing risk assessment measures. In 1993, a French law was enacted, establishing the first hemovigilance system under the auspices of the Health Products Safety Agency (HPSA) as a national system of surveillance and alert, from blood collection to the follow-up of the recipients, gathering and analyzing all adverse events of blood transfusion in order to prevent their recurrences. [3, 4]

Another early system was established in 1996 in the United Kingdom through the efforts of transfusion medicine professionals as a voluntary reporting system focused on Serious Hazards of Transfusion (SHOT). This programme is headquartered at the National Health Service Blood and Transplant's Manchester Blood Centre, but is separate from it and covers the whole of the UK. SHOT began as a voluntary system affiliated to the Royal College of Pathologists, and without any requirement to report to the UK regulator for blood, the Medicines and Healthcare Regulatory Agency (MHRA). With the transposition of the EU Blood Directive into UK law as the Blood Safety and Quality Regulations in 2005, MHRA established its own reporting system, SABRE. A joint group between SHOT and SABRE created a single on line portal for reporters, to avoid the need for duplicate reporting. The types of incidents, which are required to be reported to SHOT and SABRE, overlap but are not identical. Such hybrid reporting can run the risk of '2 sets of numbers' in circulation, and is not recommended as an optimal way to establish a national haemovigilance system. Further work is therefore ongoing between SHOT and MHRA to generate a joint data repository, and the SHOT annual report for 2011 contained for the first time a chapter with analysis of incidents reported to the MHRA.

Participation in SHOT improved from 69% in 2001 to over 90% of UK hospitals in current years. [5, 6] In a parallel initiative, the UK Departments of Health established the Better Blood Transfusion seminars and Health Care Circulars to health care staff. This work included the establishment of hospital regional and national transfusion committees and development of protocols for the process of transfusion and participation in SHOT. The UK has trained a cadre of nurses and laboratory scientists as specialized practitioners of transfusion, based in hospitals who generally take the lead in reporting haemovigilance events.

Subsequently, systems have been created and implemented in most developed nations as a hybrid of these approaches. Some of these reside within and derive reporting mandates from a national ministry of health [7, 8] while others are primarily organized through professional societies or the country's blood collection system with sharing of data to all concerned parties. [1, 9-11] The European Community currently requires implementation of a haemovigilance system in each member state with reporting to a central office. [12, 13] Although each country's system has characteristics unique for its own healthcare and transfusion systems, they bear multiple similarities and have yielded similar results. The differences from country to country have been recently reviewed. [14]

3. Current Approaches
(France, Canada, USA, Australia)

In 2006 a French law was enacted which states that any individual who observes an adverse event relate to blood collection or transfusion (including inappropriate transfusions without any observed effect) must immediately notify health care safety agencies. Imputability scores are assigned to indicate the likelihood of an adverse event being associated with a particular blood component. Their focus is on more serious transfusion events such as bacterial transmitted infections, transfusion related acute lung injury (TRALI) and ABO blood type incompatibility. Cooperative working groups are used to analyze data and assistant in solving problems that are identified. An example is the reduction in the incidence of transfusion associated bacterial infections and improving the selection of blood donors. [15]

In Canada, all blood products are regulated by Health Canada through its Biologics and Genetic Therapies Directorate. Distribution is managed through two separate agencies, HemaQuebec and Canadian Blood Services; the provincial and territorial governments of Canada fund both. Under Canadian law, the only reportable events are deaths occurring within 24 hours after transfusion and serious events that take place withing15 days. However, a voluntary national surveillance system known as Transfusion Transmitted Injuries Surveillance System (TTISS), overseen by the Public Health Agency of Canada (PHAC), collects all adverse events. The Blood Safety Surveillance and Health Care Acquired Infections Division of PHAC manages TTISS. This effort was established in response to the Report of the Commission of Inquiry in Canada (1993-1197), once again in response to infectious disease transmissions. TTISS was piloted in 1999 in four provinces and has since been expanded to all of Canada. Hospitals report through provincial and territorial blood coordinating offices either electronically or in written form. This information is then forwarded. Adverse events are graded for both severity and imputability. Since reporting to TTISS is different from mandatory reporting of deaths and severe reactions to the Blood Agencies, reports have to be reconciled.

Within Canada, Quebec is a model for provincial activity. The Quebec haemovigilance system is modeled on the French system using similar data elements and case definitions, grading of severity and determination of likelihood of association with transfusion for adverse events. There are also transfusion safety officers in each of the hospitals responsible for reporting. In addition to adverse events, the system also monitors transfusion incidents without adverse consequences such as 'incorrect blood component transfused' (IBCT) and near-miss events. Accurate rate estimates are possible through the collection of denominator data on the number of blood products transfused. [8]

In the United States, haemovigilance efforts have been more recent. [16] In a cooperative effort between the public and private sectors, efforts to establish haemovigilance were expanded to the broader term of 'Biovigilance' to incorporate cells, tissues and organs. Under the auspices of a U.S. Biovigilance Task Force managed by the American Association of Blood Banks (AABB), modules were identified that included haemovigilance for recipients and donors. [17] The AABB Biovigilance Task Force recommended a public-private partnership using CDC's National Healthcare Safety Network (NHSN) as the surveillance system that could most closely meet the data requirements for a national surveillance system for blood transfusion adverse reaction and event tracking. The NHSN is a secure, Internet-based surveillance system, which collects data from participating healthcare facilities in the U.S. to estimate the adherence to practices known to be associated with prevention of healthcare-associated infections and the magnitude of adverse events among patients. A primary purpose of this voluntary and confidential system is to assist participating facilities in developing surveillance and analysis methods that permit timely recognition of patient safety problems and prompt intervention with appropriate measures. The system encourages reporting adverse events for data collection and quality improvement purposes, and dose not impose penalties against facilities for reporting adverse events.

AABB, with collaboration from the Department of Health and Human Services (DHHS), conducts nationwide surveys to assess the amount of blood collected and transfused in the U.S. (NBCUS). The facilities surveyed include all non-hospital-based blood collection centers, a statistically representative sample of hospitals from the American Hospital Association database and a similar sampling of cord blood banks. In addition to blood collection and utilization data, some data on adverse events, defined as numbers of events that require diagnostic or therapeutic intervention, are also collected.

Blood collection centers operate their own reporting systems. [18] ABC, through its alliance of independent blood centers, conducts a variety of surveys among its members on a periodic basis and share outcomes and best practices through online reports to its participating members who participate. Some members of ABC are also transfusion services that collect and monitor adverse reactions in a similar fashion as hospital based transfusion services. [21] These activities however are for internal use and quality control and are, in general, not shared publicly. Individual blood centers also collect reports of adverse events and report these Biologic Deviations to FDA as required through regulation. Donor fatalities must be reported to FDA (21CFR606.170 (b)) within seven days after a thorough investigation (21CFR606.170 (a)). Aspects of this process are clarified in Guidance for Industry. Regulatory oversight of donors includes determination of donor eligibility and extends to protections of donor health and safety.

The 35 ARC regional blood centers actively solicit reports of infectious and noninfectious complications in recipients of blood components. In the ARC, when reactions are reported, investigations are carried out to determine the likelihood that such reactions are caused by the transfusion. Regional medical directors direct investigations and probability scores are assigned. Outcomes are compiled and entered into the Donor and Recipient Complications Program (DCRP) database. This provides the ability to track and analyze trends in complications at each region and across the ARC system to provide opportunities for process improvement. Specific outcomes are also published periodically through peer-reviewed journals. [19]

The U.S. Donor Haemovigilance System was conceived to collect and analyze data on donor reactions to improve the outcomes for blood donors. [17] The Donor System development was funded by grants from the US Department of Health and Human Services (HHS) and the Department of Defense. This effort is still in development with trial centers participating. Expert representatives from these participating centers, are designing and implementing routine and focused analyses of the donor reaction data, and will oversee analyses of data from the system. The group will consider and select interventions to improve outcomes and will design systems to monitor the success or failure of the interventions.

In conclusion, there are a number of different models of organisation which can all work. The next section discusses the properties of a good haemovigilance system.

4. What Should a Haemovigilance System Include?

A good haemovigilance system should include data collection (including both numerators and denominators), analysis by experts, production of recommendations to improve practice, communication back to the front line, and education. Good denominator data is essential, and should include as a minimum on an annual basis:

- Number of donations collected (whole blood and aphaeresis procedures)
- Number of donors attending in the year
- Number of units issued of red cells, platelets and FFP/cryoprecipitate

Analysed data should be available on the following, in ways that permit analysis of trends over time, and which allow the impact of any preventative measures to be clearly identified:

- Rates of positive tests for virus markers in blood and platelet donors, and the risk factors if these can be obtained through donor counseling
- Rates of recognised complications of donation: faints, bruises, re-bleeds.
- Rates of serious complications of donation: admission to hospital e.g., with chest pain, delayed faints leading to injury, nerve damage and other injury at the vene-puncture site.
- Rates of serious outcomes in patients, discussed further below

Rates of errors and incidents, which although no harm resulted, had the potential to cause serious harm.

5. Serious Outcomes in Patients

The following types of incident have been included in SHOT and most other haemovigilance systems from the outset:

1. Receiving blood either intended for another patient or which does not meet the patient's special requirements, categorised together as 'wrong blood to patient'. Further classification of such errors can demonstrate whether they occurred on the ward or in the laboratory, and whether problems with IT systems contributed.
2. Transfusion-transmitted infection: viruses, bacteria, prions, protozoa e.g., malaria.
3. Acute reactions: haemolytic, allergic or anaphylactic.
4. Haemolytic events
5. Transfusion-related acute lung injury (TRALI)

6. Transfusion-associated graft-versus-host disease (TA-GvHD).

Other categories have since been added:

- Near miss events, where errors have been detected in time to avoid a mis-transfusion
- Cases where the transfusion was clearly inappropriate e.g., based on a haemoglobin result from a sample upstream of an intravenous infusion of clear fluid
- Handling errors eg using platelets which have been put in the refrigerator
- Complications of autologous transfusion and cell salvage.
- Transfusion-associated circulatory overload.

Table 1. Table of definitions used in the SHOT 2011 report

CATEGORY	DEFINITION
Incorrect blood component transfused	An episode where a patient was transfused with a blood component that was intended for another patient or which was of inappropriate specification and did not meet the particular requirements of the patient e.g. phenotyped, CMV negative, or irradiated.
Inappropriate, Unnecessary or Under/Delayed Transfusion	Transfusions given on the basis of erroneous, spurious or incorrectly documented laboratory testing results for haemoglobin, platelets and coagulation tests. Transfusions given as a result of poor understanding and knowledge of transfusion medicine, such that the decision to transfuse either puts the patient at significant risk, or was actually harmful. Under-transfusion or delayed transfusion resulting in morbidity.
Handling and Storage Errors	An episode in which a patient was transfused with a blood component or plasma product intended for the him/herself, but in which, during the transfusion process, the handling and storage may have rendered the component less safe for transfusion.
Adverse Events Relating to Anti-D Immunoglobulin	An adverse event relating to anti-D Ig is one where the prescription, administration or omission of anti-D Ig has the potential to cause harm to the mother or fetus immediately or in the future.
Acute transfusion reactions	Acute transfusion reactions are defined as those occurring at any time up to 24 hours following a transfusion of blood or components excluding cases of acute reactions due to incorrect component being transfused, haemolytic reactions, transfusion related acute lung injury (TRALI), TACO, TAD or those due to bacterial contamination of the component.
Haemolytic Transfusion Reactions (HTR) and Alloimmunisation	Haemolytic transfusion reactions are split into two categories: acute and delayed. Acute reactions are defined as fever and other symptoms/signs of haemolysis within 24 hours of transfusion, confirmed by one or more of: a fall in Hb, rise in lactate dehydrogenase (LDH), positive direct antiglobulin test (DAT) and positive crossmatch. Delayed reactions are defined as fever and other symptoms/signs of haemolysis more than 24 hours after transfusion; confirmed by one or more of: a fall in Hb or failure of increment, rise in bilirubin, positive DAT and positive crossmatch which was not detectable pre-transfusion. Alloimmunisation (reporting to SHOT is optional) is defined as demonstration of clinically significant antibodies post transfusion which were previously absent (as far as is known) and when there are no clinical or laboratory signs of haemolysis.
Transfusion-Related Acute Lung Injury	Transfusion-related acute lung injury (TRALI) is defined as acute dyspnoea with hypoxia and bilateral pulmonary infiltrates during or within 6 hours of transfusion, not due to circulatory overload or other likely causes.
Transfusion-Associated Circulatory Overload	TACO includes any 4 of the following that occur within 6 hours of transfusion: Acute respiratory distress Tachycardia Increased blood pressure Acute or worsening pulmonary oedema Evidence of positive fluid balance
Transfusion-associated dyspnoea	TAD is characterised by respiratory distress within 24 hours of transfusion that does not meet the criteria of TRALI, TACO or allergic reaction. Respiratory distress should not be explained by the patient's underlying condition or any other known cause. This will allow haemovigilance systems to classify all reported pulmonary reactions without the need for exceptions or inappropriate assignment.

Table 1. (Continued)

CATEGORY	DEFINITION
Post-Transfusion Purpura	Post-transfusion purpura is defined as thrombocytopenia arising 5-12 days following transfusion of red cells associated with the presence in the patient of antibodies directed against the HPA (human platelet antigen) systems.
Transfusion-Associated Graft-Versus-Host Disease	Transfusion-associated graft-versus-host disease is a generally fatal immunological complication of transfusion practice, involving the engraftment and clonal expansion of viable donor lymphocytes, contained in blood components in a susceptible host. TA-GvHD is characterised by fever, rash, liver dysfunction, diarrhoea, pancytopenia and bone marrow hypoplasia occurring less than 30 days following transfusion. The diagnosis is usually supported by skin/bone marrow biopsy appearance and / or the identification of donor-derived cells, chromosomes or deoxyribonucleic acid (DNA) in the patient's blood and /or affected tissues.
Transfusion-Transmitted Infection	A report was classified as a transfusion-transmitted infection if, following investigation: the recipient had evidence of infection following transfusion with blood components and there was no evidence of infection prior to transfusion and no evidence of an alternative source of infection; *and, either:* at least one component received by the infected recipient was donated by a donor who had evidence of the same transmissible infection *or:* at least one component received by the infected recipient was shown to contain the agent of infection
Cell salvage and autologous transfusion	Any adverse event or reaction associated with autologous transfusion including intraoperative and postoperative cell salvage (washed or unwashed), acute normovolaemic haemodilution or pre-operative autologous donation.

Clear definitions are essential, and it is critical that each case is examined carefully by experts to answer the following:

1. Does it meet the definition for the category? How severe was the outcome? SHOT uses the following categories: death, serious morbidity (e.g., admission to Intensive Care, acquiring an infectious agent), minor morbidity (e.g., fever, skin rash) and 'no harm'. The definitions used in the SHOT report of 2011 are shown in Table 1.

2. How certain is it that the transfusion was the cause of the clinical features – this is termed imputability. It can be difficult, in a very sick patient, to sort out the cause of common features like fever and breathlessness. Different haemovigilance schemes use different classifications eg highly likely/probable/possible/unlikely.

Data can also be analysed according to age, and SHOT has found it useful to publish a paediatric chapter followed up by a manuscript in a paediatric journal. A similar analysis is now done for patients with haemoglobinopathies.

It is controversial whether a haemovigilance reporting system can really capture good data on appropriate use of transfusions. This is an important consideration as part of good clinical practice, but most countries have regarded this as a separate activity from haemovigilance. Clinical audit against national guidelines can be used. This topic is not discussed further in this chapter.

6. Outcomes and Contributions to Quality of Performance and Management Improvement

The data emerging from SHOT over the years now demonstrates the characteristics of an optimal haemovigilance system ie an increase in the number of reports overall, but a reduction in serious events (Figure 1). The SHOT scheme has made many recommendations to improve the safety of transfusion, including that further research should be carried out into information technology solutions for safer transfusion, and into new strategies for reducing bacterial contamination and transfusion-related acute lung injury (TRALI). [20] Recognition of the magnitude of the problem posed by TRALI and the high frequency of association of TRALI cases with the plasma of female donors, prompted the UK's Blood Services to reduce the number of plasma (and platelet) donations from female donors, with a subsequent marked reduction in the number of deaths attributable to TRALI. [21] This also led to an international acceptance of this approach as a new standard in reducing the risk of TRALI. [22, 23]

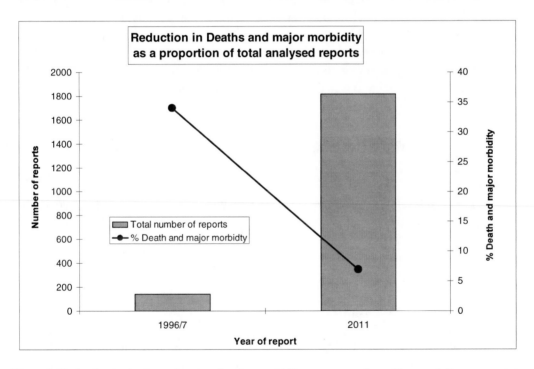

Figure 1. Reduction in deaths and cases of major morbidity as a proportion of haemovigilance reports to UK serious hazards of transfusion between 1996 and 2011.

Furthermore SHOT reported that the most frequently occurring adverse event, accounting for 1832/2628 (70%) of incidents reported, is IBCT in which the patient received a blood component that did not meet the correct specification or that was intended for another patient. [24] This has also led to the incidence of ABO incompatible transfusions showing a downward trend, suggesting the emergence of a safety culture in the UK. Achievement of this depended on a number of different agencies working together. Professional groups leading the work of laboratory scientists highlighted ABO typing errors as an issue, and made recommendations to reduce them. [25] A similar focus on laboratory errors highlighted mistakes in providing CMV negative or irradiated components to those who need them.

It was recognised, however, that most ABO errors arise at the bedside, either when the blood sample for grouping is taken, or when the blood is transfused. Mistakes in blood sampling were not previously recognised as being a main source of error. However, the practice of pre-labelling tubes before filling them with blood means that blood from Patient A might be added to a tube labelled with Patient B's details. If patient B has not been grouped before, there is no way that the error will be detected, and incompatible blood will be provided. Errors of identification also occur when blood is removed from the hospital refrigerator, when the wrong blood may be collected. The bedside check should pick this up, but checking units of blood against accompanying paperwork, but away from the patient, was a common finding. Unless the blood is checked against the patient's wristband, there is potential for hanging the wrong unit. Formally asking the patient to give their name and date of birth is best practice, but many patients will be too ill or confused to comply.

In addition to benefits to patients resulting from haemovigilance system reporting, data collection on donor reactions and interventions can also provide valuable quality improvements. A recent example of data assisted intervention actions used the analysis of the time course of syncope reactions among 500,000 whole blood donors to show three distinct periods of risk for vasovagal reactions before, during and after phlebotomy. [18] From this data, they described interventions that have been useful in controlling these reactions.

7. Communication of Haemovigilance Data and Recommendations

One criticism levelled at regulator-led systems is that the production of data and a report to achieve compliance with regulation is seen as an end in itself. In contrast, professionally led systems have as a key aim production of recommendations to improve transfusion practice, and communication of these recommendations back to the transfusion community. Formulation of recommendations requires careful analysis of several years worth of data, in the knowledge that haemovigilance data cannot claim to have the robustness of prospective clinical trials. In addition, such recommendations need to be clearly targeted towards a lead group for implementation, and practical enough to have the buy in of those who have to implement them. At the same time, they have to have sufficient independence to have credibility.

Haemovigilance systems should therefore put effort into a communications plan, to include an annual launch of the latest findings, widespread dissemination on line and in summarised paper form, and have the resource to undertake educational events throughout the year, ideally across the country.

Finally, a recent Consensus Conference addressing risk-based decision-making for blood safety, addressed the question of necessary next steps to agree upon and implementation of such a process. One of their recommendations included:

"Investment in assessment, evaluation and monitoring, such as an expanded system of haemovigilance. In order to monitor potential risks associated with blood transfusion in a proactive manner, active prospective biovigilance/haemovigilance systems should be established, as are being developed for pharmacovigilance. An effective haemovigilance system should be focused on improving recipient outcomes. An active system of haemovigilance will be of great value in documenting who receives blood, why they are prescribed and how this affects their clinical outcome". [26]

Conclusion

The overarching aim of haemovigilance reporting is to improve safety for donors and transfusion recipients. The data should be used:

- To identify trends in adverse events and reactions in donors and patients
- As an early warning system for new hazards eg infections, or for unexpected side effects of new components such as pathogen inactivated platelets
- To inform policy at national/blood service level
- To improve practice in target areas
  - o By production of clinical guidelines
  - o By education to raise awareness of transfusion hazards and their prevention
  - o By detailed audit and research.

8.1. Message to Take Home

Collection and analysis of high quality information regarding transfusion events and errors is a powerful tool in achieving and maintaining quality in transfusion medicine.

References

[1]   Faber J-C. Work Of The European Haemovigilance Network (Ehn). *Transfus Clin Biol* 2004; 11:2-10.

[2]   Faber J-C. Worldwide Overview Of Existing Haemovigilance Systems. *Transf Apher Sci* 2004;31:99-110.

[3]   Andreu G, Morel P, Forestier F, Et Al.. Hemovigilance Network In France: Organization And Analysis Of Immediate Transfusion Incident Reports From 1994 To 1998. *Transfusion,* 2002;42:1356-1364.

[4]   Rebibo D, Hauser D, Slimani. A, Herve P, Andreu G. The French Haemovigilance System: Organization And Results For 2003. *Transfus Apher Sci,* 2004;31:145-153.

[5]   Murphy Mf, Edbury C, Wickenden C, Survey Of The Implementation Of The Recommendations In The Health Services Circular 1998/224 'Better Blood Transfusion'. *Transfus Med,* 2003;13:121-125.

[6]   Stainsby D, Williamson L, Jones H, Cohen H.. 6 Years Of Shot Reporting--Its Influence On Uk Blood Safety. *Transfus Apher Sci,* 2004;31:123-131.

[7] Michlig C, Vu Dh, Wasserfallen Jb, Spahn Dr, Schneider P, Tissot D. Three Years Of Haemovigilance In A General University Hospital. *Transfus Med,* 2003;13:63-72.

[8] Robillard P, Nawej Ki, Jochem K. The Quebec Hemovigilance System: Description And Results From The First Two Years. *Transfus Apher Sci,* 2004;31:111-122.

[9] Engelfriet Cp, Reesink Hw, Brand B, Levy G, Williamson Lm, Menitove Je, Heier He, Jorgensen J, Politis C, Seyfriend H, Smit Sibinga Cth, Faber Jc, Vesga Ma, Selivanov E, Danilova T, Tadokoro K, Krusius T, Hafnerv, Snopek I, Realig, D'amelmeida Goncalves J. Haemovigilance Systems. *Vox Sang,* 1999;**77**:110-120.

[10] Beckers Ea, Dinkelaar Rb, Te Boekhorst Pa, Van Ingen He, Van Rhenen Dj. Reports Of Transfusion Incidents: Experiences From The First Year Of Hemovigilance In The Region Of The Former Zwn (South West Netherlands) Blood Bank In Rotterdam. *Ned Tijdschr Geneeskd,* 2003;147:1508-1512.

[11] Espinosa A, Steinsvag Ct, Flesland O. Hemovigilance In Norway. *Transfus Apher Sci,* 2005;32**:**17-19.

[12] Faber J-C. Haemovigilance Procedure In Transfusion Medicine. *Hematology J,* 2004;5 (Suppl 3):S74-82.

[13] Faber J-C. The European Blood Directive: A New Era Of Blood Regulation Has Begun. *Transfus Med,* 2004;14:257-273.

[14] Wiersum-Osselton Jc. Schipperus Mr. Response To The International Forum On Haemovigilance. *Vox Sang,* 2006;91:278-279.

[15] Carlier M, V̇o Mai Mp, Fauveau L, Ounnoughene N, Sandid I, Renaudier, P. Seventeen Years Of Haemovigilance In France: Assessment And Outlook. *Transfus Clin Biol,* 2011;18:140-150.

[16] Aubuchon Jp, Whitaker Bi. America Finds Hemovigilance! *Transfusion,* 2007; 47: 1937-1942.

[17] Strong Dm, Aubuchon J, Whitaker Bm, Kuehnert M. Biovigilance Initiatives. *Isbt Sci Ser,* 2008;3:77-84.

[18] Wiltbank Tb, Giordano Gf, Kamel H, Tomasulo P, Custer B. Faint And Prefaint Reactions In Whole-Blood Donors: An Analysis Of Predonation Measurements And Their Predictive Value. *Transfusion,* 2008;48:1799-1808.

[19] Eder Af, Kennedy Jm, Dy Ba, Notari Ep, Weiss Jw, Fang, Ct, Wagner S, Dodd Ry Benjamin Rj. Bacterial Screening Of Apheresis Platelets And The Residual Risk Of Septic Transfusion Reactions: The American Red Cross Experience (2004-2006). *Transfusion,* 2007;47:1134-1142.

[20] Murphy Mf. Surveillance Of Transfusion Errors: Putting Data To Use In The U.K. *Dev Biol (Basel),* 2005;120:179-187.

[21] Chapman Ce, Stainsby D, Jones H, Love E, Massey E, Win N, Navarrete C, Lucas G, Soni N, Morgan C, Choo L, Cohen H, Williamson Lm. Ten Years Of Hemovigilance Reports Of Transfusion-Related Acute Lung Injury In The United Kingdom And The Impact Of Preferential Use Of Male Donor Plasma. *Transfusion,* 2009;49:440-452.

[22] Wendel S, Biagini S, Trigo F, Fonatao-Wendel R, Taaning E, Jorgensen J, Rilsom K, Krusius T, Koskinen S, Kretschmer V, Karger R, Lawlor E, Okazaki H, Cjarlewood R, Brand A, Solheim Bg, Fiesland O Letowska M, Zupanska B, Muniz-Diaz E, Nogues N, Senn M, Mansouri-Taleghani B, Chaman Ce, Massey,E, Navarrete,C, Stainsby D, Win D, Williamson Lm, Kleinman S, Kopko,Pm, Silva M, Shulman I, Holness L, Epstein Js. Measures To Prevent Trali. *Vox Sang,* 2007;92:258-277.

[23] Funk Mb, Guenay S, Lohmann A, Henseler O, Heiden M, Hanschmann, Km, Keller-Stanislawsik B. Benefit Of Transfusion-Related Acute Lung Injury Risk-Minimization Measures - German Haemovigilance Data (2006-2010). *Vox Sang* 2012;102:317-323

[24] Stainsby D. Abo Incompatible Transfusions--Experience From The Uk Serious Hazards Of Transfusion (Shot) Scheme Transfusions Abo Incompatible. *Transfus Clin Biol,* 2005;12:385-388.

[25] Milkins C. Performance And Practice In Uk Hospital Transfusion Laboratories. *Transfus Apher Sci,* 2007;36:129-131.

[26] Stein J, Besley J, Besley J, Brook C, Hamill M, Klein E, Krewski D, Murphy G, Richardson M, Sirna J, Skinner M, Steiner R, Vanaken P, Devine D. Risk-Based Decision-Making For Blood Safety: Preliminary Report Of A Consensus Conference. *Vox Sang,* 2011;101:277-281.

In: Quality Management in Transfusion Medicine
Editor: Cees Th. Smit Sibinga

ISBN: 978-1-62618-665-1
© 2013 Nova Science Publishers, Inc.

Chapter VII

Event Management: A Total Organization Commitment to Quality and Safety and the Tools and Techniques Available to Achieve This Goal

James R. Stubbs[*1], *Gwen D. Jones*[†2],
Cheryl A. Nimtz[‡1] *and Valerie W. Halling*[§3]

[1]Division of Transfusion Medicine, Department of
Laboratory Medicine and Pathology, Mayo Clinic, Rochester, MN, US
[2]Department of Process Improvement,
Institute of Transfusion Medicine, Rosemont, IL, US
[3]Operational Support Unit, Division of Transfusion Medicine,
Department of Laboratory Medicine and Pathology, Mayo Clinic,
Rochester, MN, US

Abstract

A commitment to safety is a fundamental aspect of a quality culture. In such a culture, employees practice safe behaviours to protect patients every day. Event

* James R. Stubbs, MD, Chair, Division of Transfusion Medicine, Department of Laboratory Medicine and Pathology, Mayo Clinic, 200 First St. SW, Rochester, MN 55905 US, Tel: +1-507-266-4821 Fax: +1-507-284-1399, Stubbs.james@mayo.edu,

† Gwen D. Jones, Department of Process Improvement, Institute of Transfusion Medicine, 5505 Pearl Street, Rosemont, IL 60025 US, Tel: +1-847-736-2163, gjones@itxm.org

‡ Cheryl A. Nimtz, Laboratory Operations Manager, Division of Transfusion Medicine, Department of Laboratory Medicine and Pathology, Mayo Clinic, 200 First St. SW, Rochester, MN 55905 US, Tel: +1-507-266-2580 Fax: +1-507-284-1399, Nimtz.cheryl@mayo.edu

§ Valerie W. Halling, Supervisor, Operational Support Unit, Division of Transfusion Medicine, Department of Laboratory Medicine and Pathology, Mayo Clinic, 200 First St. SW, Rochester, MN 55905 US, Tel: +1-507-538-4718 Fax: +1-507-284-1399, Halling.valerie@mayo.edu

management systems play a central role in advancing safety. Such systems use information obtained from the detection, reporting, and analysis of errors to improve performance and enhance safety. The greatest potential for success exists when event management systems are designed to encourage and reward complete error reporting, including self reporting. A number of tools and techniques that can be used to improve the effectiveness of event management systems are described in this chapter. They range from being largely technology-driven to being founded on an understanding of human capabilities. The use of these techniques will help organizations develop and maintain effective event management systems, which will help drive organizations towards higher levels of safety and performance.

Keywords: Error management, Event management, Quality Systems, Culture of Safety, Just Culture, Process Improvement, Quality Management, Quality Principles, Process Control, Process Sustainability, Process Efficiencies, Root Cause Analysis

1. Introduction

Error detection and reporting (event management) is a vital component of any organizational system that embraces and practices ongoing continuous improvement. The primary purpose of event management is the detection, reporting, and analysis of errors so that organizations can learn how processes are affected by errors and/or what impact processes have on errors. The objective is to prevent errors from recurring, with subsequent enhancement of the quality of products and services provided to healthcare recipients. The purpose of event management cannot simply be to satisfy the requirements of the Food and Drug Administration (FDA) or any other regulatory or accrediting agency. The principal motivation of a patient-centred event management system is continuous improvement in the quality of patient care rather than simply compliance[1].

The term, error, has a wide array of definitions. In Laboratory Medicine, an error is usually characterized as a failure to follow or a deviation from accepted policies, processes and procedures. When one considers the complexity of many medical processes, which often involve numerous standard operating procedures (SOPs) and multiple personnel to carry out a large number of often complex process steps, it is not surprising that errors occur. When establishing an event management system, there are some general principles to keep in mind regarding errors. First, it has long been known that the ability of humans, no matter how knowledgeable and well-trained, to repeatedly perform defined, simple tasks without committing an error is limited. [1, 2] Data from the Mayo Clinic suggest that the "human limit" for error free performance is approximately 1 in 10,000 tasks at best. [2] The error rate might be more frequent in settings where individuals are overworked, distracted, multi-tasking, tired, or inadequately trained. Second, because human errors are certain to occur, it is crucial to have systems to identify errors that occur at any stage of a process. Errors provide a major opportunity for organizations to learn and improve, particularly if there is complete and full error reporting. Third, performance improvements occur through the understanding of the causes of errors. Improvements do not occur by simply telling employees to be more careful in their work. The ability to detect, characterize, and analyze all errors in a consistent manner

---

[1] See Chapter 9 – Patient Safety and Quality Management at the Clinical Interface.

allows for the development of logical, effective preventive strategies and performance improvements. Fourth, reductions of error rates occur when the self-reporting of errors is positively reinforced. In other words, error reporting should always be strongly encouraged. People reporting errors should never be punished. A non-punitive approach is critical to successful event management because it establishes an atmosphere of full, open disclosure and discussion of errors.

So, how can a culture that maximizes the benefits of event management be created? Such a culture cannot be successfully created or sustained without genuine buy-in and involvement of leadership. Leaders establish the overall working climate for organizations. The fundamental principles and values of an organization are shaped via the directives and the actions of its leaders. Leaders must have a clear understanding of an organization's vision, mission, and core values and they must be able to concisely and accurately convey these concepts. Leaders must understand and embrace quality principles so that organizations achieve a culture where 'all transactions are understood completely and accomplished correctly each time'. [3] An environment where every employee feels compelled to assume responsibility for the quality of the products and services provided is created by such a culture. Effective event management programs arise in such Quality Cultures. This turns out to be a mutually beneficial relationship – the appropriate culture and environment stimulates the establishment of an effective event management system and an effective event management system fuels positive changes and continuous performance improvements, which strengthens the Quality Culture of an organization.

Crucial components of effective event management systems include detection, internal reporting, investigation, causal analysis, risk assessment/criticality, description, classification, external reporting, improvement/corrective action, change control, effectiveness assessment, and data analysis/trending. This chapter will describe some of the tools and techniques organizations can use to build and support these crucial components.

2. Deviations and Non-Conformances

The United States Food and Drug Administration (FDA), as well as accrediting organizations such as the AABB, require blood banks and transfusion services to develop and implement policies, processes, and procedures that ensure that deviations that fail to meet specified requirements are monitored, captured, assessed, and investigated. [4, 5] The investigation of such deviations must include, when applicable, an assessment of effects on donor eligibility, donor safety, and patient safety. Blood banks and transfusion services must define who is responsible for the review of non-conforming blood components, tissues, derivatives, critical materials and services as well as who has the authority for the disposition of non-conforming products. Deviations, non-conformances, and adverse events must be reported as defined by requirements, which may include reporting to outside agencies, such as the FDA. Laboratories with effective and compliant systems for reporting deviations and non-conformances typically have built such systems on a foundation of strong event management programs. Such programs have well defined processes for error reporting and analysis, the internal sharing of information regarding errors, corrective and preventive actions to improve processes and performance, and the provision of feedback to staff on how error reporting has resulted in process improvements.

3. Event Management

Event management, which includes the analysis of near-miss and adverse events, is an important facet of continuous improvement and the goal of ever increasing the safety of the health care environment. To achieve success, individuals within the health care environment must be able to openly, honestly, transparently, and completely report their own errors and errors of others. Self-reporting is the cornerstone of a successful error prevention, detection, and management programme. Under reporting of errors, however, persists in many health care environments. Many reasons have been cited for such under reporting. Humans are fallible, especially when operating under cognitively complex conditions. In such settings, they may face communication challenges, frequent interruptions, knowledge deficiencies, and heavy workload. Staff may not recognize errors, or fail to perceive that individual workarounds, omissions, or non-conformances with standard operating procedures (SOPs) are events that necessitate reporting. Some individuals rely on their own judgment regarding whether an error is significant enough to report; this is especially true if the error was a near-miss and no harm resulted. Unfortunately, others may feel that reporting events does not make a difference anyway, so why waste the time and effort to generate such reports?

Errors may go unreported because self-disclosure of an error or event might increase an individual's feelings of self-doubt, guilt, or inadequacy. There may be a reluctance to report on co-workers because of the stigma of being portrayed as a tattle tale or a fear of reprisal. If the atmosphere surrounding error reporting is punitive in nature, individuals might be reluctant to self-report near-misses or events because of the fear of receiving disciplinary actions. Thus, it is very important that event reporting occurs in a non-punitive environment, so that open and transparent discussion of errors can occur in the absence of fear of consequences. One approach to overcome such fear is an event management system that allows for confidential or anonymous reporting. This may facilitate an increase in event reporting. [6]

Individuals respond to and learn from their participation in an event management programmes in different ways. Some may respond to errors constructively while others may respond defensively. Ideally, individuals will learn from errors and use the knowledge gained to prevent future harm. The key is to create an environment where people feel comfortable addressing errors in a constructive manner.

In addition to the above-mentioned behavioural issues that impact error reporting, under reporting may also occur if event reporting is viewed as too onerous by the individuals expected to participate in the process. Workers may feel that they already have difficulty managing all of their current job-related duties; therefore, they have no additional time for the added workload necessary to fully investigate and report errors. Some workers might even hope that if they wait long enough, someone else will report events for them. No matter what the underlying causes of under reporting in an event management system are, the end result is missed opportunities to improve important processes within an organization.

In order for event management to be maximally effective, any existing culture of under reporting must be changed. All members of an organization must understand that improvements cannot be made if the processes that result in near-misses or enable individuals to do the wrong thing are allowed to persist. Moore and Foss have summarized the philosophy in the following manner: *"We believe a critical step in this strategic framework is the firmly held conviction that each individual employee is privileged to participate in the care of the patient, however far removed from direct patient contact the employee may be (e.g. laboratories). To help ensure the long-term, consistent motivation necessary to maintain the needs of the patient come first culture, each employee must be trained to consider the care of every patient to be equivalent to that they would ardently wish for if that patient were their own child, parent, or spouse."* [7] When employees adopt the philosophy that the work they perform could affect the care of family members or the care they could receive as patients, this should help them take more timely, active, and complete roles in reporting breaches of SOP compliance, errors, and near-misses.

In the same publication, Moore and Foss further elucidated the concept of a Quality Culture. [7] It was emphasized that, when it comes to event management, organizations must create and maintain an environment that makes it clear that *"quality is not the prerogative of a few dedicated quality technologists or a quality team, but it is the responsibility of each employee."*

The approach to errors must be non-punitive in order to maximize reporting and to facilitate the generation of frank and open discussion of such errors for root cause analysis (RCA) and corrective action planning. All members of an organization should enthusiastically embrace the concept that error detection and data analysis is a major opportunity for process and practice improvements and enhanced safety. To be truly successful, this Quality Culture, which includes a transparent event management programme as an integral component, must be embraced, endorsed, preached, and practiced by leaders throughout an organization, including those individuals who hold the loftiest positions. Key leaders cannot simply philosophically endorse a Quality Culture; they must also make sure that the resources necessary to achieve the quality goals of the organization are provided.

A commitment to safety (behaviours and principles) should not be looked at as work that must be one 'in addition' to the current workload. Rather, it should define how work is done, how employees interact, and how people respond to errors when they occur. A commitment to safety requires a tenacious and enduring willingness to practice safe behaviours and to actively pursue opportunities to improve patient care every day.

Over the years, process improvements and technological advances have contributed to a reduction of errors and improved laboratory practices. For example, quality control, the process of on-going performance checks of laboratory tests, allows for the detection and correction of major problems or errors within the test system. Technologies such as bar coding and laboratory information systems (LIS) have had a significant impact on the incidence of errors by providing, among many features, safeguards such a warning messages that prompt users to verify critical information relevant to patient care. Despite these advances, human errors still occur in the health care setting, and it is crucial that these errors are reported and analyzed.

4. Culture of Safety

Valentin described the development of a safety culture as the evolution from a 'culture of denial', where errors never happen, to a 'reactive culture', where actions are taken in response to errors, to a 'proactive culture', where the management of risks has become an integral part of the everyday thinking of all individuals involved in an organization. [8] To successfully evolve into a proactive safety culture, there must be acceptance of the fact that humans are imperfect and making errors is part of the human condition that cannot be totally prevented. Therefore, the key question to be answered is 'what might go wrong?'. [8] The key question should not be 'who is guilty?' This proactive approach encourages individuals and organizations to think about errors that could potentially occur during various processes, thereby providing opportunities for prevention of such errors prior to their occurrence. Although it is always desirable to minimize the number and severity of errors occurring in the workplace, when errors occur, it is most constructive to consider them as learning opportunities. The reporting of near-misses should be considered commendable behaviour and thus rewarded as critical steps in future prevention of errors.

Data collected on errors must be analyzed and, when opportunities for improvement are identified, effective changes must be implemented in a timely manner. Quality staff, senior staff, and management teams all have critical roles in guiding and pushing quality improvement efforts out to the work unit and bench levels. The presentation of detailed information about the causes, outcomes, and prevention of errors to the work units keeps staff engaged and allows personnel to collectively learn from events.

Safety can be embraced and applied at the institutional level through the use of a team-based and multifaceted process that embeds safe behaviours throughout the organization. At one of the authors' institutions this process has been established as the 'Commitment to Safety.' The core of the Commitment to Safety is five essential safe behaviours that should be embedded into daily work. The following sections outline these behaviours.

4.1. Pay Attention to Detail

To avoid errors, there must be an intentional focus on the specific task being performed. The importance of focus becomes ever increasing as tasks become more complex because the risk for human error is known to positively correlate with task complexity. The risk of errors also increases when external (environmental) or internal (worries or preoccupations) distractions compete or impede an individual's or a team's focus on a task. Individuals should be mindful about the task to be performed, avoid internal and external distractions, obtain and use accurate task-related information, have the necessary materials to perform the task, take appropriate actions to perform the task, and review and evaluate the appropriateness of the action. The consequences of human error can be quite variable, but there are situations where human errors do have substantial adverse affects. Even the smallest details, if not addressed appropriately, can have a significant impact on outcomes. Developing a culture where attention to detail becomes imprinted in the thoughts and behaviours of individuals within an organization can result in a significant decrease in the risk of human errors. [9]

4.2. Communicate Clearly

Exchanges of verbal, written, or electronic information must be accurate and delivered in a manner that guarantees comprehension. Communications must be intentional (an identifiable process where everyone involved knows that a communication event is occurring), respectful, non-intimidating, and non-judgmental. Opportunities must be provided for clarification and verification of the accuracy and understanding of the information being exchanged. Individuals involved in information exchanges should also be observant of body language and the overall tone of a communication event and use these cues to assess the effectiveness of the episode and whether more discussion, explanation and/or clarification is necessary to achieve success. Applying these principles to the communication process will help prevent misunderstandings or erroneous assumptions that could result in incorrect decisions or actions. [9]

4.3. Have a Questioning and Receptive Attitude

Individuals within an organization must be allowed and encouraged to ask questions when concerns arise. There should be an open and respectful environment created for addressing such questions, and there needs to be demonstrated responsiveness to concerns that are raised. Key features characterizing this approach include:

- Allowing individuals to speak frankly, openly, and honestly;
- Providing positive reinforcement when questions are raised;
- Appreciation for and deference to expertise wherever it may be found;
- Maintaining a focus on mutual purpose and an atmosphere of mutual respect;
- Demonstrating respect for everyone's competence;
- Caring for one another as people who are important;
- Trusting one another's intentions;
- Understanding and managing one's own emotions and the emotions of others;
- Assure that time is available to adequately address all questions.

Adoption and application of these principles will have a positive impact on problem identification and resolution. [9]

4.4. Hand Off Effectively

There needs to be a real-time interactive process for the conveyance of information from one individual to another or one team to another that accompanies a transfer of responsibility. Such a process ensures that complete and accurate information is transmitted to individuals assuming responsibility so that no important information or duties are misunderstood or overlooked. Key attributes of the process include interactive communication (i.e., face-to-face or voice-to voice communication), focus and engagement in the handoff process, encouragement of questions and clarification prior to handoff completion, avoidance of distractions and interruptions during the activity, maintenance of the applicable level of confidentiality, and assuring that concerns pertaining to patient safety are effectively and appropriately communicated up the chain of command. [9]

4.5. Support Each Other

In order to achieve maximal patient safety and the highest achievable organizational quality, a culture must be created that promotes teamwork, collaboration and cooperation across all professions and at all staff levels within an organization. Attributes associated with a supportive work environment include common goals and shared vision throughout an organization, a deference to expertise no matter where it is found, inter-professional collaboration (e.g., physicians and nurses), shared expectations with regard to psychological safety and mutual respect, a constant readiness and flexibility to adapt as part of multiple teams to meet common goals, and a mutually supportive behaviour that implies 'you are not alone and together we will prevent harm'. The message must be clear that every employee within an organization is highly valued and his/her input is absolutely essential. In this environment, every employee is empowered to ask questions and voice and act upon concerns about issues or situations that could compromise safety. Team members are expected to observe and report on the work practices of other team members. Hierarchies are flattened by design to enable all to be equally and comfortably vigilant and observant for any signs of diminished quality, inadequate patient care or any other forms of potential harm. It is expected that individuals within organizations will respond appropriately and completely to those signs. The chances of this occurring are maximized if all employees support each other via open communication. Coaching and praise are important practices that foster a supportive work environment. The creation of a supportive work environment facilitates efforts to consistently deliver safe, high quality patient care and increase the probability that harm will be prevented. [9]

5. Managing Errors with Event Management

Successful event management systems must have well planned and properly implemented strategic goals and strategies, and an administrative infrastructure which effectively provides functional support. Event management is an integral part of the Quality Plan that is required by many regulatory agencies. [10] Error detection and reporting is one of the Quality System Essentials (QSE), and it plays a crucial role in a system of ongoing continuous improvement. [10] The principal reason for an event management system is to facilitate the discovery, reporting, and analysis of errors in order to learn how they affect processes and how processes affect errors. The goal is the prevention of recurrent errors, which results in the improvement of the products, services, tests, and care provided. Key elements of an event management program include detection, internal reporting, investigation, causal analysis, risk assessment/criticality, description, classification, external reporting, improvement/corrective action, change control, effectiveness assessment, and data analysis trending (Figure 1).

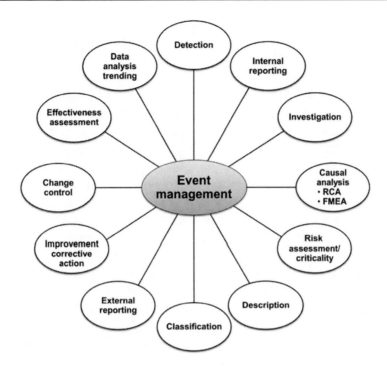

Figure 1. Event Management Programme.

It is important to clearly delineate and communicate the organization's expectation of employees regarding the reporting and documentation of errors, deviations, and non-conformances. Errors should be recorded in a consistent, structured manner, which should lessen the burden of the reporting process. The error reporting process should be an integral part of new employee training, and the process should be reviewed as a 'refresher' on a periodic basis (e.g., staff meetings etc.) for the benefit of all employees. The training materials for the error reporting process must contain clear instructions on 'what', 'when', 'where' and 'how' to properly report events, where 'who' is everyone in the organization. To sustain participation and enthusiasm for the event management process, successful reporting and follow-up of system failures, errors, events, and near-misses should be positively reinforced and publicly celebrated within an organization. In order to successfully create a culture that encourages safety awareness and the identification of improvement opportunities, event reporting cannot be linked to punitive actions or processes.

Errors can be the result of technical issues and human fallibility. In laboratory testing, it is important to remember that errors can occur during any phase of the testing cycle. The potential for errors encompasses the time from decision to perform a test through the final interpretation of the test and any clinical actions taken based on the test results. While it is important to focus on key phases of a process that occur within the laboratory, it is equally important to capture process-related errors occurring outside of the laboratory that involve other services that intersect with the laboratory. This allows for the construction of a much more complete picture of the process under analysis and maximizes the opportunities for significant performance improvements. In addition to applying event management principles to the actual work performed, it is often valuable to capture and analyze customer service-related issues. Such analyses may also identify process improvement opportunities.

In addition to helping in the determination of whether events are preventable, effective event management systems should also be able to assign risk/severity assessment scores to events. Accurate assessment of severity and/or potential to cause harm is an important factor that can be used to identify the events that need to be addressed the soonest. Centres looking to include risk/severity assessment in their event management system need to be aware that the various commercially available risk assessment tools utilize different parameters in their risk score assessment, and it is important to choose a tool that best fits the specific goals and needs of the organization.

Event management programmes are more likely to be successful when resources are dedicated at levels that assure that the process is ongoing and effective. There must be adequate personnel who are given sufficient time to address error reports and identify and follow-up on improvement plans. Adequate training (e.g., statistics) must be provided to enable personnel to properly utilize multiple performance improvement tools.

Although errors cannot be totally eliminated, they can be reduced by adopting a non-punitive system of accountability that encourages error reporting in the interest of patient safety. The event management system must encompass the full extent of an organization's processes. In the clinical laboratory for example, this means that all individuals involved in testing processes (i.e. all stakeholders) inside and outside the laboratory must collaborate in the event management process as it pertains to such testing. Such an approach increases the likelihood that significant process improvements can be achieved.

5.1. Reporting System for Event Management

A robust error reporting process enables organizations to identify, through appropriate error analyses, important trends or patterns, leading to activities such as root cause analysis (RCA) and implementation of corrective/preventive actions (CAPA) when appropriate. Whether event tracking is performed on paper, with simple computerized databases, or with sophisticated commercial software programs, the process chosen must be sufficient to effectively and efficiently meet the needs of an organization. The primary considerations when creating or choosing an event tracking system are flexibility and configurability. The event tracking system should be capable of tracking and trending unique events at the local level as well as enable broad tracking and trending at higher organizational levels. Additional important aspects of successful error management programmes are the devotion of sufficient time to seek and gather input from key stakeholders in the process or processes under evaluation and the development of standardized categorization and documentation of events so that consistent, accurate reports can be generated.

Many event reporting systems have not incorporated near-miss events into their data collection and analysis processes. This represents a lost opportunity to most effectively improve practices and safety. One reason for not capturing near-miss events is the labour intensiveness of many event reporting systems. End users may view their process of event reporting as cumbersome and time-consuming. A process characterized by the completion of detailed forms, their submission up the chain of command for review, and required interviews and meetings has served as a deterrent in some organizations, resulting in the reporting of only the most egregious errors. Event reporting often exists in a world of competing time management priorities, increasing workloads, and complex processes and procedures. It is not surprising that in such busy and complex environments, many event management systems are not as robust as they could be and errors continue to go undetected or unreported.

An effective event management system allows individuals filing reports to document events punctually, easily, and quickly. While a majority of event reports pertain to a single event, the event management system needs to be robust enough to handle event reports that involve two or more errors. Users should have a clear understanding (via training, and procedures) on how to use the system. The inclusion of informational prompts during the reporting process can help guide the user regarding the critical information to be included in reports. Printed material or drop-down boxes defining types of events or providing explanatory text can help facilitate standardization of terminology and event categorization. Preferably, the event reporting mechanism allows the initial reporter to simply provide enough key details of the event to allow the next level reviewer to easily determine the next steps in the investigation. For continued success, it is important to close the communication loop so that all staff appreciate that reported events result in process improvements and their efforts had a positive impact on the quality of the products and services provided. Performance improvements and increased safety will not result from simply reporting errors. For positive changes to occur, error reporting must be combined with systematic analyses, proper feedback to personnel, and appropriate actions taken as a result of the analyses.

An event management system that relies on a paper-based error reporting process has intrinsic shortcomings, such as having a limited means to optimally track and trend events. The use of an electronic, computer-based error reporting system will result in a reduction in the number of lost reports, enhanced communication, and more efficient movement of reports between members of an organization who write, review and analyze the documents. An electronic reporting process directs the reporter to include key pieces of information and forces users to provide the information required (i.e., required fields) before allowing that portion of the reporting process to be considered complete. This decreases the incidence of incomplete reports. Electronic reporting systems reduce the time required for completion of reports, which allows for the application of more timely interventions to facilitate process improvements.

A relational database is a useful tool for the recording and extraction of data. This type of database can be structured to reflect the work-flow at each individual work unit and have search capabilities. Additional considerations when developing or evaluating a computerized event management system include: Interfaces, tiered access to programme functionality and data, hardware needs, required fields, standardized dictionaries, risk assignment, automated alerts, security (passwords), free text fields, ability to modify reports when additional investigation is completed, and ability to generate CAPA. The electronic reporting system should be systems oriented with a focus on robust reporting capabilities that usefully support data assessment and process improvement activities. Additional potentially desirable characteristics of an electronic event management system include capabilities for automatically generated reports, *ad hoc* reports, and trending tools. Oversight reports that allow for the monitoring of turnaround times and of reports needing completion add to overall timeliness and efficiency of the event management process.

5.2. Corrective and Preventive Actions

CAPA are well known practices utilized in association with Current Good Manufacturing Practices (CGMP). In the *Guidance for Industry –Quality Systems Approach to Pharmaceutical CGMP Regulations* from the FDA, a number of principal concepts regarding events and CAPA are presented from the perspective of the federal oversight agency. [11] The document focuses on the importance of proper investigation, understanding, and correction of discrepancies, failures, and deviations in the manufacturing process with an additional emphasis on prevention of recurrences. The guidance describes CAPA as being composed of three distinct activities. First, there are remedial corrections of existing problems. Second, there are RCA with corrective actions where an understanding of the causes of discrepancies, failures, and deviations is gained. RCA are followed by actions or interventions taken to prevent recurrences of similar problems. Third, there are preventive actions, which are taken to avoid occurrence of potential problems that have been identified.

Regardless of the nature of an identified problem, when a decision is made to proceed with further evaluation and investigation, the steps in the process that follow: root cause analysis, actions, verification, implementation, and effectiveness checks, are quite uniform. RCA is used to identify the causes of discrepancies, deviations, or failures as well as generate ideas for corrective actions that will prevent recurrences or preventive actions to prevent similar or related events in the future. CAPA are critical components of a continuous improvement programme. Discrepancies, deviations, or failures can be identified in multiple ways such as internally by employees, through processes utilized by the event management programme, through document reviews, or by recommendations by external auditors. Corrective actions are considered to be a reactive response to problems requiring correction. Examples of corrective actions include: SOP updates, redesign of forms, employee training modifications and improvements, and error proofing an existing process. Preventive actions are proactive steps taken to prevent potential discrepancies, deviations, or failures prior to their occurrence. Examples of preventive actions include: software or equipment validations, increasing the frequency of (preventive) maintenance, or implementing a second check on a key process. To ensure that CAPA are effective, one can evaluate these actions periodically through a systematic approach called Plan-Do-Act-Check. [12]

6. Human Factors

There are a number of models that describe the manner in which humans process information. Figure 2 [13] illustrates a model constructed by Wickens and colleagues. This model consists of several parts:

- Sensory processing – This is input provided by stimuli that come from all human senses
- Short term sensory store – This prolongs the stimulus for a short time after its occurrence
- Perceptual encoding – Stimuli are assigned to a perceptual category

- Memory – A stimulus goes into working memory after it has been perceptually encoded
- Decision and response selection – A decision regarding what to do with a stimulus
- Response execution – A response (action) carried out, which depends primarily on human movement
- Feedback – The consequences of the action are monitored
- Attention resources – A decision regarding where to focus one's attention while performing a task

This information is of great value when utilized in approaches to mistake-proof processes that have been shown to pose risk for errors. Errors are natural. Defects are not. Defects can be removed through the use of performance improvement tools. Errors, on the other hand (memory lapses or mistaken observations), are natural and integral parts of the human condition that will occur. The challenges are to understand how to modify processes or systems to reduce the risk of harm or to realize that some process defects or errors cannot be eliminated or reduced and strategies to cope with this inevitable likelihood must be developed.

Wickens' Model of Human Information Processing*

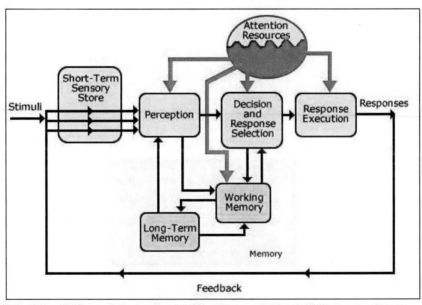

*adapted from Wickens, C.D., _Engineering Psychology and Human Performance_, Harper Collins, New York, 1992

Figure 2. Wicken's model of human information processing.

Human Factors (HF) is the study of human capabilities and limitations. It focuses both on areas where people excel as well as areas where they perform poorly in terms of thoughts, actions, and the processes used to perform tasks and functions. Those principles are applied to the design of tools, systems, tasks, jobs and environments to optimize the settings in which humans must function. The objectives of HF principles are to reduce errors, increase safety, increase reliability, increase system performance, reduce fatigue and physical stress and increase ease of performance of duties. In order to achieve these objectives, human capabilities and limitations must be taken into account. Errors can be reduced by understanding the interaction of humans and their work. No matter what fixes are introduced to reduce errors, humans will still have to perform tasks, so cognition, ergonomics, capabilities and limitations, heuristics and biases must be taken into account. An environment must be established where it is 'easy to do the right thing and hard to do the wrong thing'. The goal is to understand what is currently happening in current processes and why such things are happening. Once that understanding is gained, if processes require improvement, there are techniques to achieve the desired enhancements.

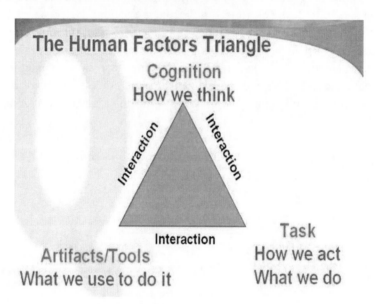

Figure 3. The Human Factors triangle.

The Human Factors Triangle [14] serves as one conceptual approach (Figure 3). Understanding the relationship between cognition (how people think), the task (how people act and what they do) and the artifacts or tools (what people use to perform tasks), allows for a better understanding of human capabilities and limitations.

6.1. Cognition

An important aspect of cognition and its impact on the ability to do work is that human attention has finite limits. Niebel defines attention as *"the amount of cognitive capacity devoted to a particular task or processing stage"*. [15] When a person's attention is divided between several tasks, a decrease in performance and productivity often occurs in comparison to the performance of a single task. It is important to minimize multitasking to the greatest extent possible because this is the setting in which the majority of errors occur. Another important factor is how people maintain attention and performance over long periods of time. Frequent rest breaks, task variation, feedback regarding performance, and internal (caffeine) or external (music, white noise) stimulation may help people to maintain their attention over extended time periods. [15]

6.2. Tasks

Tasks are the activities or jobs that people perform. How do tasks take into account human capabilities and limitations? Do some tasks exceed human capabilities (e.g., from the context of ability to remember or complexity of activities)? Does a task pose a heavy physical load to the body- perhaps exceeding a person's limitations? For the tasks themselves, how do people know what to do next? Are people relying on memory? What other things influence a person's ability to do the task? Are the work layouts for conducting tasks adequate? Are there poor environmental conditions impeding task performance (too hot, too cold, too dark, too bright, too cluttered, etc.)? With regard to memory, as shown in Figure 2, received stimuli go into the sensory store where they reside for a very short time. Although a large number of stimuli might be coming into a person at any given point in time, only a small amount of that information gets encoded and sent to working memory (i.e., short-term memory). There is a limit to the amounts of time and information that can be kept in working memory (7 ± 2 items at one time). [15] The likelihood of information loss is increased when there are a larger number of items in working memory because of the longer time necessary to process this volume of material. Wickens, Gordon, and Liu (1997) recommend the following to minimize errors on tasks that require working memory. [14]

- Minimize memory load, in both capacity and time to maintain recall
- Utilize chunking (storing items as a unit in long-term memory – an area code for example is not three items to be stored, but a single chunk), in terms of meaningful sequences and use of letters over numbers
- Keep chunks small, no more than three or four items in a chunk
- Keep numbers separate from letters
- Minimize confusion of similar sounding items

Once information is transferred from short term memory to long term memory, retrieving the information is more difficult unless there is frequent activation of the information or there are associations with previous knowledge that can be utilized. This is particularly important when a person needs to complete a task that is complicated or performed infrequently. SOPs or job aids help to decrease the load on long term memory, and thus decrease the likelihood of errors due to memory. Grout et al. stressed the point that, in healthcare, an infrastructure has been built that relies on memory, including lengthy procedures that instruct people on how to perform tasks. [16] The authors wrote *"These procedures are not intended to be consulted during the actual performance of the task, but rather to be committed to memory for later recall"*. [16] As previously discussed, when information in long term memory is not used frequently it is harder to retrieve; therefore, a procedure-based approach that relies on memory requires ongoing training to reduce the likelihood of errors. When events occur, there is a tendency to take actions that change the content of the worker's memory, either by retraining or by making procedural changes, and often the changes to the procedures make them even more complex and lengthy! In regard to this issue, Grout has written, "*If SOPs become simpler and help reduce the cognitive load on workers, it is a very positive step. If the corrective responses to adverse events are to lengthen the SOPs with additional process steps, then efforts to improve patient safety may actually result in an increase in the number of errors*". [16] When events occur, efforts should be directed at making it hard (or impossible) to do the wrong thing and easy to do the right thing during that process in the future.

6.3. Tools

The third component of the Human Factors Triangle is tools. Tools are what we use to perform tasks. There needs to be an understanding of the tools people use and the extent to which they match up with their capabilities and limitations. What tools are people given and how easy or difficult are they to use? Are people given the tools they need to perform their assigned tasks? Do the tools provided effectively assist personnel in the performance of their tasks? Regarding the equipment used to perform tasks, there are a number of additional factors that can impact human performance. How easy is it to read displayed information? How is aural and visual information presented? How is information organized? Is equipment located so it is easy to use? One approach is to mistake-proof processes.

7. Use of Human Factors in Problem Solving

Many approaches are employed in event investigations. It appears, however, that very few event investigations take into account the impact of human factors. Human Factors considerations can be incorporated into standardized basic problem solving approaches. Examples of where this has been done include the airline industry and the military. [25] At the institution that employs some of the authors of this chapter, a multidisciplinary team of management and staff members are asked to silently brainstorm possible causes of events using the Human Factors Analysis and Classification System (HFACS™) checklist. [26] The (HFACS™) used is a modified taxonomy for healthcare checklist that has been divided into four categories: Actions, Preconditions for Actions, Oversight/Supervisor Factors, and Organizational Influence. The team then reviews and votes on the silent brainstorming ideas that have been presented to the group. The possible causes that receive the most votes are moved to the next phase, solutions identification (if further investigation or root cause analysis are judged not to be required). In the next phase, the team uses the Human Factors Intervention Matrix (HFIX™) checklist to identify potential solutions to the problems or issues identified. [27] This checklist has also been modified to best address the main causes of human errors and the categories consist of: Task/Procedure, Technology/Engineering, Technical/Physical Environment, Human/Team, Team Interaction/Communication and Organization /Supervisory. Potential solutions are then prioritized through the use of voting by team members. The HFIX™ solution tool is used to score the top five to seven ideas for feasibility, acceptability, cost, effectiveness and sustainability. The Human Factors contributing to events can be identified using this approach. Depending on the human factors identified, it may be necessary to implement more than one solution. The use of a standardized rating scale helps maximize the likelihood that the most effective solutions for each event are identified and implemented. Furthermore, the process makes sure that the employees who most regularly work with the processes are part of the solutions, which increases their acceptance of any changes that are made. The use of Human Factors analysis as part of event management results in more thorough investigations and the choice of solutions that decrease the likelihood of recurrences. This process ensures that the tools, systems, tasks, jobs, and environments are safe, effective, and comfortable, and align with human capabilities and limitations.

8. Mistake-Proofing

Mistake-proofing is defined as making it hard (or impossible) to do the wrong thing and easy to do the right thing, keeping errors/mistakes from causing defects/harm, and/or making your processes resilient against inevitable errors. The best mistake-proofing strategies have the following characteristics:

- They are devised by the people closest to the work
- They provide immediate feedback to people performing the tasks
- They compel countermeasures to avoid or prevent mistakes
- They either shut down a process to avoid errors or deliver a warning (audible or visual) about the potential for errors
- They should be simple and inexpensive

Two different mistake-proofing approaches can be used to address process defects. The first approach is prevention-based mistake-proofing. In prevention-based mistake-proofing, there is a sense that an error or event is going to occur and actions are taken to prevent the occurrence while the process continues to move forward until all required elements are present and correct. The second approach is detection-based mistake-proofing. In detection-based mistake-proofing an abnormality is discovered at the time of its occurrence and corrective action occurs at the point of origin. Four priorities in mistake-proofing have been identified [17]:

1. Eliminate – Concentrate on eliminating non-value added steps in a process rather than mistake-proofing them.
2. Prevent – Remove the root cause of a defect. If defective step(s) cannot be eliminated then:
   a. Replace the steps with new steps that lack defects
   b. Simplify processes to reduce the possibility of errors
   c. Seize opportunities to automate processes
   d. Integrate inspections into work flow
   e. Standardize processes as much as possible
   f. Integrate visual management into processes

When redesigning tasks, efforts should focus on finding ways to minimize operator requirements that require a high demand on working memory, minimize stress, simplify complex tasks (e.g., remove complex calculations), minimize the need for exact recall of specific complex details, and reduce the number of tasks that require high levels of physical or mental endurance. Process design should always take into account human capabilities. When the requirements necessary for task performance are considered, do the considerations include the capabilities and limitations of the humans who will be performing such tasks?

The prevention of errors related to the use of technology involves choosing types of equipment and using this equipment in such a way that perceptual confusion is minimized. Do the icons convey exactly what they mean? Are people already familiar and comfortable with the symbols in use? Is there easy discrimination of the buttons, knobs etc such as distinct colours, distinct shapes, and adequate spatial separation to minimize the risk of errors? Have un-needed usage modes been disabled?

3. Detect – Detect errors when they occur and have methods in place to prevent or minimize adverse outcomes

Shutdown methods stop process errors from occurring. Warning methods employ active visual or audio signals to alert operators or users that an error has occurred. Sensory alert methods (e.g. bells, alarms, lights) make the errors obvious; however, success depends on the operator performing the checks. Checklists guard against the possibility that individuals will forget critical steps or aspects of processes or procedures. Crosschecking is often used as a method of error detection. Although they are useful for error detection, one must be aware of some of the pitfalls associated with crosschecks. First, it has been demonstrated that as the numbers of crosschecks increase, quality decreases. Second, when individuals know that other people will be 'double-checking' their work, there is the temptation to be less diligent or thorough when performing tasks.

4. Manage – Defects identified within the value stream

The priority here is the identification and separation of defects prior to the occurrence of the next process step. This is a setting where crosschecks can be used to identify and isolate defects and remove them from processes. Another method of managing defects is to utilize devices that will stop a process when a defect has occurred. When mistake-proofing the root cause of errors, it is important to remember two important concepts:

- The simpler the processes, the fewer the errors
- Improvements that complicate processes are not really improvements

9. Fair and Just Culture

When events occur, organizations must make a choice as to the approach to such events. Should this be an opportunity to learn or should this be an opportunity to assign blame? In order to achieve the highest quality of goods and services, organizations must create an environment where staff are encouraged and feel uninhibited about reporting problems, errors or misunderstandings because there is a clearly delineated shared goal to identify, analyze and improve through the knowledge gained from such reports. In a Fair and Just Culture (FJC), errors are approached in a fair-minded manner, with productive conversations, and the creation of effective structures that help organizations learn from events and errors. Frankel and colleagues recently described three initiatives to improve patient safety, and one of these three initiatives was a Fair and Just Culture. [18] An organization with a FJC has a willingness to equally divulge its weaknesses and its areas of excellence. In this environment, employees feel secure bringing forth safety issues resulting from their actions or the actions of others. The atmosphere is one where employees feel 'safe and emotionally comfortable' performing their jobs. This enables them to work at peak capacity with the knowledge that at any time they can disclose 'weakness, concern, or inability.' They are encouraged to request assistance when concerns about quality and safety arise. [18]

In Figure 4, three behaviours that result in errors are shown [19]:

1. *Human error/Inadvertent Action* – This is when individuals inadvertently perform duties or tasks in a manner different from the way they should have been performed (slips, lapses, mistakes) [19].
2. *Risky Behaviour* – This is when individuals make a conscious choice to deviate from policies, procedures, rules, or protocols or when people make behavioural choices that increase risks where such increases in risks are not recognized, or the choices to increase risks are mistakenly believed to be justified. [19]
3. *Reckless Behaviour* – This is when individuals consciously disregard substantial and unjustifiable risks. [19]

Organizational responses should be correlated to the behaviours associated with the events or near-misses. Isolated human errors/inadvertent actions should be addressed as opportunities to correct process weaknesses (e.g., making drug labels more readily distinguishable from one another in order to minimize medication errors). Individuals making human errors/inadvertent actions should be consoled rather than disciplined. Risky behaviours may be a signal that system or process flaws are present and that these flaws need to be addressed. However, individuals engaging in risky behaviours should be coached so that they gain an understanding of the risks they have taken. Disciplinary actions may be justified in response to reckless behaviours.

The actions taken must alleviate the risk of future reckless behaviours; therefore, it may even be appropriate to remove individuals engaging in reckless behaviours from the organization altogether. [18] If individuals repeatedly make the same errors, this could be a sign of process issues; however, it may also indicate employee performance problems, especially when employees do not demonstrate performance improvements following coaching or additional training.

Recurrent errors may signify that certain individuals are not able to perform at the levels necessary to meet the demands of their current jobs and the best solution might be for them to find jobs that better fit their skill sets. [20]

Fair and Just Culture

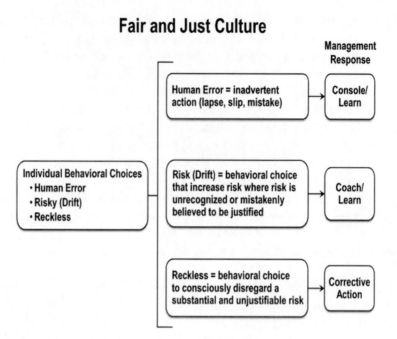

Figure 4. Fair and Just Culture.

9.1. Accountability

In a Fair and Just Culture, individuals understand that will be held accountable for their actions. However, these same individuals also realize that blame will not be assigned to them when it is evident that processes or systems are not properly designed to allow them to safely and effectively perform their duties. A FJC enables organizations to develop an environment characterized by consistent accountability of all employees. Marx asserts that there is a need for a different kind of accountability in the workplace. [21] This different kind of accountability is one where employees are expected to raise their hands in the interest of safety. Marx further emphasizes that the 'greatest evil of all' is when individuals do not report their errors, thereby depriving the 'system and others' of an opportunity to learn.

10. Effective Teamwork and Communication

Effective teamwork and communication are critical features of successful event management programs. The Joint Commission has reported ineffective communication as the number one cause of sentinel events in health care. [22] Some of the authors of this chapter are part of an organization where an employee training programme entitled 'Teamwork is Real' has been developed to improve teamwork and communication (Figure 5). [23] The curriculum, facilitated by an allied health employee and a physician, includes didactic presentations, audience participation, and role playing as methods to deliver its messages. The training has allowed employees to obtain knowledge of and skills in:

- Reflective listening skills, to ensure the understanding of others;
- The PEARLS model (Partnership, Empathy, Apology, Respect, Legitimization, Support), to integrate the use of effective communication;
- The SBAR (situation, background, assessment, and recommendation), model to communicate clearly;
- Positive assertion skills to raise concerns by saying, "*I need a little clarity*";
- Effective team communication to protect patient safety and increase collaboration.

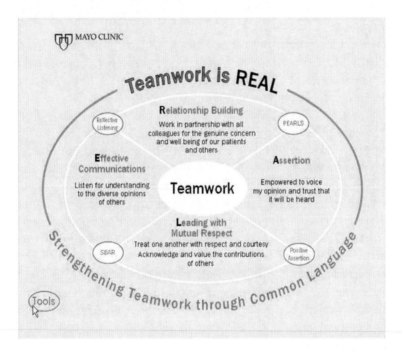

Figure 5. Teamwork model

The following should be considered when events resulting from lack of teamwork or communication occur:

- Can communication processes be modified in ways that ease the burden on individuals while ability to complete the tasks is maintained or improved?
- Can briefings or planning sessions be developed or improved so that proper attention is paid to critical process steps and safety issues?
- Can communications procedures be improved or standardized in order to reduce the risks of miscommunication (e.g., standardized read back procedure for critical value notification)?
- Can procedures that improve employee interactions be developed (e.g., describe tasks that foster teamwork, communication, and inter-employee safety checks)?
- Can the responsibilities of each member of a working team be more clearly defined?
- How can each member of a team be positively supported for having a focus on safety?

11. Performance Management

Performance management (PM) is a scientific approach that utilizes the principles of applied behaviour analysis to maximize human performance in the workplace. [24] The core concept of PM is that the provision of positive reinforcement for desired behaviours increases the frequency of such behaviours. The use of positive reinforcement leads to performance changes because the receipt of such reinforcement motivates employees to 'want to' perform at a higher, desirable level rather than feeling like they 'have to'. In other words, positive reinforcement promotes discretionary effort.

Discretionary effort comes from consequences, such as positive reinforcement, and not from antecedents. Applied behaviour analysis incorporates a model known as the Antecedents, Behaviour, and Consequences (ABC) model. [24] Antecedents precede behaviours and prompt behaviours to occur. The primary function of antecedents is to communicate information about behaviours and their consequences (i.e., 'if you do that, this is what will happen'). Antecedents are often presented in a manner where people are informed what their tasks are, when the tasks will be done, and how these tasks will be performed. When antecedents work, it is because of the desired behaviours have been associated with previous consequences. When antecedent-prompted behaviours do not produce anticipated consequences, these antecedents quickly lose the ability to produce desired behaviours. Behaviour is primarily and much more strongly driven by the actual consequences of one's actions. In many organizations, the majority of time is spent on antecedents, and then additional time is spent on the actions that need to be taken because people are not performing as instructed. Delivering consequences to guide behaviour is a much more efficient and effective use of organizational time. Consequences result in increases of desirable employee behaviours (through the appropriate use of positive and/or negative reinforcements) and decreases of undesirable employee behaviours (through the appropriate use of punishment or extinction techniques). The Consequence Matrix is depicted in Figure 6. [24] As can be seen, the ideal consequences for people are positive, immediate, and certain.

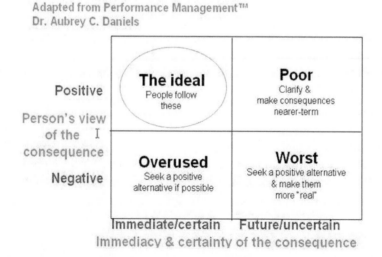

Figure 6. The consequence matrix.

11.1. Performance Management Applied to Event Management

The first step when applying PM to event management is the identification of the specific desired behaviours that will be cultivated. For example, two behaviours that are essential to an effective event management system are prompt, full reporting of events and timely follow-up, investigation, and identification of solutions to prevent event recurrences. These are behaviours that can be fostered by PM. Once the desirable behaviours are identified, specific, measurable goals must be established to allow for the identification of satisfactorily performing individuals. Next, there must be a plan regarding how feedback on these behaviours will be provided. The feedback provided should specifically pertain to the targeted behaviours sought from employees. Such feedback must be timely. It should be delivered at least daily and as soon as possible after employee performance. The feedback can be delivered verbally or visually. Finally, the types of reinforcements valued by employees must be identified and utilized. It is important to regularly use individualized, immediate, positive reinforcers (i.e. positive and meaningful consequences) and to habitually recognize and reward positive, desired behaviour. One effective technique is to attempt to catch employees doing the 'right thing' and providing immediate, real-time positive reinforcement. PM utilizes two distinct, important activities to enhance the effectiveness of the discipline – feedback and reinforcement. Feedback consists of instructions or suggestions while reinforcement is the provision of encouragement and motivation. Feedback and positive reinforcement work synergistically to effectively change and improve behaviours.

12. Causal Tree Analysis

Causal Tree Analysis (CTA) is a method that focuses on adverse events with the purpose of determining all the elements or factors that must be present to allow the adverse events to occur. [28, 29] CTA can visually show how relationships between equipment failures, human errors, and other external events combine to cause adverse events. CTA is used commonly to investigate all potential mechanisms leading to adverse events. It has been useful in the investigation of the reliability and safety of complex systems, particularly when there are significant human safety concerns. CTA is used extensively in the nuclear and aerospace industries; however, it has not been widely used in healthcare to date. [28, 29] In healthcare, areas where CTA might be beneficial include medication errors, infusion pump errors, patient falls, wrong blood given or transfusion-related deaths. An important point to take note of with CTA is that only one top event can be analyzed with a single causal tree. Tools utilized to conduct CTAs include brainstorming, cause and affect analysis, and/or failure mode and effect analysis (FMEA). For example, CTA can be used with FMEA to focus on the most critical failure mode.

Many different approaches can be used to facilitate a CTA. A very common CTA method is summarized as follows:

1. Define the adverse event (bad outcome) – this is termed the top event;
2. Draw a box at the top and list the top event inside;
3. Analyze the system to identify all the events that contribute to the top event – these are termed intermediate level events;

4. Continue until the lowest level of possible causes is reached – these are termed the basic level events;

5. The 'AND' and 'OR' gates constitute the major characteristics of the fault tree. AND gates are present when all the input events contribute. OR gates are present when one or more input events could contribute;

6. Analyze the CTA to determine ways to eliminate the intermediate events that led to the top event. The analysis should start with the highest failure probability and severity;

7. Finally, an action plan is prepared, the plan is implemented, and the CTA is updated.

Errors tend to occur when several lines of defense fail. Most serious adverse events, therefore, are the result of breakdowns at multiple levels rather than a single error. CTA is a tool that can be used to identify root causes of events that pose safety risks. It can be used to identify all causes of a single event.

13. Sustainability after Implementation of Process Improvements – Six Sigma is Our Friend!

Long term sustainability of improved processes can be difficult. However, with the right tools in place and consistent vigilance, the difficulties of sustaining improvements eventually subside. Nevertheless, even when desired specifications are consistently achieved, monitoring of processes remains a vitally important activity that should never diminish.

Through the application of Six Sigma principles, several tools may be used within the 'control' phase of the methodology that provides great confidence that improvements are sustainable. [30] Some of those tools are control plans, reaction plans, communication plans, training plans, audit plans, and statistical process control (SPC).

13.1. Control and Reaction Plans to Sustain Improved Results

Control plans are used to monitor and control processes so that gains can be sustained long-term. It is a detailed assessment and guide for maintaining control of process characteristics and associated variables to ensure capability of meeting established specification limits. Most standard control plans describe for a process owner the crucial procedure and process steps to monitor, the project baseline (initial output), the expected results post improvements (the specification limits), how and where improvements are measured, the frequency for which results are monitored, who is responsible for monitoring results, tools utilized to monitor results (i.e. reports, control charts, SOPs, etc.) and clear and concise steps to control and sustain improvements. Data falling outside of defined specification limits warrant actions that are outlined in control plans (Figure 7).

Reaction plans are referenced in control plans, and they are activated when control plans do not drive expected results. Reaction plans instruct users to drill down to root causes, contributing factors and necessary corrective actions in order to drive processes back into control.

Six Sigma Process Control Plan

Process Name:	2R Reduction in Discard Rate	
Customer:	Process Owner	Int/Ext 7873
Location:	Control Plan Ave, Illinois	
Area:	Operations	

Prepared by:	6.26.12	Black Belt
Approved by:	Process Owner signature	
Approved by:	Project Champion signature	
Approved by:		

Sub Process	Sub Process Step	CTQ KPOV	CTQ KPIV	Specification Characteristic	Specification/ USL LSL	Measurement Method	Sample Size	Frequency	Who Measures	Where Recorded	Decision Rule/ Corrective Action	SOP Reference
Vein Selection	Rate veins in designated area. Document rating on record. Review and assess. Determine best possible vein based on rating to ensure successful venipuncture	Best possible Vein selection and phleb selected to handle the degree of difficulty	Most suitable vein for successful venipuncture	All Staff trained to utilize SOP to select the best possible vein based on anatomy and phlebotomy skill levels to have successful venipuncture	USL of 4.5% controllable discards	Cognos 8 Report for monitoring discards. Assess discard type, number of discards, by location and individual	Weekly Collection total	Daily, weekly, monthly	Operations/ Process Owner	Management report and Operating stats	USL exceeded for the Dept. begin evaluation of cause (location, volume, individual, discard type) to determine root cause and C/A. If individual found to be having difficulty, go back to training plan, assess knowledge of XYZ process and proper utilization. Perform observations as needed. Refer to the reaction plan if spec. is not met on continual basis.	New SOP- XYZ SOP- XXXXXX rev. 0
SOP for vein selection	Assessment of the donor's veins in both arms using XYZ process	Guide phleb. in appropriate vein selection for successful venipuncture	Assist in pairing phleb with veins of the appropriate difficulty for his/her skill level	All staff trained and signed off on SOP and documented observed performance of use. SOP found in document control system for reference	USL of 4.5% controllable discards	Cognos 8 Report for monitoring discards. Assess discard type, number of discards, by location and individual	Weekly Collection total	Daily, weekly, monthly	Operations/ Process Owner	Management report and Operating stats	USL exceeded for the Dept. begin evaluation of cause (location, volume, individual, discard type) to determine root cause and C/A. If individual found to be having difficulty, go back to training plan, assess knowledge of XYZ process, proper utilization, and clarity of SOP. Determine if SOP revisions are warranted.	New SOP- XYZ SOP- XXXXXX rev. 0

Figure 7. Control and reaction plan format.

Essentially, reaction plans serve as trouble shooting guides. Typically, they are derived from details the Black Belt (trained practitioner on Six Sigma methodology) and the project team responded to and tweaked in processes during their pilot phases until desired results were generated and sustained.

13.2. Working on Control Plans – Pitfalls

When working with process owners on the use of control plans, the process owners may very well understand all of the control plan elements as they are being explained, but that does not guarantee clear understanding beyond the training and review process steps. This will not be known until control plans are turned over to process owners, when it will become evident that the processes are beginning to go out of control. It is important to be a healthy sceptic going into control plans. Never assume that process owners will fully understand all of the moving parts of control plans or how to completely use them.

Following training on control plans, reaction plans and implementation of improved processes, it sometimes becomes obvious that staff did not achieve full understanding of their roles in control or reaction plans. Although improvements are implemented based on statistically proven and successful pilot results, and staff are trained on those improvements, sometimes specification limits are not met.

The root cause for not meeting statistically proven results can sometimes be perplexing. An example of one approach taken was to have the Six Sigma Black Belt meet with the process champion, the process owner and the leadership team to determine the reasons why the process did not result in the expected improvements. The decision was made to have the process owner and the Black Belt conduct field visits to identify the reasons why control plan expectations were not being met.

Staff observations and feedback resulted in the identification of several contributing factors that led to unexpected post-process implementation results. Utilization of the control plan and monitoring of results were not fully understood to be a daily part of the process to control and sustain results. Staff lacked clear understanding that the control plan was used to control and sustain the process improvements, and the reaction plan was used if the process drifted out of control (i.e., exceeded specification limits). Staff was unaware of the impact on results that would occur if the process improvement steps, which were implemented on the basis of defects identified in the Six Sigma project, were not followed.

Several 'aha moments' were experienced during the field visits with staff. First, staff often does not understand that Six Sigma is an integral part of the 'fabric' of the organization. Second, it was apparent that continued management reinforcement was not robust enough to ensure that the control plan was optimized to yield expected results. It is critical that staff performing the improved process is acutely aware of the process changes, the specification limit(s) for which they are held accountable and resources and tools used for monitoring performance.

A clear 'take home' message from this scenario is that there is a great need for the Six Sigma Black Belt to remain involved until it is clear that the process owner has full understanding of the dynamics of using the control plan by way of sustained improved results.

Another method to gauge the understanding of process owners and leadership teams is through a defined mechanism for reporting results outlined in a communication plan.

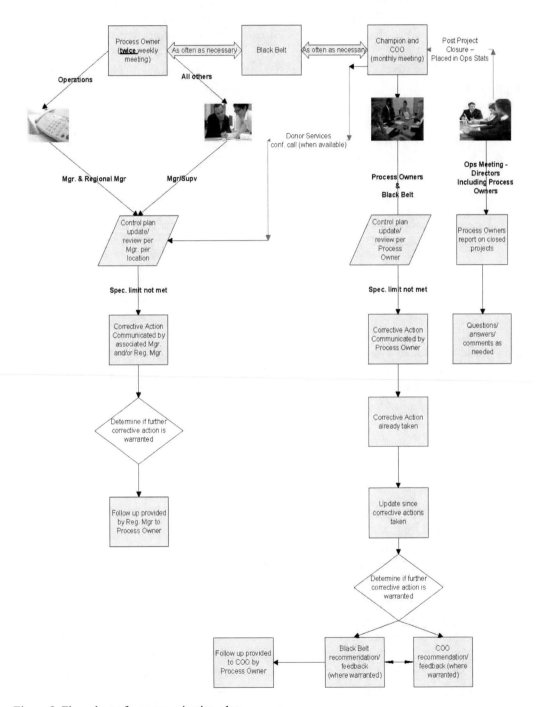

Figure 8. Flow chart of a communication plan.

13.3. Communication Plan for Robust Reporting

Communication plans clearly outline the frequency of reporting results against established specification limits, the corrective actions if metrics fall outside of range, the necessary support required to remove any barriers that prevent adherence to specification limits and the follow up actions when warranted. These plans also identify the forum in which reporting will occur; via live meetings, video conferencing, and/or conference calls (Figure 8).

Typically, Executive Directors or Chief Operating Officers have been considered the project champions process owners should report to. Project Champions provide oversight and management of each critical element of Six Sigma projects.

When creating communication plans, working with project champions and process owners to determine the date, time, frequency, and the expectations of control plan meetings should be set to assure that the important stakeholders will be able to participate. It is crucial to keep the reporting commitment per the communication plan to ensure visibility throughout the organization. Ensuring visibility helps drive the necessary accountability as well as the assurance of management engagement. This helps to keep Six Sigma culture alive.

13.4. The Importance of Having a Robust Training Plan

It is expected that there will be some turnover within an organization, which means there will be new employees to be trained. To assure proper and on-going training, it is highly recommended that training plans are put in place for any improved process. Without such training plans, sustainability of improved results can be compromised (Figure 9).

Having robust training plans in place provides the security of knowing that training will be performed in a consistent manner as long as the plans are followed, regardless of who is conducting the training. All standard operating procedures and policies should be documented within training plans. Much like any other training, there should be verification by way of sign-off from both trainers and trainees acknowledging full understanding and training completion. Observations of performance of new processes with sign-off may also be warranted.

There are times when staff previously trained on improved processes may be identified as not meeting specification limits on a consistent basis. Often, control plans are written so, that in such instances, employees are sent back to be retrained on the processes and then observed, monitored and evaluated. Training plans ensure that training on improved processes is consistent, which makes it easier to identify when employees have deviated. Once retraining is performed and all questions answered and observations are successfully performed, employees are usually back on track with successful process performance.

Training plans along with all other aforementioned plans should be assessed for revisions based on, but not limited to continuous process improvement, changes mandated by regulatory agencies, or policy changes. All Six Sigma plans are considered to be living and breathing documents. It is extremely important to make sure that revision numbers are captured for document control in accordance with current organizational quality control document systems. The best way to assess the need for changes is through comprehensive audit plans.

BASIC ELEMENTS OF A TRAINING PLAN

☐ New SOP

☐ Revised SOP

Rationale for New/Revised: ....

SOP(s)/Policies Impacted: _____

SOP Implementation Date: _____

1. **SOP(s), policies & training materials**

- New or revised SOP(s)/policies
- Training tools/guides
- Identify where/when in the process should the training occur
- Training checklist, competency exam and/or observation checklist
- Target date for SOP/training materials completion

2. Train the trainer

- Date & time needed for training
- Who are trainer(s) being trained
- Training conducted by

3. Training for Group A

- Size of each group
- Number of sessions required
- Timeframe (start/end) training completion
- Time required for each sub groups within group A
- Training conducted by

4. Training Completion

- All staff fully trained
- Training checklist, competency exam and/or observation checklist accurate and complete
- All staff deemed competent per the new/revised process

Figure 9.

13.5. What are the Elements of Audit Plans?

Audit plans focus on the key control points of improved processes. Audit plans can determine whether the integrity of improved processes remains intact. Elements of improved processes are based on validated and quantifiable data. Audit plans define which documents will be reviewed to monitor improved processes and the frequency of such reviews. Audits document the consistency of adherence to improved processes following their implementation. As such, audit plans help in the evaluation of processes that have deviated from targeted improvements.

As described in the earlier discussion regarding the moving parts of training plans, audit plans are also used to assure process owners that control, reaction and training plans are currently linked, which ensures compliance and process improvement sustainability. It also ensures that current metrics are measured accurately (Figure 10).

AUDIT PLAN FOR XYZ PROCESS

- **Daily Audit**

  - ✓ **Each Record will be audited to ensure that the XYZ process is documented on the record indicating XYZ utilization.**

- **Monthly Audit**

  - ✓ **Financial audits based on XYZ process results are conducted to ensure that financials are in order based gain from process.**

- **Annual Audit**

  - ✓ **SOP audit/review will be performed to ensure that the SOP does not warrant a revision based on any findings, changes and/or mandated revisions.**
  - ✓ **Annual staff competency is performed to ensure performance according to SOP/compliance by way of observations**

    - ▪ **Inability to pass will result in retraining and repeating annual competency**
    - ▪ **If inability to pass after retraining, next steps are determined by management**

  - ✓ **Annual staff competency is performed to ensure understanding of SOP/processes by way of written exams**

    - ▪ **Inability to pass will result in retraining and repeating annual competency**
    - ▪ **If inability to pass after retraining, next steps are determined by management**

Figure 10. Audit plan for a process.

Audit plans are typically written by Black Belts or Green Belts (Trained Six Sigma Practitioner on a smaller scope than a Black Belt). The responsibility for audits resides with process owners. Process owners may select auditors at their discretion; however, audit plans should be followed precisely. Audit results must be documented and the results reported back to process owners and/or process champions. Results from audits highlight any deviations for those responsible for taking corrective actions.

13.6. Statistical Process Controls (SPC)

There are times when variation exists within processes, some more than others depending on the process types. Statistical Process Controls (SPC) are very powerful tools that can be used to monitor and control process variations. Some of the benefits found when using SPCs are the stabilization of out-of-control processes, the monitoring of the consistency of processes, and the minimization of process variations that affect the quality of products or services.

Control charts are a type of SPC in common use. When performing analyses of the overall health of processes, control charting is a quick and easy way of determining the performance of the inputs and outputs used to monitor and control the performance of processes.

When viewing control charts, Six Sigma methodology teaches two types of variation: special cause variation – which indicates something out of the ordinary has caused a process to go out of control; and common cause – this results from the normal operation of a process and is dependent on process design.

It is typically easier to identify and fix special cause variations, due to the ability to identify unique process deviations and track isolated causes. When control charts indicate common cause variations, this typically means that the process itself is broken, and it is much more difficult to determine the inputs causing process variations and failures.

Advantages of using control charts are; a simple method to monitor the behaviour and performance of process inputs or output measures, a simple method to assist in knowing when to take actions, provides insight on trends and other process performance indicators, assess when changes made to processes yield desired results, and enables ongoing and continuous view of process performance.

14. The Power of Process Mapping

Process mapping is a graphical representation of the steps within processes. Mapping of processes can be useful for many reasons, but, primarily, it is used to increase overall performance within an organization. Often times, simple flow charts or 'high level' process maps are used to ensure a clear and concise understanding of processes, and also to drive standardized operational definitions of processes for staff. This increases the chances of having consistent output. The level of magnification of process mapping is determined by the objectives. However, to increase efficiency, productivity, and the identification of defects within processes, 'detailed' process maps are more beneficial.

When completing detailed process maps, it is critical to have a team of process experts. Typically, process experts are operations employees who perform such tasks on a daily basis. It is important that the team presents 'fearless candor' to each mapping session to derive the true picture of how processes are currently being performed. It is equally as important that the team feels valued as process experts, mapping objectives are clear, and expectations are set for both the mapping facilitator and team.

When instructing on how to map out processes, it is a good practice to ensure the team understands that steps that they provide are actual steps performed, and not steps quoted from standard operating procedures, as these may differ. The rationale for encouraging staff to provide the actual steps performed is to enable identification of real defects, wasted steps, possible non-conformances within processes, and steps not outlined in SOPs that should be.

Each identified process step will have an output (expected outcome). The operations team provides the expected outcomes for each process step. If steps are not yielding expected outcomes based on their specifications, defects within those process steps may be present. It is important to highlight or document questionable steps to identify potential defects, and ensure that necessary focus on such steps is paid when walking through the actual processes. After process outputs are identified, the team should be instructed to provide current inputs for each process step. In other words what inputs (resources) are used for each step within processes to yield the current outcomes?

To further drill down into processes with the mapping team, it might prove valuable to classify inputs by type. There are three input types: Controllable, which are variables that can be adjusted or controlled; Noise, which are variables that cannot be controlled (i.e. weather, humidity, etc.), and lastly; SOP, which are variables specifically defined and written to be part of processes. Non-conformances should be communicated to both the process owner and the quality management unit.

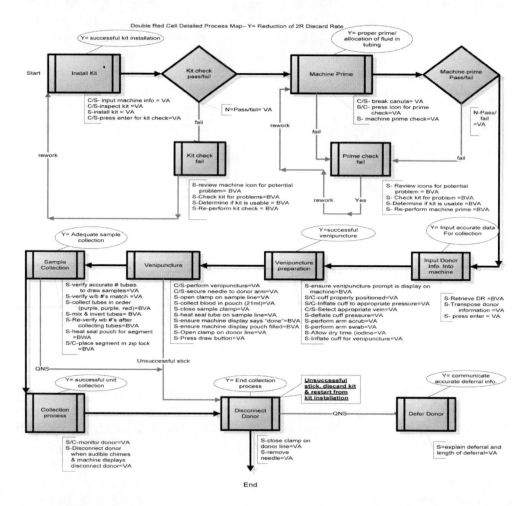

Figure 11. NVA activities flow.

Once input types are identified, to better understand the value of each input and/or to assist in spotlighting waste within processes, inputs may be labelled by their 'activity type'. There are three input activity types: Value added (VA) which are activities that, when left out of processes, will result in a failure to achieve expected outcomes. Business value added (BVA) inputs are mandated activities required by regulations and/or laws. The third activity type is non-value added (NVA). NVA activities do not add value to processes nor do they have an impact on outputs. It is probably safe to say that NVA activities are considered waste and depending on the identified inputs, they may have an impact on cycle times, costs for supplies and/or associated labour costs (Figure 11).

Following completion of process maps, the next step is to carefully walk through processes step by step in the actually operational units to ensure that the maps are accurate. It is important to identify any steps that were not stated to be part of the processes during the mapping sessions. It is also important to inquire about steps, already present or needed in addition, in order to obtain an understanding of input types and activities. Once identified and understood, all necessary steps should be added to detailed process maps accordingly.

While walking through processes, evaluate the steps previously identified as NVA steps. Determine and confirm that NVA steps have no impact on outputs. It is important to measure current impact (i.e. current cycle times). This will allow for more accurate assessments of the impact of process improvements. It is advisable to consult with process owners and propose the elimination of wasted steps and the data associated with such changes (e.g., time savings) to clearly illustrate increases in productivity.

Following the elimination of wasted steps, pre- versus post-cycle times and/or productivity (output) should be measured. The specifications (benchmark) for monitoring and sustainability of cycle times should be established.

Although process mapping can be used as a standalone tool to identify and eliminate waste and to determine the functions of process input and outputs, it is also used when applying Six Sigma principles. To further drill down on process breakdowns and true root causes, detailed process mapping lends itself to the initiation of techniques such as the Cause and Effects (C&E) Matrix, FMEA, and the development of control plans.

14.1. Cause and Effects Matrix

At times, repeated errors or events occur within processes when the root causes of those failures have not been definitively identified. Usually, such processes are not as robust as necessary to provide repeatability and reproducibility of expected outcomes. There are times when process owners feel that there is not enough time to more extensively pursue the identification of the true causes of process failures. With Six Sigma principles, Black Belts or Green Belts can further drill down to the causes of process failures by using the teams that were formed for the mapping of processes.

The C&E Matrix is used to determine the importance of process inputs to the ability to meet expected outcomes. The process inputs and outputs are derived from detailed process maps. It is helpful to visualize and prioritize the relationships and level of importance between several inputs versus several outputs. The C&E matrix uses a scoring system to determine that level of importance. A 1 through 10 scoring system, with 1 being the least important and 10 being the most important, is an example of such a scoring system; however, any scoring system can be used as long as it is comprehensive and understood by team members.

The C&E matrix identifies those inputs that have more or less of an impact on process outputs. When driving the use of a C&E matrix, the key question posed to team members is, "*How important is this input to that output*" by way of the scoring system. A simple example is, "*How important is gasoline to driving a car?*" Clearly, gasoline is necessary to successfully drive almost all automobiles; therefore, this question is likely to be scored very high by the team.

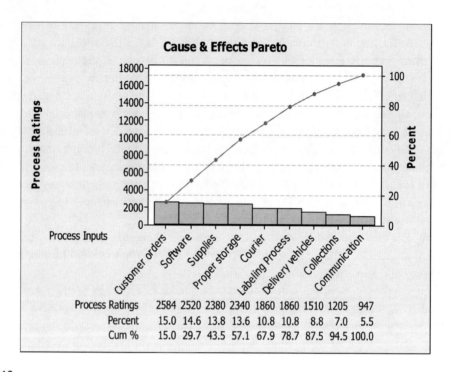

Process Ratings	2584	2520	2380	2340	1860	1860	1510	1205	947
Percent	15.0	14.6	13.8	13.6	10.8	10.8	8.8	7.0	5.5
Cum %	15.0	29.7	43.5	57.1	67.9	78.7	87.5	94.5	100.0

Figure 12.

Scores are based on the opinions of the process experts (team); therefore, they are subjective assessments. It is not the expectation that the scores will be reproducible; however, scores provided by true process experts can be remarkably similar in terms of the relative importance of the inputs being assessed. When a cross-functional team is used, scores may differ based on the assessed importance of inputs from each of the unique personal perspectives on the team. In such cases, rather than just averaging those scores, it is suggested that the differences be discussed and reconciled so a consensus score can be generated.

To eliminate the inputs that are not likely to impact on expected outcomes, a Pareto chart may be used with the principle that, after establishing the scores, 20% of the inputs affect 80% of the expected process outcomes (Figure 12). This allows teams to focus on the inputs that appear to have the highest impact on the failure of process outputs. Using these critical inputs, teams can focus their attention on possible failure modes, the effects of those failure modes, and the causes of those failures.

After identifying and exhausting the causes for failure of noted process inputs, teams are now in position to work on fixes. Once fixes are identified, it is highly recommended that pilot studies be conducted to measure pilot performance and compare results to initial performance baselines to assure that performance has improved. If improved performance is not realized, it may be necessary to perform FMEA.

14.2. Failure Mode and Effects Analysis

Failure Mode and Effects Analysis is used in a manner similar to the C&E diagram. Using the inputs previously identified as having the highest degrees of impact on process outputs, the team next identifies the ways in which inputs can go wrong (i.e., input failure modes).

After identifying possible failure modes, the team focuses on identifying possible failure effects and the causes of the failure modes. At this point, it may be necessary to provide examples of failure modes and failure effects. These can be confusing concepts and it is worthwhile to make sure the team understands the differences. An example of a failure mode is not manufacturing enough products. An example of a failure effect is not meeting customer demands. The cause of the failure mode and effect might be an inadequate number of employees. Typically after a few examples, the team understands the concepts and it becomes easier to repeat the steps while assessing the remaining inputs.

After identification of failure modes, failure effects and causes, the team is guided through a scoring exercise which ranks the severity of failure modes to customers (internal/external), the likelihood of their occurrence, and how well the causes of failure modes can be detected. Scoring allows for the delineation of the severity, frequency of occurrence, and the level of difficulty in detecting the causes of failures.

If standard spreadsheets are used when conducting FMEAs, the formulas used to calculate scores should be included in the spreadsheets for the three ratings (severity, occurrence, and detect ability) in order to arrive at a risk priority number. Risk priority numbers reflect the odds that causes of failure will not be caught until after failure modes and effects have occurred. The causes that drive risk priority numbers help determine what actions will be taken to correct the failures. The recommended actions should be documented on FMEA spreadsheets. The recommended actions should be piloted and post-implementation performance should be measured against baseline to gauge improvements. The actions piloted should be adjusted until significantly improved performance measurements are achieved on a consistent basis.

Conclusion

Event management is an organizational system that utilizes the information derived from the detection, reporting, and analysis of errors to improve performance and safety. It is an important component of the QSEs. A constructive approach to errors provides a major opportunity to gain knowledge (impact of errors on processes and vice versa) and foster continuous improvement. A major goal of event management is the prevention of recurrent errors.

Event management systems are most effective in organizations that incorporate and value the concepts of a Quality Culture. Such a culture is created when all levels of an organization, from leadership at the highest levels on down to the front-line personnel, all share the same commitment to quality. An environment where every employee assumes responsibility for the quality of the organization's products and services can thus be created. Organizations with a maximally functioning Quality Culture view error detection, analysis, and the actions taken from this information as a major opportunity for performance improvements and enhanced safety. It is important for organizations to clearly communicate to employees the expectation that errors, deviations, non-conformances and failures will be reported and documented promptly upon discovery.

Strong event management systems have well-defined processes for addressing errors that allow organizations to use the information for performance improvement. A feature that is critical to the success of such systems is the creation of an atmosphere that fosters open, honest, and complete error reporting, including self reporting. This necessitates that error reporting programs be non-punitive. Complete reporting will only occur if employees are allowed to take the appropriate actions without fear of adverse personal consequences.

A commitment to safety can be adopted as a crucial component of an organization's Quality Culture. Organizations with a commitment to safety have employees driven to practice safe behaviours to protect patients every day. As part of the safety culture, much attention is paid to errors that could potentially occur, which provides an opportunity to be proactive and prevent their occurrence. Furthermore, a culture of safety encourages the reporting and analysis of near-misses, as these also serve as a 'fertile ground' of information that can be used to enhance performance and safety. The lack of inclusion of near-misses in event management represents a significant lost opportunity for improvement. The core of a commitment to safety consists of five safe behaviours: Pay attention to detail, communicate clearly, have a questioning and receptive attitude, handoff effectively, and support each other. If all employees are committed to practice the five safe behaviours, a culture of safety becomes an integral part of an organization.

In addition to the cultures of quality and safety, many organizations have implemented a Fair and Just Culture. In a Fair and Just Culture, individuals are held accountable for their actions, the assignment of blame is typically avoided, and the type of behaviour exhibited in association with errors or deviations dictates the type of follow-up actions undertaken. There are three categories of error-related behaviour in a Fair and Just Culture: human error/inadvertent action, risk behaviour, and reckless behaviour. The type of behaviour drives the organizational response to the employee (ranging from consolation, to coaching, to disciplinary actions).

There are a number of tools and techniques available to enhance the effectiveness of event management systems.

- Electronic reporting systems direct the users to provide important information, decrease the incidence of incomplete reports, reduce the time required for report completion, improve data searching capabilities and report generation, and enable process improvement interventions to be more timely.
- CAPA consists of three activities: remedial corrections of identified problems, root cause analyses with corrective actions, and preventive actions that play critical roles in event management;

- Human Factors, the study of human capabilities and limitations, can be used to reduce errors, increase safety, and increase overall employee performance. A fundamental goal of HF is to create an environment where it is 'easy to do the right thing and hard to do the wrong thing';
- Mistake-proofing consists of techniques designed to keep errors from causing harm or to make processes resistant to errors. Prevention-based mistake-proofing utilizes actions taken to prevent anticipated errors while a process moves forward. In detection-based mistake-proofing, abnormalities resulting in errors are discovered at the time of their occurrence and corrective actions occur as a response;
- Performance Management focuses on consequences of behaviour, in particular the use of positive reinforcement, to influence human performance in the workplace. PM techniques stimulate employees to 'want to' perform at higher, desirable levels;
- Causal Tree Analysis is used to identify all the factors that must be present for events to occur. CTA illustrates how relationships between these factors (e.g., human error + equipment failure) come together to cause events.

Event management-related process improvements can be difficult to maintain long-term unless appropriate actions and activities are utilized to keep them going. Control plans, reaction plans, communication plans, training plans, audit plans, and statistical process control are tools that can help sustain improved processes over the long run. The success of these tools hinges on continued management reinforcement of process changes and the specification limits to which employees will be held accountable. Employees also require a clear understanding of the tools used for monitoring performance. Effective communication is a crucial component of long-term sustainability of process improvements. The chances of success are also increased when Six Sigma becomes an integral part of an organization's everyday operations.

Process mapping, a graphical representation of process steps, is another important tool available for use in event management. Mapping processes often result in process improvements. There are three types of activities identified though process mapping: value added, business value added, and non-value added. Deeper investigations of the root causes of process defects can lead to the use of Cause and Effects Matrix, Failure Mode and Effects Analysis, and the construction of a control plan.

15.1. Message to Take Home

Event management is a crucial component the quality programs in organizations committed to safety and continuous performance improvement. Effective event management requires a top to bottom philosophical and resource commitment in order to be successful. Sustained success will not occur without such commitment. In those organizations driven to achieve sustained success in the area of event management, there are many tools and techniques outlined in this chapter that can be used to achieve maximal organizational safety and performance. Constructive event management systems help to drive organizations towards higher levels of safety and performance, which advances the overall quality of patient care. It is the right thing to do. Please join our cultures of quality and safety!

References

[1]   Taswell HF, Sonnenberg CL. Error analysis: types of error in the blood bank. In: Smit Sibinga CTh, Taswell HF eds. *Quality Assurance in Blood Banking and Its Clinical Impact*. Dordrecht: Martinus Nijhoff Publishers; 1984:227-237.

[2]   Motschman TL, Santrach PJ, Moore SB. Error/incident management and its practical applications. In: Duckett JB, Woods LL, Santrach PJ, eds. *Quality in Action*. Bethesda MD: American Association of Blood Banks; 1996:26-37.

[3]   Crosby PB. Keeping neat records of noncompliance is not quality. ASQ-Quality Progress; 1997 May [cited 2012 August 7]. Available from: URL: *http://asq/qualityprogress/past-issues/index/index.html?fromYYYY=1997&fromMM= 05&index=1.*

[4]   21 CFR 606.171(b) in: *Code of Federal Regulations, Title 21,* Food and Drugs. National Archives and Records Administration, Office of the Federal Register. US Food & Drug Administration. Silver Spring, MD: 2012

[5]   Standard 7.0. In: *Standards for Blood Banks and Transfusion Services*, 28th edition. AABB. Bethesda, MD: 2011: pages 79-83.

[6]   Kiekkas P. The role of non-blaming culture in learning from errors. *Nurs Crit Care.* 2011; 16:3-4. doi: 10.1111/j.1478-5153.2010.00439.x.

[7]   Moore SB, Foss ML. Error Management: Theory and Application in Transfusion Medicine at a Tertiary-Care Institution. *Arch Pathol Lab Med.* 2003; 127(11):1517-22.

[8]   Valentin A. Patient safety – an essential paradigm in intensive care medicine. In: Flaaten H, Moreno R, Putensen C, Rhodes A, (eds), *Organization and Management of Intensive Care*. Berlin: 2010 Medizinisch Wissenschaftliche Verlagsgesellschaft, 351–358.

[9]   Mayo Clinic Commitment to Safety: Safe Behaviours. Rochester (MN): Mayo Foundation for Medical Education and Research; c2010 [cited 2012 Aug 1]. Available from: *http://intranet.mayo.edu/charlie/commitment-to-safety/safety-habits/* *[internal access only]*

[10]   Foss ML, Stubbs JR, Jones, G. Integrating Quality, Education, Lean, and Performance Management into a culture of continuous improvement. *Transfusion* 2011; 51:1598-1603.

[11]   Guidance for Industry - Quality Systems Approach to Pharmaceutical CGMP Regulations. Rockville (MD): Food and Drug Administration: Pharmaceutical CGMPs. 2006. Available from: *http://www.fda.gov/downloads/Drugs/GuidanceComplianc eRegulatoryInformation/Guidances/UCM070337.pdf*

[12]   Plan-Do-Check-Act (PDCA) Cycle. Milwaukee (WI): American Society for Quality. Excerpted from Nancy R. Tague's The Quality Toolbox, Second Edition, ASQ Quality Press, 2004, pages 390-392. Available from: *http://asq.org/learn-about-quality/project-planning-tools/overview/pdca-cycle.html*

[13]   FAA Human Factors Awareness Web Course: Wickens' Model of Human Information Processing. US Dept. of Transportation, Federal Aviation Association; c2010 [cited 2012 Aug 20] Available from: *http://www.hf.faa.gov/webtraining/Cognition/Cog Final008.htm*

[14] Wickens CD, Gordon SE, Liu Y. In: Wickens cd, Gordon se, Liu Y, eds: *An Introduction to Human Factors Engineering*. Harlow, NY: Pearson Longman. 1997: p.275.

[15] Freivalds A, Niebel B. Design of Cognitive Work In: Freivalds and Niebel (eds): *Niebel's Methods, Standards, and Work Design.* 12th edition McGraw-Hill Science/Engineering/Math; 2008: pages 273-317.

[16] Grout J. Mistake-proofing the design of health care processes. (Prepared under an IPA with Berry College). AHRQ Publication No. 07-0020. Rockville, MD: Agency for Healthcare Research and Quality; May 2007. Available at*: http://www.ahrq.gov /qual/mistakeproof/mistakeproofing.pdf*

[17] Mayo Clinic Quality Academy: Mistake Proofing. Rochester (MN): Mayo Foundation for Medical Education and Research; c2012 [cited 2012 Aug 22] Available from: *http://mayoweb.mayo.edu/quality-learning/tc-dmaic.html [internal access only].*

[18] Frankel AS, Leonard MW, Denham CR. *Fair and Just Culture, Team Behaviour, and Leadership Engagement: The Tools to Achieve High Reliability. Health Serv Res.* 2006 August; 41(4 Pt 2): 1690–1709. doi: 10.1111/j.1475-6773.2006.00572.x

[19] Mayo Clinic Commitment to Safety: Fair and Just Culture Overview. Rochester (MN): Mayo Foundation for Medical Education and Research; c2012 [cited 2012 Aug 1]. Available *from: http://intranet.mayo.edu/charlie/commitment-to-safety/files /2011/09 /Overview.pdf* [internal access only].

[20] California Hospital Patient Safety Organization: Just Culture. c2012 [cited 2012, Aug 1] Available from: *http://www.chpso.org/just/index.php.*

[21] Marx D. *Patient Safety and the "Just Culture": A Primer for Health Care Executives.* Medical Event Reporting System for Transfusion Medicine. New York: Trustees of Columbia University in the City of New York; c2001. [cited 2012 Aug 16]. Available from: *http://www.unmc.edu/rural/patient-safety/tools/Marx%20Patient%20Safety%20 and%20Just%20Culture.pdf.*

[22] Leonard M, Graham S, Bonaum D. *The human factor: the critical importance of effective teamwork and communication in providing safe care. Qual Saf Health Care.* October 2004; 13(Suppl 1): i85-i90. doi: 10.1136/qshc.2004.010033

[23] Mayo Clinic Program in Professionalism and Ethics: Teamwork is REAL. Rochester (MN): Mayo Foundation for Medical Education and Research; c2012 [cited 2012 Aug 1]. *Available from: http://mayoweb.mayo.edu/professionalism/teamwork-real.html* [internal access only].

[24] Daniels AC. Performance Management: Improving Quality Productivity through Positive Reinforcement. In: Daniels AC, ed. *Performance Management Publications*; 3rd edition Tucker (GA): 2004: 23-24.

[25] Institute for Healthcare Improvement: Improving Patient Safety by Incorporating Human Factors. Circa 2006 [cited 2012 Aug 20]. Available from: *http://www.ihi.org/IHI/Topics/PatientSafety/MedicationSystems/ ImprovementStories/ImprovingPatientSafetybyIncorporatingHuman Factor .html*

[26] Shappell SA; Wiegmann DA. Human Factors Analysis and Classification System. c2000 [cited 2012 Aug 1]. Available at: *http://www.nifc.gov/fireInfo/fireInfo_ documents /humanfactors_classAnly.pdf*

[27] Shappel S, Wiegmann D. Developing a Methodology for Assessing Safety Programs Targeting Human Error in Aviation. Federal Aviation Administration. Nov 2006 [cited 2012 Aug 20]. Available from *http://www.dtic.mil/cgi-bin/GetTRDoc?AD=ADA461400*

[28] Risk-Based Decision-Making Guidelines, Volume 3: *Procedures for Assessing Risks: Applying Risk Assessment Tools,* Chapter 11: Fault Tree Analysis (FTA). Circa 2007 [cited 2012 Aug 20]. Available at: *http://www.ceet.niu.edu/tech/asse/tech482 /Chapter_11_Fault_Tree_Analysis.pdf*

[29] Lalli VR, Packard MH. NASA, Lewis Research Center Office of Safety, Environmental & Mission Assurance: Design for Reliability. Circa 2000 [cited 2012 Aug 1]. Available from: *http://paso.esa.int/5_training _materials/training_09_reliability%20course.pdf*

[30] *Institute of Transfusion Medicine Six Sigma Program – Chicago, IL/Pittsburgh PA. Circa 2007* [cited 2012 Aug 24] Internal access only.

In: Quality Management in Transfusion Medicine
Editor: Cees Th. Smit Sibinga

ISBN: 978-1-62618-665-1
© 2013 Nova Science Publishers, Inc.

Chapter VIII

Organizational Roles, Responsibilities and Change Management in Support of Quality Systems[1]

Th. Hein Smit Sibinga[*1] *and Jay S. Epstein*[†2]

[1]Constitution Medical, Inc., Boston, MA, US

[2]Office of Blood Research and Review, Center for Biologics Evaluation and Research, Food and Drug Administration, Rockville, MD, US

Abstract

Protection of patients against the inherent risks of blood transfusion necessitates a comprehensive system of science-based safeguards. Consequently, in the more developed countries, blood banking has evolved to become either a highly regulated enterprise, which operates under well-defined standards and controls [1-7] or fully under government control as part of a national healthcare system. Consistently, in many countries, blood collection and processing are regulated on the pharmaceutical model of drug manufacturing rather than treated as a practice of medicine. [2-10] This includes requirements for standard operating procedures, document control, process validation, and outcome measurements, including quality control testing. [2-10] Within the blood bank, a Quality Programme plays an essential role to assure compliance with applicable standards and regulations. Furthermore, it provides the framework in which change can be managed without compromising the integrity of the blood system. The Pyramid Model of Quality Management defines five key roles that ensure an organization will deliver outputs consistent with expectations. These roles include Operations, Quality Control,

---

[1] Note: This chapter reflects the views of the authors and should not be construed to represent the views or policies of the US Food and Drug Administration.

[*] Director, Product Development, Constitution Medical, Inc., 186 Lincoln Street, 3rd Floor Boston, MA 02111, US, E-mail: smitsibinga@yahoo.com, Tel: +1-781 704 3321

[†] Director, Office of Blood Research and Review, Center for Biologics Evaluation and Research , Food and Drug Administration, HFM-300 ,1401 Rockville Pike, Rockville, MD 20852, US, Tel: +1-301-827-3518, E-mail: jay.epstein@fda.hhs.gov.

Quality Assurance, Audits and Compliance/Regulatory. The case for change and the programme for change are addressed in the context of the quality system.

Keywords: Blood banking, cGMPs, Quality management, Quality Pyramid Model, Change programme

1. Introduction

Blood transfusion is an essential therapy that saves lives in acute emergencies, improves quality of life in numerous medical conditions and enables many complex medical and surgical procedures. The banking of blood components for use in transfusion permits maintenance of a relatively stable blood inventory to address expected needs, rather than a system based on urgent collections driven by medical emergencies. Over the past several decades, blood banking in developed countries has evolved from small-scale hospital based collections to more centralized blood collection systems in which millions of blood units collected from altruistic volunteers unrelated to specific patients are shipped to multiple hospitals where the blood is stored pending release for transfusion. [1, 11, 12] In some cases, blood collection was established for military needs. [11, 12] In addition, the procedures for selection of low risk donors, safety testing of donations, blood collection per se, processing into components, storage conditions, labelling, blood grouping and cross-matching for transfusion all have greatly evolved. [2-7]

Recognition of the need to control the inherent risks associated with products manufactured for blood transfusion has prompted some countries to require blood banks to adopt a pharmaceutical approach to blood products, whereby the steps in preparation of blood components are seen as manufacturing steps subject to standardization and quality control within an overall system of quality management. [2-7] Today blood collection includes donor education and consent; donor selection based on epidemiologic risk factors for blood borne infections; laboratory testing at a minimum for HIV, hepatitis B and C, and syphilis (and other infectious risks such as HTLV, Chagas disease and West Nile Virus in some regions); processing of blood into multiple components including a variety of manipulations to reduce risk (e.g. leukocyte reduction, pathogen reduction in some jurisdictions, irradiation); quarantine of units pending results of donor screening and testing; quality control testing; investigation of process failures; comprehensive data management for traceability; and haemovigilance monitoring and reporting. [2-7] Current Good Manufacturing Practices (cGMPs) have been applied to blood establishments throughout their operations including the collection and processing of blood and blood components. [2-7] National laws and regulations provide a general framework for cGMPs in blood collection. [2-7] More specific information on how to comply with cGMPs most often is provided in guidance.

Achieving consistent quality across the organization depends to a large degree on achieving a quality focused culture, well documented processes and systems, and implementation of an organizational model designed to support the organization's quality needs. Supporting programs such as those based on Six Sigma, Lean, continuous education and performance management then drive the entire organization towards continuous improvement.

Error detection, Corrective and Preventive Action (CAPA), issue prevention, education, regulations, Six Sigma and daily productivity all need to be balanced for the blood centre to consistently meet its objectives. To do so effectively, a clear infrastructure with well-defined roles and responsibilities needs to be established and maintained. The most appropriate structure and operating principles depend on the organization's needs, maturity, culture and many other factors. An overarching quality management strategy that describes how the organization will achieve its mission and vision with respect to quality management is central to establishing and maintaining continuous improvement. This chapter reviews organizational quality management considerations and provides insight in the steps needed to successfully build-out an integrated quality improvement infrastructure. Additionally, we will examine key organizational considerations and change management principles required to establish a sustainable quality management culture.

1.1. Evolution of Quality Management in Blood Banking

Early in its history, transfusion was viewed primarily as a medical practice used by physicians to treat their patients. As a result of medical needs arising from World War I and World War II, collection and transfusion of blood and blood components became more widespread. [11, 12] Physicians returning from the war expected blood to be available for transfusion in the civilian setting. [11, 12] Over time, centralized community-based blood collection centres were established that could meet the demands of multiple hospitals, lessening the burdens on individual hospitals while creating specialization in donor recruitment, blood collection and component preparation. [1, 11, 12] Standards for blood collection and processing were established. In many countries existing drug laws were applied to blood collection, while in other countries new laws specific to blood collection were introduced. [2-10] National authorities have issued regulations or general standards for blood collection, as well as guidance documents explaining these requirements and how they should be met. [2-10] In addition, professional organizations representing blood collectors or transfusion services were established. [12] These organizations also issued standards and accredited blood banks. [12] Advances in technology resulted in the availability of new blood collection systems and new types of blood components. The advances also resulted in greater complexity in blood collection, including new donor screening tests and testing systems. Additionally, many blood centers have expanded their business models in recent years. In particular, many blood collection centers now are involved in preparation of haematopoietic stem cells by aphaeresis of peripheral blood and in banking of cord blood. [13]

Quality management has also evolved in blood banking. In the US, during the 1980s, a blood bank's quality management was comprised mainly of quality control functions (e.g. performance of in- process controls and equipment maintenance) carried out as an additional responsibility by a technologist. As new scientific and technological advances improved the safety of transfusion products (e.g., improved assays to detect blood borne diseases; automated high through-put test platforms; computer assisted donor history taking), the understanding of effective quality management also advanced. By the mid-1990s blood bankers that formerly held that they provided a medical service were told by regulators that they were manufacturers of a drug product. Cognizant of the post World War II quality assurance advances that were applied successfully in many industrial settings, the Food and

Drug Administration began to require that quality management systems in blood establishments should go beyond just quality control functions. Blood bankers and their professional organizations were soon leading the way in the use of modern quality assurance tools such as CAPA, root cause analysis, quality assurance oversight independent of those performing the manufacturing tasks, oversight of written SOPs and of training, a focus on systems, quality audits etc.

1.2. The Need for National Blood Regulation

In the wake of the AIDS tragedy, the risk of transfusion transmitted disease has become an increasingly important public health concern. Increasingly recognized threats from hepatitis viruses and from emerging infectious diseases such as West Nile Virus and vCJD in some regions have intensified these concerns. [2-7] In response, health policy makers around the world have adopted aggressive safety measures that minimize risks. [2-7] However, though well established in some countries, global progress in blood quality, safety and availability has evolved slowly despite recognition of the need by the WHO World Health Assembly (WHA) in 1975. Most recently in 2010, the WHA adopted resolution 63.12 noting *"the unequal access globally to blood products, particularly plasma-derived medicinal products, leaving many patients in need of transfusion and with severe congenital and acquired disorders without treatment"* and that *"unsafe and/or poor-quality blood products can render patients vulnerable to avoidable risk if the blood programmes are not subject to the level of control now exercised by experienced national or regional regulatory authorities."* The WHA therefore urged Member States to *"take all necessary steps to update their national regulations on donor assessment and deferral, the collection, testing, processing, storage, transportation and use of blood products, and operation of regulatory authorities in order to ensure that regulatory control in the area of quality and safety of blood products across the entire transfusion chain meets internationally recognized standards."* Under this resolution, the global need for strengthening of national regulatory authorities to promote international standards for blood products has been recognized for the first time. In parallel, at the request of the WHO, its Blood Regulators Network developed 'Assessment Criteria for National Blood Regulatory Systems' that WHO has since published after consideration of public comments. [15] These criteria are intended to assist countries in carrying out internal or external assessments of their system.

1.3. The Role of Current Good Manufacturing Practices in Blood Establishments

A major effort of both blood establishments and blood regulators worldwide has been the development and adoption of current Good Manufacturing Practices (cGMPs) which define the quality standards for blood product manufacturing. Regulatory requirements for cGMPs in blood collection and processing exist in many countries [2-10] and a Guideline is available at a WHO website (http://www.who.int/bloodproducts/brn/en/). Under these requirements, and in a manner similar to pharmaceutical products, blood establishments must follow cGMPs in the manufacture of blood components.

cGMPs are based on statutory requirements that are further explained in regulations and guidance. [2-10] For example, under U.S. laws, blood is considered to be a drug, as well as, a biologic. [8]. Under the U.S. Food, Drug and Cosmetic Act (FD&C Act), a drug is adulterated if "*the methods used in, or the facilities or controls used for, its manufacture, processing, packing, and holding do not conform to or are not operated or administered in conformity with current good manufacturing practice to assure that such drug meets the requirements*" of the FD&C Act. [8] In the U.S., blood is subject to premarket approval as a biologic product under the United States Public Health Service Act (8) when it is introduced or delivered for introduction into interstate commerce. In addition, FDA regulated blood and blood components are subject to the general cGMPs and blood specific cGMPs. Similarly, the European Union adopted Directive 2002/98/EC setting standards of quality and safety for the collection, testing, processing, storage and distribution of human blood and blood components [3] to "*ensure that blood and its components are of comparable quality and safety throughout the blood transfusion chain in all Member states*" as well as Commission Directive 2005/62/EC of 30 September 2005. [16] The latter Directive includes standards and specifications for a quality system for blood establishments. The European and U.S. requirements show broad overlap in specifics and in intent. Other countries have also developed standards for blood collection. [4, 5]

U.S. regulations applicable to cGMP in the manufacture of drugs, including blood and blood components, can be found in section 21 of the U.S. Code of Federal Regulations (CFR) at 21 CFR Part 211 and more specific blood component requirements at 21 CFR Part 606. These provisions have the force of law and establish a framework for blood component manufacturing, providing both general and specific requirements for blood collection, processing and testing. A sampling of the applicable FDA regulations includes the following:

Section 606.20 – Personnel	Includes requirements that personnel involved in blood collection must be adequate in number and have the educational background and training to perform their assigned functions
Section 606.40 Plant and facilities	Includes requirements that the facility must be of suitable size, location and construction for its purpose
Section 606.60 Equipment	Equipment includes requirements that "*equipment shall be observed, standardized and calibrated on a regularly scheduled basis as prescribed in the Standard Operating Procedures Manual and shall perform in the manner for which it was designed so as to assure compliance with the official requirements prescribed in this chapter for blood and blood products.*"
Section 606.100 Standard Operating Procedures	Includes a requirement for written standard operating procedures to be maintained "*for all steps to be followed in the collection, processing, compatibility testing, storage, and distribution of blood and blood components for transfusion and further manufacturing purposes.*" It also requires that these "*procedures be available to the personnel for use in the areas where the procedures are performed.*"
Section 606.120-122 Labelling standards	Includes labelling requirements for the container label and the circular of information
Section 606.140 Laboratory controls	Includes a requirement for "*scientifically sound and appropriate specifications, standards and test procedures to assure that blood and blood components are safe, pure, potent and effective.*"
Section 606.160-171 Records and reporting responsibilities	These sections include requirements for concurrent records for each step in the production of the component, records of product distribution, and records of adverse events including the investigation of the event. These sections also require reporting to the FDA donor or transfusion related fatalities as well as product deviations related to distributed product.
Sec. 211.22 Responsibilities of quality control unit	Requires that manufacturers of drug products, such as blood for transfusion, have a quality control unit with "*the responsibility and authority to approve or reject all components, drug product containers, closures, in-process materials, packaging material, labelling, and drug products, and the authority to review production records to assure that no errors have occurred or, if errors have occurred, that they have been fully investigated.*"

1.4. Managing Change in Blood Banking

In order to ensure blood safety, many regulatory authorities have established a multi-layered system of protections in blood component manufacturing. In addition to component processing standards per se (i.e. skin disinfection, sterile collection containers, functionally closed system separations, etc.), these safeguards include donor selection, laboratory testing for transfusion transmissible viruses, and quarantine inventories pending a final determination of product suitability. However, blood banking is an evolving science and practice in which changes take place inevitably. Changes occur for many reasons including new collection equipment, new types of blood components, new infectious disease tests, facility or information systems changes, and new methods for blood grouping, typing, and compatibility testing. Many of the changes that have occurred in blood establishments have been the result of changes in donor screening criteria, donor testing for markers of transfusion transmissible infections and automation.

Blood establishments must assure that the changes accomplish the intended goals without unintended consequences, which might adversely affect the ability to provide safe blood when and where it is needed. The implementation of new test methods, information systems, and new or modified manufacturing processes all share common change control challenges – document control; validation; training; and monitoring via outcome measures. In addition to self-initiated changes, there are many parties outside the blood establishment with the authority to mandate change, including government regulators, third-party payers, certifying organizations, or additional authorities within the larger health care organization. Some changes require regulatory agency notification or amendment to a product approval prior to implementation, as is the case in the US. [17] Regardless of the source or circumstance that dictates the need for change, the change itself must be managed effectively.

Many countries have laws regarding the procedures to be followed when making changes to an approved blood product. In this sense, regulatory oversight is part of a system of change control in blood banking. More specifically, blood regulations often require that blood establishments should have and maintain a quality management programme within which change can be implemented in an orderly manner that assures validation of new or modified processes, proper implementation and complete documentation. The importance of quality management cannot be disregarded when it comes to maintaining blood product safety. Quality management ensures appropriate management, standardization of processes, and a cultural expectation of continuous improvement. [18]

A significant challenge in the midst of all these developments has been how to manage and control changes. Change control processes must ensure a smooth, well-documented transition from the old to the new. During preparation for the change, the execution of the change and after the change there should be sufficient supporting data to demonstrate that the revised process will result in a product of the desired quality, consistent with the approved specifications. [19]

The core requirements for managing change in the blood bank include:

- Document control,
- Validation, and
- Training.

Document Control

The highly regulated world of blood banking dictates that all processes are documented concurrently with the performance of the task ('say what you will do and do what you say'). Thus, any change in a process must be accompanied by a change in the written documentation with a history of all changes. To accomplish this, there needs to be a system in place for how documents are modified or created. Most facilities will even have a procedure on how to write a procedure including the following elements:

- Proper format – what is the document lay-out?; what sections are required?; how are review and approval documented (both initial and periodic review)?
- Change control – who can request a change?; how could the change impact other processes (i.e., risks of unintended consequences)?; who approves the change?; and how is the change request processed and evaluated?
- Version control – what mechanism is employed to ensure that the current version of the document is available?; and how and for how long are obsolete documents archived?
- Implementation – how are the changes made effective? This step is the culmination of all the other activities, and defines the official transition to the new or modified procedure.

Validation

Validation is the "confirmation, through the provision of objective evidence, that the requirements for a specific intended use or application have been fulfilled". [20] Validation is not a one-time activity but a series of activities taking place over the lifecycle of a process. Documented procedures are required to address validation activities in respect to evaluation of effects of a change and the extent of revalidation. Many approaches to process validation are divided into three stages:

- Develop the process design;
- Validate the process design through process qualification to determine if it is capable of reproducible results without negatively affecting other processes;
- Continual monitoring and evaluation to verify that the process remains in a state of control.

The goal of process design is to develop a process that can consistently deliver a product that meet its quality attributes. Documentation should include essential activities and decisions made in regard to the process. This information is beneficial during the process qualification, and continual monitoring and evaluation stages.

The process must be validated to ensure that the desired outcome is achieved without any unintended consequences. A crucial step in this stage is to determine the criteria that will be used to determine a successful qualification. This qualification stage is usually performed prior to full-scale implementation of the new or changed process. During this stage, the actual facility, equipment, procedures, and trained personnel, are utilized to conduct the validation – hence this step tests the entire process in the production environment. A successful qualification will confirm the process design and demonstrate that the process performs as expected.

Before implementation of the process organization-wide, a formalized program for the collection and analysis of data related to product quality must be implemented. Quality indicators that can be used to verify that the process remains in control include use of release criteria and monitoring trends and recognizing drift before things are out of control. Statistical trending and review of the quality indicators should be accomplished by trained personnel and reported to the appropriate personnel within the organization. Appropriate action should be taken based on the analysis of the data to promote continual process improvement and to re-enforce management's commitment to quality assurance. Monitoring product quality ensures that a state of control is maintained throughout the process lifecycle. This provides assurance of the continued ability of the process and in-process controls to meet the desired quality of the product and to identify changes that may improve the process. [21,22]

The output of continual monitoring and analysis of collected data are the process's outcome measurements. A robust measurement process that focuses on the critical steps of a process is integral to knowing where to allocate resources and also provides an indication of where change is necessary. A viable measurement process provides real-time data on how processes are operating, and offers indications of problem areas and areas for improvement. Without objective data, effective continual improvement is a 'shot in the dark'. A quality measurement process can encompass different tools, depending on the maturity of the quality assurance program.

Training

Training is a critical process in managing change. It is not appropriate to hold personnel accountable for a new or modified process without first providing adequate training. As has been mentioned previously, all processes should be documented and training is no exception. When establishing a training program, the following should be considered:

- Method of conducting the training – when is traditional classroom training required?; is training via self-study acceptable for a minor change?; and who determines the method of training?
- Document / track training – who is responsible for recording and tracking completed training?; what mechanism (i.e., electronic or paper) is used to track the training?; and does a supervisor need to review and approve all completed training prior to a person being considered 'competent' to perform the task?
- Determine competency – how is competency demonstrated (i.e., written quiz, observation of task, verbal questions)?; what is an acceptable passing score for competency?; who administers the competency test; and who determines acceptability?

Resistance to Change

Those that undertake the task of a 'change agent' must recognize that it is human nature to resist change. Success in managing change requires attention to the human factors operating in the workplace. A significant proportion of changes that are introduced do not reach their full potential – that is, they are not fully implemented or do not produce the benefits envisioned. Changes usually don't fail because of technical reasons, such as something inherently flawed about the change itself. They usually fail for human reasons: the change agent did not take into account the real and predictable reactions of people to alteration of their routines. People don't resist change' so much as they resist 'being changed'. [23]

Therefore, the charge of change management relies heavily on clear and open communication (listening empathetically, convincing others of the need for change). Communicating the goals of the change and the benefits to the affected people will hopefully cultivate readiness instead of resistance to the change. Equally important is having people become integrally involved in designing and implementing the change thereby promoting ownership of the change. [24]

1.5. Design and Implementation of the Quality Programme

Various chapters in this book cover the how and why of key quality programmes which are required for a successful quality management programme. In most cases, one will find that a comprehensive programme is warranted that integrates a wide array of quality management tools and initiatives. This chapter focuses on the roles and responsibilities that are essential to a comprehensive quality management programme.

In order to achieve an effective and sustainable quality programme, the management team should consider whether a holistic approach to quality management is warranted, and if so, whether this can take the form of implementing select topics, or a more fundamental change programme is warranted. Examples of questions to consider include: is the reporting structure effective, are the information management systems appropriate for the needs of the organization (even if paper-based), is there an appropriate quality culture, how good is the organization and preventing recurrence of error.

What should the quality management structure be, what should it 'feel' like, and what initiatives will be needed to transform the current organization towards the future state. Are there intermediate steps, short and long term programmes? How will the organization build and celebrate success? Which projects allow the organization to try out new quality management tools and build expertise and ownership?

2. The Pyramid Quality Management Model

In the medical device, diagnostics and pharmaceutical industries, various organizational models for quality management are in use. The specific needs of the organization, culture, mission and organizational structure help determine how the quality system is structured. The Pyramid model (Figure 1) is a common depiction of the quality management roles within an organization. To better reflect the supporting role of quality and compliance, we have drawn the pyramid with the point down; The Quality, audit and regulatory functions are there to help the organization consistently meet its performance and productivity goals.

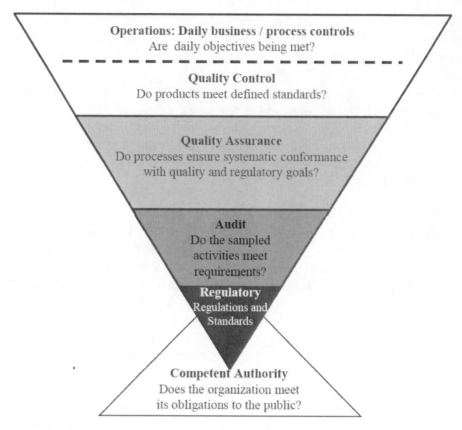

Figure 1. The Quality Pyramid model.

The Pyramid model defines five key roles involved in ensuring that the organization delivers to expectations. Each of these will be discussed in more detail below.

- Operations, which deploys business and process controls to achieve the daily objectives of the organization;
- Quality Control, either integral to operations or as in the form of an independent function, helps ensure that quality and safety of individual products and services are safeguarded for instance through batch release or statistical/time based sampling;
- Quality Assurance is typically independent from operations, and has a more strategic perspective than Quality Control. The Quality Assurance unit typically takes a leadership role in analysing trends, coordinating improvement initiatives, assuring that processes are documented and adhered to by trained personnel;
- Audit function is often, but not necessarily integral to quality assurance. This function evaluates whether the organization performs in accordance with both documented processes and accepted industry standards;
- Compliance/Regulatory is responsible for managing the interface with regulatory bodies and ensuring that new rules and regulations are implemented in a timely manner.

Depending on the company or department, two or more of these functions may be grouped together. In most industries, the Quality Assurance and Audit functions are independent from Operations.

- Operations oriented functions (whether recruitment, the laboratory or distribution) form the basis to delivering to expectations. To perform consistently operations need qualified personnel, infrastructure and defined processes. From a quality metrics perspective, operations should be focused on managing efficiency, effectiveness and productivity related objectives. Depending on the nature of the business, cost, speed and quality need to be brought into balance.

- Quality Control: *"The operational techniques and activities undertaken to verify that the requirements for quality of the process related activities have been fulfilled"*[2]

- Quality Control helps ensure that each delivered product meets quality and compliance requirements. Depending on the nature of the process, quality control may be integral to operations or be independent from operations, possibly reporting through Quality Assurance. For instance batch release of pharmaceuticals is often controlled through an independent QC group, whereas in-process quality controls for medical device manufacturing are frequently controlled by manufacturing.

In the blood centre, the approach to quality control might vary by department. For instance quality control for donor motivation may be integral to the motivation function, whereas final release of product is governed by quality assurance.

- Quality Assurance: "Planned and Systematic activities to ensure that the process is performed and documented in compliance with applicable standards and regulations" Quality Assurance is typically independent from operations. The mission of quality assurance is to ensure that processes ensure systematic conformance with internal quality and external compliance goals. For this reason, quality assurance organizations tend to have a strong focus on improving operations processes. Six Sigma [25], TQM and Lean [26] all evolved from the continuous drive towards process improvement[3]. In addition to it's core responsibilities, most quality assurance organization also cover key roles such as administration of training programmes and documentation control.

- Audit: "Independent examination to determine whether the sampled process related activities were conducted, recorded, analyzed and reported according to applicable rules and regulations."
  In small to medium size organizations, audit is integral to the Quality Assurance group, whereas large organization may have a separate, Audit and Inspection management. Through detail examination of recorded evidence, it provides an

---

[2] Definition from the International Conference on Harmonization (ICH) of technical requirements for registration of pharmaceuticals in human use - Good Clinical Practice (GCP) guidelines (ICH-GCP) definition.

[3] Total Quality Management dates back to the 1980s and early 1990s. It is often seen as a predecessor to Six Sigma. Six Sigma incorporates a series of structured, data driven tools and techniques aimed primarily at improving success through continuous improvement of quality. Lean on the other hand finds its roots in a drive to reduce waste, whether in the form of resources, effort or time. Lean and Six Sigma are not mutually exclusive, when used together in the form of lean six sigma, a sustainable balance between cost and efficiency can be found.

indication of whether the organization is operating in compliance with applicable standards, rules and regulations. Within the context of this chapter, we will reserve the term Audit for internal audits, performed by or on behalf of the organization itself. We will use Inspection for Audits performed by Inspectors on behalf of a Competent Authority, a government agency such as the FDA or blood industry body such as the AABB.

- Regulatory is often organized as a separate function from Quality Assurance and Audit, but this is not a requirement. The regulatory function helps ensure that the organization understands applicable laws, and ensures that the organization maintains the licenses, clearances and approvals required to operate in accordance with the letter and intent of local as well as national or global regulatory expectations.

3. Roles and Responsibilities of Quality Assurance

Fundamentally, quality assurance (QA) is there to support operations in such a way that there is a high degree of confidence that operations can consistently deliver to expectations. Depending on your organizational model, quality control, audit, regulatory and/or administration of training programs may be part of responsibilities of the quality assurance organization. For the purpose of this discussion, we will focus on the core responsibility of quality assurance: ensuring that processes systematically meet quality and compliance standards.

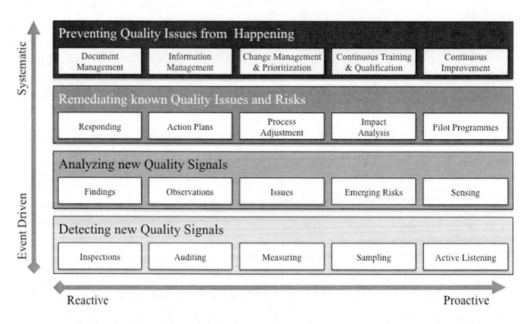

Figure 2. Elements of a Quality Management programme.

Quality cannot be assured by focusing on adherence to defined policies, procedures and processes alone. Consistent quality follows from combining well-defined processes with an appropriate organization, and infrastructure and effective tools. The more challenging side of quality is driving organizational and cultural behaviour. Quality Assurance in cooperation with the management team organization needs to construct a programme to continuously improve process, peoples' attitudes and skills and systems in unison.

Although any quality assurance organization is responsible for a myriad of activities, the responsibility can be narrowed down to four distinct responsibilities, Detection, Analysis, Remediation and Prevention (Figure 2).

- **Detecting** new Quality Signals. Quality signals can be generated from review of batch records, audits, in process measurements, periodic sampling and by listening to employees, customers and suppliers. To achieve effective issue detection consider factors such as:
  - Creating awareness of quality and coordinate oversight of Inspections and Internal audits.
  - Establish periodic and real time measures for tracking of quality/compliance process performance
  - Establish local presence; actively participate in leadership meetings as a Quality Steward; active listening to all levels of the organization, inside and outside the organization (investigators)
- **Analyzing** Quality Signals. There is no question that each quality issue must be addressed in a timely manner. However, quality assurance needs to continuously look at all signals in order to look for broader trends. What are the real issues that should be addressed? What are the symptoms, and what might the underlying root-cause(s) be? Roles to consider for Quality Assurance include:
  - Collaborating in the understanding the cause and effect of Findings, Observations, Issues and Risks.
  - Gaining appreciation for and full understanding of emerging risks and quality issues.
  - Participating in internal and external forums for maximum exposure to the changing environment.
- **Remediating** known Quality Issues and Risks. Remediation needs to focus on more than addressing the observed symptoms. Quality Assurance needs to help the organization determine the root cause of the issue. Once the corrective actions have been implemented, quality assurance should follow up over an extended period of time to determine whether the observed issues have truly been addressed. Quality Assurance has a key role in driving implementation of solutions including appropriate corrective actions:
  - 'Diagnosing and Treating' known quality issues, irrespective of source.
  - Driving accountability for development and realization of solutions.
  - Continuously challenging existing processes.
- **Preventing** Quality failures from happening. Quality Assurance should be a primary driver in helping the organization implement the infrastructure and systems needed to prevent issues from happening in the first place. This ranges from document

management practices to training and driving continuous improvement programmes. Here Quality Assurance has a key role in building the foundation needed for sustained improvement:
- Developing and deploying of scalable document and information management.
- Creating awareness and ensuring compliance to Change Management processes.
- Fostering a Continuous learning and improvement mindset.

It is worthwhile to realize that the term CAPA (Corrective And Preventive Action) follows a similar pattern, though CAPA programs are *de facto* focused on addressing a specific observed (quality or compliance) issue. A good organization wide CAPA programme relies on the organization's ability to discover issues, analyze them, implement one or more corrective actions to keep the issue from recurring in the near term, typically followed by more systematic improvements to prevent the issue from occurring in the future. Within the Six Sigma tool-set there is a similar principle, referred to as DMAIC (Define, Measure, Analyze, Implement and Control). The *Define and Measure* stages tend to focus on understanding the nature, size, scope and impact of the issue. In the *Analyze* phase, root causes are determined and hypotheses formulated and preliminary solutions tested. The *Implement* phase brings the implementation of the preventive actions, whether all at once or gradual in a controlled manner. The last, and often overlooked stage is to *Control*; to measure whether the change actually has the desired impact.

Accepting that the quality function fundamentally has the broad scope of detection, analysis, remediation and prevention of issues, inherently means that it needs to continuously reach out across the entire organization to nudge and drive all personnel, volunteers, suppliers and customers forward.

4. The Challenge for Quality Assurance

If fundamentally the role of Quality Assurance is Detecting, Analyzing, Remediating and Preventing Issues, then the question for the head of Quality Assurance is how to fulfill these roles to drive the entire organization towards being increasingly proactive and systematic in improving overall performance of the organization.

How proactive is the organization in dealing with quality issues? Consider how quality issues are generally addressed. For instance, is a majority of effort devoted to reacting to fixing past issues found during audits, or is the organization good at preventing problems and ensuring that products and services meet minimum requirements?

How systemic does the organization tend to be? Or consider to what degree quality related activities are focused on addressing individual issues versus providing systemic solutions aimed at error prevention, simplification or safe-guards?

Striving for proactive, systematic approaches will generally help drive the entire organization towards sustained excellence. This is not to say that in all cases, a strongly proactive, systematic approach is the optimal answer for the organization.

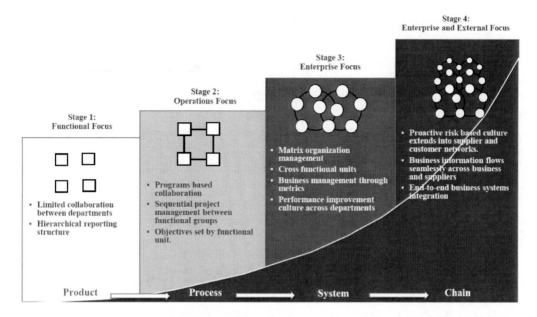

Figure 3. A Four-Stage Business Maturity Model.

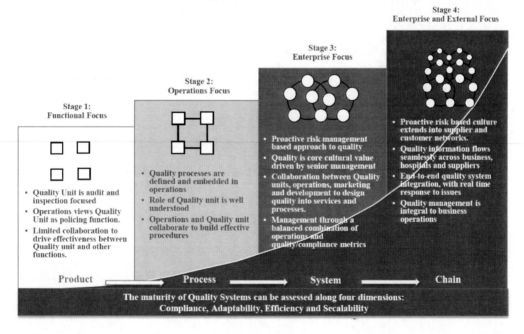

Figure 4. Maturity Model applied to Quality Management. To be effective, the organization's approach to quality management needs to be in line with the overall culture. For instance, a Quality Assurance organization striving for a highly collaborative approach may work well in an environment where matrix style management is well engrained. Yet in a strongly autocratic, departmentalized organization a highly collaborative approach to quality management may prove challenging.

5. Maturity of Quality Management

Organization maturity models may be applied to quality management. One common model states that any organization moves between four stages of maturity (Figure 3, organization maturity model). This model is readily applied to quality management, resulting in the considerations depicted in figure 4. As quality management matures, errors reduce, compliance with standards and regulations becomes inherent, overhead reduces and the organization becomes increasingly efficient in applying it's resources, both by reducing waste of effort (Lean Principles) and by through reducing waste through quality (Six Sigma principles).

In short, unless the entire organization evolves along with quality management, it will have difficulty maintaining momentum towards continuous improvement.

7. Building the Case for Change

Implementation of quality initiatives at the level of the organization requires a clearly stated, reasoning supported by the entire management team. Audit or compliance will provide a compelling, but not adequate case for change. Bringing about sustainable quality improvement often requires change to culture, business processes, roles and responsibilities. The platitude that quality is everyone's business is all too true; the Quality Group is wholly dependent on all management, staff and volunteers to drive continuous improvement.

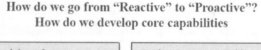

How do we go from "Reactive" to "Proactive"?
How do we develop core capabilities

We need to develop capabilities for:
- Early detection of quality issues
- Effective management of information
- Proactive improvement of processes and methods
- Understanding and communicating cause and effect
- Continuous training and education of our staff and partners
- Selecting staff with right "quality" mindset
- Leveraging trust and cooperation on all levels
- Build a model which is applicable on all levels (mobile/HQ)

Quality Assurance enables:
- Proactive and systematic **Detection** of performance, quality and compliance issues.
- **Analysis** of issues to raise awareness and enable action
- Interaction across organization to enable effective and sustainable **Remediation**
- Provides coaching, awareness and systems needed to **Prevent** issues from recurring

Figure 5. Example of transformation activities.

The management team will benefit from formulating a joint vision of how they believe good quality management will help transform the organization and summarize this in no more than a few clearly worded paragraphs. Once this is understood, a mission statement for the programme is then usually readily verbalized by describing the key objectives of the quality management program in action-oriented language (Figure 5). Consider questions such as:

- What will be achieved by implementing a comprehensive quality management programme?
- Is it to become a world-class leader, is it to consistently exceed industry standards, to better serve blood donors and patients, reduce waste and improve efficiency?
- Why does it matter to all staff involved? How will the programme benefit them?
- How will we measure progress and success?

8. Building the Change Programme

Having gained a clear perspective of what the organization needs to achieve and what key programmes need to be deployed leaves one often under-appreciated but essential aspect. Continuous improvement and building an environment where Quality, Service and Efficiency go hand in hand means that broad changes are requested of staff and volunteers. More often than not, there is no reason to doubt their commitment to doing the best possible. However, change is always difficult.

It is well accepted that for change to be embraced, it typically takes multiple exposures to new expectations. Common wisdom is that it takes at 4-7 progressive touch points for staff to understand and integrate behavioural change (Figure 6)

This means that management needs be actively engaged in managing change, create visibility, celebrate success and actively demonstrate the behaviour expected from staff. The programme needs a well developed plan including such elements as:

- High level time scale; what quality initiatives will be piloted where and when;
- How will the overall program be communicated, not only at the start but also at key milestones throughout implementation;
- Who will act as 'ambassadors' for the programme;
- How will progress and improvement be measured. Consider both temporary metrics designed to measure progress towards the programme's goals and quality metrics to be included in daily operations and monthly reporting;
- How will both the documentation and the cultural aspect of change be managed.

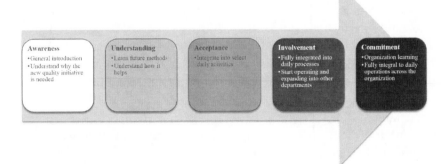

Figure 6. Phases of creating change.

Conclusion

The establishment of a comprehensive quality culture and quality system is essential in the setting of blood banking where the control of inherent risks of blood necessitates a manufacturing process that operates consistently under well-defined standards. The Quality Assurance organization supports the organization by providing improvement programmes, documentation services, analytical support and most importantly the continuous emphasis on doing the right thing, the right way at the right time. Arriving at a desired quality culture not only requires effective programmes aimed at such critical aspects as deviation management, CAPA and continuous improvement, but requires the organizational change programmes and organizational structure needed to bring the entire organization along on the journey towards ever improving performance. In the interest of transfusion safety, and consistent with their role, it is incumbent on all managers of blood banks to exercise leadership in implementing effective quality programmes.

References

[1]   AuBuchon JP, Linauts S, Vaughan M, Wagner J, Delaney M, Nester T. Evolution in a centralized transfusion service. *Transfusion.* 2011 ; 51:2750-2757 *http://www.ncbi.nlm. nih.gov/pubmed/22150685m*

[2]   Epstein JS. Best practices in regulation of blood and blood products, Biologicals 2012; 40: 200-204.

[3]   Directive 2002/98/EC of the European Parliament and of the Council of 27 January 2003 setting standards of quality and safety for the collection, testing, processing, storage and distribution of human blood and blood components and amending Directive 2001/83/EC. *Official Journal of the European Union,* 2003; 33

[4]   Seitz R, Heiden M, Nübling CM, Unger G, Löwer J. The harmonization of the regulation of blood products: a European perspective *Vox Sang* 2008; l94:267–276

[5]   Health Canada Good Manufacturing Practices (GMP) for Schedule D Drugs, Part 2, Human Blood and Blood Components in Good Manufacturing Practices (GMP) Guidelines 2009 edition, Version 2 (GUI-0001) *http://hc-sc.gc.ca/dhp-mps/compli-conform/gmp-bpf/docs/gui-0001-eng.php*

[6]   Epstein J, Seitz R, Dhingra N, Ganz PR, Gharehbaghian A, Spindel R, Teo D, Reddy R. Role of Regulatory Agencies. *Biologicals* 2009; 37:94-102.

[7]   Slopecki A, Smith K, Moore S. The Value of Good Manufacturing Practice to a Blood Service in Managing the Delivery of Quality. *Vox Sang* 2007; 92:187-196.

[8]   21 USC 301 et. seq. (US Federal Food, Drug and Cosmetic Act): 42 USC 262 (Regulation 0f Biological Products) Part 211 Current Good Manufacturing Practice for Finished Pharmaceuticals; 21 CFR Part 606 Current Good Manufacturing Practice for Blood and Blood Components

[9]   Kendrick DB. Blood Program in World War II. Office of the Surgeon General, Department of the Army, Washington D.C. 1989. *http://history.amedd. army.mil /booksdocs/wwii/blood/default.htm*

[10] Shoos Lipton K, Otter J. AABB and FDA: a shared history of patient safety *Transfusion* 2010; 50:1643-1646.

[11] US Department of Health and Human Services National Blood Collection and Utilization Survey 2007.

[12] AABB: annual report summary for testing in 2010. Prepared by the Relationship Testing Program Unit *http://www.aabb.org/sa/facilities/Documents/ rtannrpt10.pdf*

[13] WHA28.72 *Utilization and supply of human blood and blood products*. 1975 *Handb. Res., Vol. I, 1.5.2.2; 8.2.4* Thirteenth plenary meeting, 29 May 1975.

[14] WHA63.12 *Availability, safety and quality of blood products*. 2010. Sixty-third WHA, Eighth plenary session of the WHA 21 May 2010

[15] Assessment Criteria for National Blood Regulatory Systems. http://www.who.int/entity/bloodproducts/NationalBloodRegSystems.pdf

[16] EudraLex The Rules Governing Medicinal Products in the European Union; Manufacture of Medicinal Products Derived from Human Blood or Plasma, annex 14, Manufacture of Medicinal Products Derived from Human Blood or Plasma. *http://ec.europa.eu/health/files/eudralex/vol-4/annex14_rev30-03_2011_en.pdf*

[17] U.S. FDA, Guidance for Industry: Changes to an Approved Application: Biological Products: Human Blood and Blood Components Intended for Transfusion or for Further Manufacture   2001. *http://www.fda.gov/BiologicsBloodVaccines/GuidanceComplianceRegulatoryInformati on/Guidances/Blood/ucm076729.htm*

[18] Vyas GN, Williams AE, Editors. Advances in Transfusion Safety. International Association for Biologics. 2005; volume 120

[19] TS066 -- *Use and Quality Assurance of Blood Components*, Chapter 1 – Principles of a Quality System for Blood Establishments, European Directorate for the Quality of Medicines & HealthCare (EDQM), Council of Europe, 16th Edition, 2011

[20] Sharma G, Parwai AV, Raval JS, Triulzi DJ, Benjamin RJ, Pantanowitz L. Contemporary Issues in Transfusion Medicine Informatics. *J Pathol Inform*. 2011;2;3-11

[21] ReVelle JB. *Quality Essentials: A Reference Guide from A to Z*. ASQ Quality Press, 2004, pages 8–9.

[22] Palmer B. *Making Change Work: Practical Tools for Overcoming Human Resistance to Change,* 2004, ASQ Quality Press, Milwaukee, MI, USA, pages 7–9.

[23] Pyzdeck T. *The Six Sigma Handbook: The Complete Guide for Greenbelts, Blackbelts, and Managers at All Levels*, 2003, McGraw-Hill Companies, New York, NY, USA

[24] George ML, Rowlands D. *The Lean Six Sigma Pocket Toolbook*. 2005 McGraw-Hill Companies, New York, NY, USA

In: Quality Management in Transfusion Medicine   ISBN: 978-1-62618-665-1
Editor: Cees Th. Smit Sibinga   © 2013 Nova Science Publishers, Inc.

Chapter IX

Patient Safety and Quality Management at the Clinical Interface

Michael F. Murphy[*1], *Sunita Saxena*[†2] and *Cees Th. Smit Sibinga*[‡3]

[1] NHS Blood and Transplant and Oxford University Hospitals,
University of Oxford, UK

[2] Los Angeles County and University of Southern California Medical Center, Keck School of Medicine, University of Southern California, LAC andUSC Healthcare Network Laboratories, Los Angeles County-Department of Health Services, LAC+USC Medical Center, Los Angeles, CA, US

[3] ID Consulting for International Development of Transfusion Medicine,
University of Groningen, Zuidhorn, NL

Abstract

This chapter outlines the multiple current and emerging clinical interfaces in the transfusion chain between the blood supplier, the hospital blood bank, the clinician and the patient, and how they may be influenced to maintain and where necessary improve the quality of care and patient safety. The activities at each interface are described along with measures to assess outcomes for each type of activity and interventions to improve patient care.

[*] Michael F. Murphy, MD, FRCP, FRCPath, Consultant Hematologist, NHS Blood & Transplant and Oxford University Hospitals, Professor of Blood Transfusion Medicine, University of Oxford, OX3 9BQ, UK, Tel: +44-1-865.44.7902, Fax: +44-1-865.44.7957 E-mail: mike.murphy@nhsbt.nhs.uk.

[†] Sunita Saxena, MD, MHA. Director of Patient Safety, Los Angeles County+ University of Southern California Medical Center, Professor of Pathology (Ret.), Keck School of Medicine, University of Southern California, Director, LAC+USC Healthcare Network Laboratories, Los Angeles County-Department of Health Services, LAC+USC Medical Center, 1200 N State Street, Los Angeles, CA, 90033 USA, Tel: 323 226 6609, Fax: 323 226 3570, E-mail: saxena@usc.edu.

[‡] Cees Th. Smit Sibinga, MD, PhD, FRCP Edin, FRCPath, Professor of International Development of Transfusion Medicine, ID Consulting for International Development of Transfusion Medicine, University of Groningen, De Gast 46, 9801 AE Zuidhorn, NL Tel: +31-6-2223.4325, E-mail: c.sibinga@planet.nl.

Keywords: Patient safety, quality management, transfusion practice, monitoring, benchmarking

1. Introduction

The aim of transfusion therapy is to ensure that, when it is clinically indicated, patients receive the correct transfusion support, in a safe and timely manner. In many countries, blood for transfusion is neither safe, sufficient nor reliably available, and haemorrhage is a major direct cause of mortality. However, even in modern health care settings with adequate blood supplies, patients die from transfusion complications [1, 2], or from lack of adequate transfusion support; for example, massive haemorrhage is still one of the most common direct causes of maternal death worldwide. At the other end of the spectrum, patients are frequently over transfused and become unnecessarily at risk of transfusion-related complications. [3]

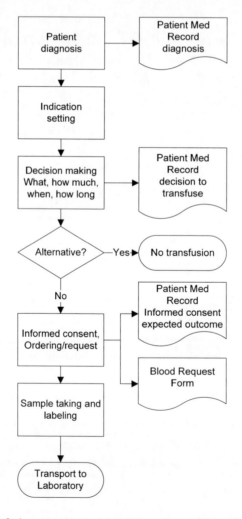

Figure 1. The hospital transfusion process: decision to transfuse and blood sample collection.

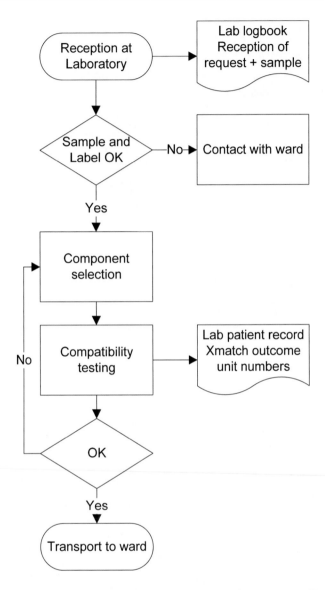

Figure 2. The hospital transfusion process: laboratory testing and the provision of blood.

Doctors in all branches of medicine and surgery, nurses and laboratory scientists are involved in some aspect of transfusion, which is an interacting sequence of three distinct in-hospital transfusion chain processes:

1) The ordering (bedside to hospital blood bank) (Figure 1);
2) The immunohaematology laboratory testing and blood product selection (hospital blood bank to bedside) (Figure 2);
3) Transfusion of blood/blood component (bedside), the monitoring of patients and the management of any adverse events (Figure 3).

There are multiple clinical interfaces in this complex chain (or pathway), which require engagement, co-operation and co-ordination by staff, and with patients, to ensure patient safety and the appropriate use of blood. In addition, there is the interface between the blood supplier and the hospital or other care setting, which is the link or gateway that connects the procurement chain with the chain in hospitals.

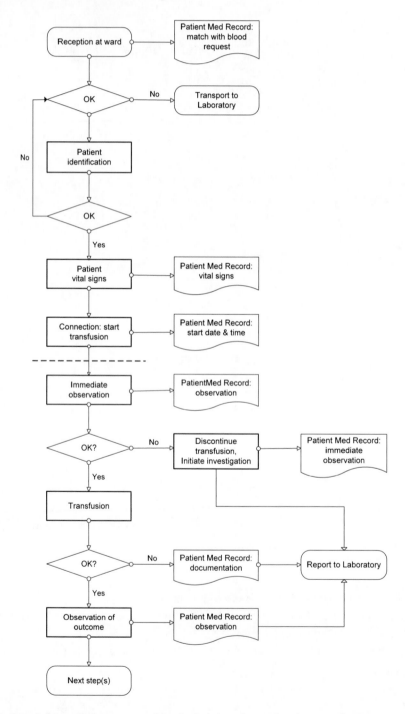

Figure 3. The hospital transfusion process: blood administration and patient monitoring.

Effective quality frameworks requiring accreditation and regulatory compliance in both the laboratory and clinical settings are needed to minimise transfusion risks and to ensure that the supply of donated blood is managed effectively. [4-6] These in turn require a patient-centred approach to transfusion, committed leadership and adequate resources.

In this chapter, we will provide an overview of the clinical interfaces in the transfusion chain from the blood supplier to the hospital blood bank, the clinician, and the patient. We will outline the type of activities at each interface, and provide measures to assess outcomes for each type of activity, as well as interventions to improve outcomes supported by evidence for their effectiveness.

2. Clinical Interfaces

This part of the chapter describes in detail the clinical interfaces in the transfusion chain in three scenarios, the first where the blood supply is the main limiting factor ('traditional transfusion chain' or 'supply driven'), the second where the transfusion chain is driven by the demand for blood by hospitals ('advanced transfusion chain' or 'demand driven'), and the third where new initiatives are being used to focus even more on patient safety and the avoidance of unnecessary transfusion ('emerging transfusion chain' or 'patient driven' practice) (Annex 1, Table 1).

Very roughly, the 'traditional transfusion chain' is found in hospitals in low, medium and even in some high human development index (HDI) countries, the 'advanced transfusion chain' in most of the high and very high HDI countries, and the 'emerging transfusion chain' in very high HDI countries[17].

2.1. Traditional Transfusion Chain (Supply Driven)

In the traditional transfusion chain, there are a number of processes with important interfaces. The first process is at the bedside with a patient seeking medical help from the clinician. This consultation might lead to a decision to include supportive haemotherapy in the treatment plan or not, and it may lead to the ordering of blood or blood components. The interfaces are 1) clinician and patient – diagnosis, considering blood transfusion and alternatives to transfusion and a decision to transfuse or not followed by informed consent; 2) clinician or ward and hospital blood bank, involving completion of the blood request and collection of a patient blood sample for compatibility testing. The requesting process should follow strict criteria established by the internal customer, the hospital blood bank (see Annex 1, Table 1 – A1 and A2).

The second major process happens in the hospital blood bank. The interfaces are 1) hospital blood bank and the external supplier of the blood and blood components to secure an adequate stock of blood components. Stock management plays an important role; 2) Hospital blood bank advising the clinician/clinical team on the appropriateness of the proposed supportive haemotherapy and issuing compatible blood components (see Annex 1, Table 1 – A3 and A4).

---

[17] See Chapter 15 – Annex 4: HDI ranking

The third major process happens at the bedside between nursing and medical staff and the patient. This involves the identification of the correct patient, the right units of blood or blood component and the right time for the transfusion. The process ends with the interface of the ward and the hospital blood bank to report back on the outcome of the transfusion and the final destination of the units of blood or blood components. In case of adverse effects, this might lead to a laboratory investigation to determine the nature of the adverse event and its cause in order to prevent re-occurrence (see Annex 1, Table 1 – A4).

When an active hospital transfusion committee (HTC) is present, there is an interface of the HTC and the prescribing clinicians in terms of local guidelines for transfusion practice based on the best available evidence. Another interface is the blood supplier and the HTC for exchange of transfusion outcome data and epidemiology of the use of blood and blood components in the hospital.(see Annex 1, Table 1 – A5 and A6).

In most situations in the traditional transfusion chain, the supply of blood drives blood usage because of shortages and inappropriate functioning of the hospital and the external interfaces. Although clearly identified, these interfaces are largely not established or developed and therefore miss the important communication function to support quality management. The major processes and their interfaces will be described in more detail below.

2.1.1. Blood Ordering Process

This follows a sequence of events that eventually guide the hospital blood bank to select an appropriate blood component for the patient (Figure 1). The critical control points of this process include:

i.   establishing the diagnosis;
ii.   a clear definition of the indication for haemotherapy;
iii.   seeking and documentation of informed consent from the intended blood recipient;
iv.   establishment of the specific blood component indicated for the patient after consideration of transfusion alternatives;
v.   ordering by fully completing a well designed blood request form, accompanied by drawing a pre-transfusion cross match sample, and
vi.   proper documentation and transportation of the blood request form and pre-transfusion blood sample to the laboratory for ABO and RhD typing and compatibility testing.

Hospitals should establish guidelines on the documentation of the above critical control points. The guidelines should include:

i.   documentation of the diagnosis in the patient's medical record;
ii.   provision of an appropriate blood request form, based on a standard operating procedure (SOP), onto which the details of the order are documented;
iii.   documentation in the patient medical record of the intended intervention and expected outcome of the transfusion;
iv.   clear and concise labelling of the sample to avoid confusion and errors (wrong blood in tube).

2.1.1.1. Diagnosis: Is there a Need to Transfuse?

The clinical and laboratory assessment of a patient provide the basis for any haemotherapy. Based on existing knowledge, the prescribing clinician characterises the need for blood into scenarios such as anticipated blood loss during an elective surgical procedure, massive blood loss resulting in impending multiple organ damage, chronic anaemia causing diminished oxygen carrying and delivery capacity of blood, and the need for prophylaxis or treatment with haemostatic and coagulation factors. These clinical impressions are followed by appropriate laboratory tests such as determination of haematocrit or haemoglobin concentration to confirm the need for red blood cell transfusion while assessment of fibrinogen level, international normalized ratios (INR), active partial thromboplastin time (APTT) and platelet counts and function tests would confirm the need for supportive haemotherapy with coagulation factors and/or platelet concentrates. [7-10]

2.1.1.2. Indication Setting: What is the Need?

Blood and blood components are collected from healthy donors after conducting a standardised selection procedure and laboratory testing. The blood components that are accessible in most developing and developed countries include whole blood, red cell concentrates, platelet concentrates, frozen fresh plasma (FFP) and cryoprecipitate. Other components that are not yet available in many transitional and low HDI countries, include apheresis derived components, leukocyte reduced and irradiated cellular blood components and plasma derivatives such as factor VIII concentrates, albumin and immunoglobulins. [11]

Red cell transfusions are indicated in the management of anaemia in normovolaemic patients to improve oxygen carrying and delivery capacity and in exchange transfusion of newborns. They should not be administered when other methods of anaemia treatment will be effective (iron substitutes, folic acid, vitamin B12 or erythropoietin). [7-9] Platelets are indicated in thrombocytopenia, for example following massive transfusion or treatment regimens of cytotoxic chemotherapy. They are also indicated in congenital or acquired thrombocytopathies and to support thrombocytopenic patients in special situations for example during neurosurgery. [10, 12, 13]

FFP should be used to treat bleeding in patients with multiple coagulation deficits. It should not be used as a source of nutritional proteins or as volume expander in preference to volume replacement fluids such as colloids or crystalloids. [14, 15]

Cryoprecipitate is indicated when there is a deficiency in clinical scenarios of acquired fibrinogen deficiency such as massive haemorrhage and disseminated intravascular coagulation (DIC), and may be used in developing countries to treat haemopilia A due to the lack of availability of factor VIII concentrates. [16, 17]

2.1.1.3. The Decision to Transfuse or Use Alternatives to Transfusion

In elective surgery, the decision to transfuse whole blood or a red cell component is based on estimates (anticipated blood loss, blood volume, haemoglobin and haematocrit estimates, cardiopulmonary and circulatory ability to deliver oxygenated blood to the peripheral tissues and their ability to extract the oxygen). [18] With all these uncertainties, clinicians are likely to over- or under-transfuse. It is therefore highly desirable to educate clinicians in good transfusion practice and provide local guidelines to assist the prescribing clinician in the optimal and appropriate use of blood. In order to achieve acceptance and adherence to guidelines, each country should generate consensus on its own national guidelines and these can consequently be harmonized at international consensus meetings. [18, 19]

Eindhoven et al. designed guidelines on perioperative transfusion which were evaluated with a case-control study in patients undergoing elective primary total hip replacement in two hospitals, one with cases (using the guidelines) and the other with controls (using the haemoglobin and haematocrit as indicators for transfusion). [20] The new guidelines led to a significant reduction in the use of allogeneic blood and a decrease in the number of patients transfused in the hospital following the guideline compared to the hospital with controls.

This compares well with the work of Yeh et al. who prospectively analysed transfusion requests and then repeated the audit three months later after the clinicians had undergone education on new transfusion guidelines. [15] They found that there was a 74.6% decrease in fresh plasma usage and a 50% decrease in inappropriate requests.

The above two situations show that an educated bedside decision making process greatly improves blood usage and provides an opportunity to the prescribing clinician to make use of transfusion alternatives as the situation warrants. Rosencher et al. in their study to assess blood management in elective orthopaedic surgery in Europe found that an accurate choice of a blood conservation strategy before the surgical procedure reduced the risk of exposure to allogeneic blood and improved the cost effectiveness of the selected method (pre-deposit autologous donation, acute normovolaemic haemodilution, cell saver or post-operative blood salvage). [21]

2.1.1.4. Informed Consent

Like any other medical or surgical intervention, blood transfusion has expected benefits but also carries potential risks to the patient. Patients therefore need to be informed of the reasons for an intended blood transfusion so that they can consent to it. True informed consent is only possible for elective or planned transfusions but not for emergency transfusions. [22]

The patient, or guardian, must be given sufficient information to make an intelligent choice. This means that the patient should be competent and free to agree or to disagree to an intended transfusion. [23, 24] Informed consent is a process not a single event [25] and consists of:

  i.   providing the information on the expected benefits and potential risks;
  ii.   providing an opportunity to the patient to ask questions;
  iii.   offering alternatives;
  iv.   advising the patient without coercion;
  v.   documentation of the consent or refusal to the proposed transfusion.

There are some contentious issues with patient consent. The Canadian expert working group in their guidelines for red cell and plasma transfusions for adults and children agreed that health care workers should inform patients about the possibility and likelihood of blood transfusion, and solicit and answer questions that patients might have. [19] However, they failed to agree on the need to discuss alternatives to transfusion during the consent process, given their inconsistent availability and varying effectiveness in averting allogeneic blood exposure. Rock et al. in their retrospective review of 1,005 patient medical records, agreed that the patients had the right to an informed consent on blood transfusion. [26] However documentation of this process was found in only 13.2% of the medical records.

Another issue of great concern in the informed consent process is how much information should be provided to patients. Holland and Schmidt indicated that, at a minimum, patients should be provided with all the reasons for a transfusion as well as the alternatives and risks, stating that any complication that would occur with a frequency of one percent or greater would be considered frequent and therefore should be disclosed. [27]

Further requirements to inform the patient are found in the recommendations of Justice Krever from the Commission of Inquiry on the Blood System of Canada where it is required that after treatment the patient is informed by the physician about the particular blood component that was used. [28]

In-service training, implementation of rational clinical transfusion practices and instituting appropriate monitoring systems, leads to tremendous improvement in the informed consent process. Saxena et al. showed an improvement on consent documentation from 80 to 100 % over a period of 5 months having employed a team of trained nurses to carry out the process of seeking consent from blood recipients in that period. [29] The professional practice of appropriate informed consent is based on well designed protocols that spell out the responsibility of the clinician for seeking, timing, frequency of, documentation of, and the environment in which informed consent should be sought. [30]

2.1.1.5. Blood Loss at Surgery

Many elective surgical procedures are accompanied by peri-operative blood loss which may necessitate intra-operative or post-operative transfusion with red cell transfusion alone to improve oxygen carrying and delivery capacity, or red cell transfusion plus plasma products and platelet concentrates as required if there is massive haemorrhage. [16]

Careful assessment and management of patients prior to surgery reduces peri-operative morbidity and mortality in situations of restricted availability of blood and blood components for transfusion. This includes identification and treatment of anaemia, identification, stabilization or treatment of medical co-morbidities, and identification and treatment of pre-existing bleeding disorders. [31, 32]

It is also important for each hospital to institute and facilitate methods that will minimise peri-operative blood loss. These should include the use of anti-fibrinolytic drugs, employing appropriate anaesthetic techniques for particular surgical procedures, use of vasoconstrictors, use of meticulous (bloodless) surgical techniques, and appropriate positioning of patients during and after surgery. Additionally, a significant amount of surgical blood loss can be tolerated as long as normovolaemia is maintained with intravenous replacement fluids (colloids or crystalloids). [18, 32]

Many elective surgical procedures rarely require transfusion. However, for some major procedures, notably orthopaedic or cardiovascular, blood should be ordered and made available in advance. Peri-operative orders and use vary between hospitals and individual clinicians due to differences in surgical and anaesthetic techniques, attitudes to use of blood, cost and availability of blood components or transfusion alternatives. Therefore, it is important for each hospital to evaluate blood loss during the commonly performed surgical procedures to guide clinicians in making appropriate and evidence based decisions in blood requesting. To measure blood loss at surgery [33-35], two methods can be used. The direct method involves measuring collected blood in swabs, drainage bags and suction bottles, while the indirect method measures blood loss by haemoglobin or haematocrit changes over the peri-operative period of time. It should be noted that the direct method does not allow for blood hidden in draping linen, in the suction tubes or evaporations during surgery. On the other hand, the indirect method is a simple, inexpensive and non-invasive method as long as the post-operative haemoglobin or haematocrit is measured in a normovolaemic state.

2.1.1.6. Peri-Operative Blood Order Schedule

Unlike emergency situations e.g., trauma, obstetric bleeding and ruptured vessels, planned surgical procedures provide an opportunity to devise a tariff of blood to be provided for each type of surgery, that is a maximal surgical blood order schedule (MSBOS). [18] Reports show that a substantial amount of blood given intra-operatively and post-operatively is transfused following demonstrable anaemia. [36, 37] Pre-operative cross-matching of blood units for surgical patients is performed in anticipation of a potential need which may not materialise and consequently many blood units cross-matched before surgery are never transfused. [38] This leads to wastage of precious blood bank resources including maintenance of an unnecessarily high blood inventory and unnecessary cross matching. It also increases the number of units that become outdated and therefore wasted.

The development and use of a MSBOS enables the identification of surgical procedures that can be accommodated by the human and laboratory resources. [18, 19, 39] It also leads to:

i.   reduction in unnecessary compatibility testing;
ii.   reduction in the returns of unused blood;
iii.   reduction in wastage due to outdating;
iv.   more efficient management of the blood inventory.

Over time, an evaluation of blood use compared with actual blood orders should be carried out for each type of surgery to determine cross match-to-transfusion (C/T) ratios that may be used to persuade surgical teams to reduce the number of red cell units in the MSBOS where excessive red cell units are being cross matched but not transfused.

2.1.1.7. Surgical Blood Order Equation

Nuttall et al. retrospectively analysed the predictors of peri-operative red cell requirements in patients undergoing major orthopaedic surgery and used these variables to develop the surgical blood order equation (SBOE). [38] The SBOE [40] is as follows:

> Haemoglobin lost – (preoperative haemoglobin – minimal acceptable haemoglobin) = units of red cells required at surgery

Values that are negative or less than 0.5 units are assigned an order to type and screen blood only, and values between 0.5 unit and less than 1 unit are rounded off to 1 unit.

The SBOE has a number of advantages [40,41]:

i.   it maximises the efficiency of blood use;
ii.   it predicts the extent of peri-operative blood use.

Nuttall et al. in a prospective double-blind randomised clinical trial compared the SBOE, with the MSBOS for ordering allogeneic red cell units for 60 patients undergoing total hip arthroplasty and found that the SBOE was more accurate (58% correct orders) than the MSBOS (7 % correct orders: p = 0.0001). [42] The SBOE had a lower C/T ratio than MSBOS (0.83 vs. 4.12). SBOE reduced the monetary costs and risks of allogeneic blood. In a related study, Guerin et al. prospectively evaluated 162 consecutive patients who underwent total hip and total knee arthroplasty for determinant factors for peri-operative blood transfusion. [37] They found that patient variables (age, weight and pre-operative haemoglobin levels) significantly determined the quantity of peri-operative transfusion. They also found that there was a considerable clinical and economic reward in using patient-based transfusion protocols in determining peri-operative red cell unit requirements.

2.1.1.8. Blood Sample Collection

From the patient perspective, pre-transfusion sample collection for ABO and RhD typing, alloantibody screening and identification, and cross-matching marks the first step on the path to actual bedside transfusion. Errors in this procedure can be devastating, because they may lead to ABO incompatible red cell transfusions. [43]

Linden et al. [44] estimated that errors in pre-transfusion sample collection accounted for 15% of ABO incompatible red cell transfusions reported in New York State. In a period of six years (1993 to 1999), Butch et al. reported an unfortunate increasing trend of total laboratory errors related to patient sample collection from 10 to 20 percent. [45] These errors are usually due to inadequate patient identification, incorrect labelling of the drawn samples or improper documentation of this procedure. At Johns Hopkins Hospital, Baltimore Lumadue et al. reported that one in every 71 samples was mislabelled and one in every 2,800 was correctly labelled but mis-collected (a properly labelled tube containing blood of another patient – 'wrong blood in tube'). [46] This would have lead to serious hazards if these errors had not been found. Development and adherence to hospital guidelines on pre-transfusion sample collection reduces the frequency of mis-labelled and mis-collected samples. [47, 48]

2.1.1.9. Blood Request Form

The blood request form (BRF) is the traditional means of communication between the clinician and the hospital blood bank. The BRF should contain the identification details of the patient, the diagnosis and indication setting for the transfusion, the required type and quantity of blood component, the previous transfusion history, and the identity of the prescriber. [49, 50]

The design of a BRF has a profound effect on the compliance of clinicians to this tool. Kajja et al. in their analysis of the design and prescriber compliance to the Mulago Hospital blood request form found that clinicians did not adequately comply with even the old blood request form in use. [51] A properly designed BRF followed by training results in improved blood usage. Hui CH et al. in their study of the impact of a new BRF that had been designed in a self educating style for the prescriber, found an improvement in appropriate use of fresh (frozen/thawed) plasma and platelets after its introduction in a large tertiary teaching hospital in Australia. [14]

2.1.2. Blood Selection Procedure

The blood selection process takes place in the hospital blood bank (figure 2) and consists of three steps: reception of the pre-transfusion sample and blood request form at the laboratory, component selection for compatibility testing and issuing of the blood component. [52]

Errors in the laboratory include;

    i.   wrong sample used for compatibility testing;
    ii.   wrong unit of blood selected for compatibility testing;
    iii. wrong unit of blood issued for the patient;
    iv. wrong transport conditions for the issued unit of blood component.

There are two critical decision making steps that emerge out of these three steps which directly determine the outcome of the whole process – 1) acceptability of the sample (integrity and volume, the accompanying patient identity on the sample label) and 2) the compatibility of the unit of blood with the patient blood sample.

To guard against errors, documentation is needed for each of the steps. It is important for laboratories to establish strict labelling guidelines and procedures for the acceptance or rejection of improperly labelled specimens. Strict adherence to labelling requirements can significantly reduce erroneous blood grouping and compatibility testing, and diminish the likelihood of transfusing ABO incompatible red cells. [46] The American Association of Blood Banks (AABB) provides details for improving the labelling of pre-transfusion testing specimens in *Guidelines for the Labeling of Specimens for Compatibility Testing*. [53]

2.1.2.1. The Cold Chain

The maintenance of quality and efficacy of blood and blood components from donor to recipient calls for sound storage and transport conditions in hospitals. There are several good reasons to ensure optimal storage and transport conditions of the blood components:

    1) preservation of the biological function of the constituents;
    2) avoidance of a reduction in metabolic activities (hibernation); and
    3) minimise the risk of bacterial growth.

The cold chain requires acquisition of appropriate equipment like refrigerators, freezers, agitators and transport boxes. A proper cold chain also requires validation, calibration of the equipment, maintenance and repair, and training of the involved personnel. Last but not least, monitoring and continuous assessment are indispensable. Lack of proper quality management affects the quality of blood.

2.1.3. Bedside Administration of Blood

Bedside administration of blood has two closely interrelated sub-processes and a number of procedures (Figure 3). It begins with the interface of the clinical area and the hospital blood bank involving the issue of the blood component, patient identification, and preparation of the patient for the transfusion (vital signs). It ends with the completion of the transfusion and documentation of the transfusion outcome.

There are critical control points in this process that need to be documented - unit identity and how this matches with patient identity, patient vital signs before starting the transfusion, the time and date the transfusion is started, patient vital signs and clinical status 15 minutes after starting the transfusion, date and time of completion of the transfusion, outcome of the transfusion and any other actions taken during or after a given transfusion. Neglect or non-conformance to standard procedures in the above process may lead to bedside errors which may have catastrophic consequences for the patient. The most commonly reported bedside error is transfusion of blood to the wrong patient followed by use of sub-standard facilities and techniques to administer blood to patients that may lead to bacterial contamination of the blood component and subsequent bacteraemia in the patient. [43] Other mishaps include poor practice in monitoring patients receiving blood transfusions, which may result in undocumented and unreported transfusion reactions. [43, 54]

In the more advanced world, Linden et al. estimated the rate of transfusion errors to be 1 in 12,000 in New York. [55] Robillard et al. report that the haemovigilance programme in Quebec identified ABO incompatible red cell transfusion as the commonest major adverse event occurring at a rate of 1 in 13,000 transfusions. [56] Andreu et al. reported similar findings from the haemovigilance programme in France. [57]

Other published studies have also reported weaknesses in performance of bedside clerical checks, like matching the blood unit label with the patient wrist band. [49,59,60] Factors put forward to explain these errors include increasing patient to nurse ratios, elimination of specialty nursing teams responsible for administration of blood, shorter lengths of hospital stays and higher nursing turn over rates. [43] However, these factors cannot be generalised for all settings.

In summary, in the traditional supply driven transfusion chain, the quality of bedside transfusion practice is affected by a number of factors which may be intrinsic to the prescribing clinician like prior medical school training and working experiences or can be external like availability of continuing medical education, peer recommendations, feedbacks from haemovigilance teams, administrative support from hospital governance, financial incentives and patient attitudes and desires. [61] However, the most prominent factor is the continued shortage of supply of blood components caused by an absence of well functioning interfaces in particular between the hospital and its blood supplier.

2.2. Advanced Transfusion Chain (Demand Driven)

Blood transfusion is an essential part of modern healthcare. However, like most therapies, it is also associated with significant clinical risks. Minimising the risks and optimising the benefits of transfusion depend on close collaboration throughout the 'transfusion chain' from suppliers to the clinical prescribers of blood and patients. The two main elements for safe and effective transfusion are good clinical practice and a sufficient supply of safe and efficacious blood. In developed countries, there is generally a sufficient supply of blood although motivation and retention of donors are significant challenges.

Good transfusion practice requires the avoidance of clinical and laboratory errors leading to 'wrong blood transfusion', appropriate decision-making about the rational use of blood based on assessment of clinical findings and laboratory parameters, and the monitoring of patients for adverse effects of transfusion and their management if they occur. Unfortunately, there is evidence of sub-optimal practice in all of these aspects of transfusion. The main themes underlying this poor practice are typically very similar, and have been described in detail elsewhere along with interventions to improve practice. [3] The latter are also considered in section C on Emerging Interfaces.

The key interfaces in the 'advanced' transfusion chain in developed countries are the HTC and clinical teams, clinicians and patients, clinicians and the hospital blood bank, the hospital blood bank and the blood supplier, and the blood supplier and the HTC (see Annex 1, Table 1).

To be effective, these clinical interfaces should operate bi-directionally; for example, clinicians make requests for blood to the hospital blood bank, and hospital blood banks provide ad hoc advice to clinicians and draw attention to local and national guidelines for good practice.

2.2.1. Hospital Transfusion Committee

The HTC is the focal point for overseeing transfusion practice in hospitals. Its role is outlined in statements from regulatory bodies like the Joint Commission in the United States [6] and documents such as the English NHS *Better Blood Transfusion* health circulars [62], and the AABB publication *The Transfusion Committee: Putting Patient Safety First.* [63] The key interfaces of the HTC are with clinical teams, the hospital blood bank and the blood supplier (see Annex 1, Table 1 – B1 and B6).

The HTC has the remit to promote best practice for the use of blood, review the safety and effectiveness of clinical transfusion practice, monitor the performance of the hospital blood bank and the blood supplier, participate in regional or national initiatives and communicate with local patient representative groups as appropriate. A chairperson with understanding and experience of transfusion practice should be appointed by hospital senior management.

To be effective and to deliver its objectives, the HTC requires support from dedicated hospital transfusion teams, at a minimum consisting of a medical specialist with scheduled time for transfusion medicine, one or more transfusion nurses (sometimes called transfusion practitioners or transfusion safety officers) and a blood bank scientist/manager. Other necessary resources include information technology (IT) and administrative support to facilitate regular meetings, data retrieval and audit. The HTC is an essential component of hospital clinical governance, so it must be incorporated into the hospital framework for clinical governance, performance and risk management, and report its findings and activities in a timely and meaningful way, accompanied by recommendations for action where necessary.

It is also essential that the HTC should have the confidence of the major blood prescribing clinical teams in their main activities of providing local guidelines for safe transfusion practice, the appropriate use of blood, blood avoidance, the use of alternatives to transfusion, and the management of adverse events.

Hospitals should adopt recommendations from authoritative professional guidelines and carefully review their content to consider whether any customisation is required for local use. This may involve developing guidelines for transfusion practice for an individual clinical team e.g. critical care or cardiac surgery as well as producing generic protocols for the management of disseminated intravascular coagulation and massive haemorrhage. These local guidelines should be disseminated with training for all involved staff, and be readily available for reference by individual clinicians e.g., on the hospital intranet.

Monitoring of practice and feedback to clinical teams (and possibly to individual clinicians) is a key role for the HTC. Feedback can be provided indirectly by issuing reports to clinical teams, but better is to provide direct feedback at an appropriate forum which also allows the delivery of education about good transfusion practice and any relevant new developments and research findings.

Audit of blood use can be conducted retrospectively, concurrently on a daily basis or prospectively in advance of the transfusion. [64] The increasing use of computer physician order entry (CPOE) facilitates audit by the collection of more reliable information on the 'reason for transfusion', can be used to alert physicians about relevant blood count data, and provides the opportunity for incorporating clinical guidelines about appropriate blood use. [65] Prospective review allied to mechanisms for 'decision support' has even greater potential to minimise unnecessary transfusions.

The interface between the HTC and hospital blood bank is essential to provide data to the HTC on transfusion practice and any problems that need to be tackled with clinical teams. Similarly, the relationship of both the HTC and the hospital blood bank with the blood supplier is important, for example to provide information on the quality of blood components, and new developments and services. Ideally, the blood supplier should also provide data on blood usage and blood wastage in comparison with other similar hospitals that might be useful for the HTC to drive local changes in transfusion practice.

The HTC has an important role in collaboration with the hospital blood bank in providing feedback to the blood supplier on the quality of its blood products and other services as well as collecting and communicating haemovigilance data.

2.2.2. Clinicians and Clinical Teams

Clinicians clearly have a key role in the safety of the transfusion process, decision-making about the use of blood and alternatives to blood, providing information to patients, and monitoring patients during and after transfusions. The key interfaces of clinicians are with patients and the hospital blood bank and the HTC (see Annex 1, Table 1 – B2 and B3).

Many patients, and indeed the general public, have a very limited understanding of the true benefits and risks of transfusion, and may consequently have considerable anxieties about transfusion. Patients who have received a transfusion often do not recall the consent process, either because they were not given full information or because they rapidly forgot it. Communication by clinicians with transfusion recipients needs to be improved. There is considerable variation in the methods used for obtaining and documenting consent to transfusion.

In California, for example, providing patients information prepared by the California Department of Health Services that describes transfusion-associated risks and benefits as well as available options for blood transfusions (Paul Gann Blood Safety Act, H&S § 1645) and its documentation is a legal requirement. [66]

In the United States, obtaining consent to transfusion is an accreditation requirement of The Joint Commission. [6] In the Netherlands, there exists already for over two decades a law regulating the medical treatment agreement aspects, which includes the obligation of the clinician and the hospital to inform patients on the intended medical treatment and interventions – a written informed consent, whereas in the UK consent is strongly encouraged and its documentation recommended without either being mandatory. [67]

Involvement of patients in decision-making about the use of blood and the safety of transfusion procedures such as blood sample collection and the administration of blood are potential important interventions to improve the quality and safety of blood transfusion and increase blood avoidance where this is appropriate. [68] However, it is as yet unclear how willing patients and healthcare staff would be for patients to engage more robustly in these activities.

There is clearly a varied emphasis on good transfusion practice by clinical teams. Some teams carry out even major procedures without blood transfusion by attention to patient care throughout the peri-operative period. It is the role of the HTC and hospital blood bank to encourage clinicians to use restrictive transfusion thresholds and other good blood management practices.

As well as providing ad hoc advice, drawing attention to local and national guidelines for good practice, the HTC and hospital blood bank can encourage clinicians and clinical teams to participate in local, regional and national audits of transfusion practice for example on the usage of blood.

2.2.3. Blood Suppliers

Blood suppliers have an essential role in the transfusion chain for the supply of standard and special blood components and products for transfusion, the provision of advice to hospital blood banks about serological problems, the investigation and management of adverse events, regulatory issues and quality management. The key interfaces for blood suppliers are with the hospital blood bank and the HTC (see Annex 1, Table 1 - B5 and B6).

Blood suppliers should also have a proactive role in promoting good transfusion practice in hospitals through clinical consultations, as well as supplying blood components and specialist services. This role may be indirect in providing education and training, support for developing guidelines and auditing practice, and the means for sharing experience. However, there are increasing numbers of blood suppliers providing more direct support for hospitals, for example by providing centralised comprehensive blood bank services for a region and specialist clinical advice. [69]

In some institutions, the Chief Medical Officer of the blood supplier is a regular member of the HTC. This allows him/her to actively participate in discussions about new components, upcoming strategies to improve the safety of blood components, and blood inventory trends with the hospital customers.

In recent years, blood suppliers in many developed countries have promoted better blood management and safe transfusion practice through national initiatives involving the creation of haemovigilance schemes for incident reporting, and the establishment of national and regional committees to improve the education and training of clinical staff prescribing blood, developing guidelines on blood usage, and providing the mechanism for reviewing blood use in local, regional and/or national audits with feedback of data to clinicians.

2.2.4. Hospital Blood Bank

The hospital blood bank has a central role in the transfusion chain between the blood suppliers and clinical teams. The key interfaces of the hospital blood bank are with them, and they are bi-directional (see Annex 1, Table 1 – B3, B4, B5 and B6). The hospital blood bank also has an essential role in supporting the activities of the HTC. These interfaces have already been briefly described above.

The hospital blood bank is dependent on the blood supplier for the supply of standard and special blood components for transfusion, scientific advice about serological problems and the investigation and management of adverse events, advice about regulatory issues and quality management, and other services e.g. stem cells, tissues, therapeutic apheresis. In turn, the blood supplier is dependent on the hospital blood bank for information on how blood is used, including any that is wasted, to assist with demand planning, and reporting of any concerns about quality or patient adverse events which might indicate a need for the supplier to review their processes or consider new developments to improve quality or minimise the risk of adverse events.

The hospital blood bank might wish to review the performance of the blood supplier in terms of the timeliness and adequacy of the supply of blood and other services, and discuss these issues either in individual meetings with the blood supplier or in joint meetings with other hospital blood banks.

In recent years, as well as providing compatible blood and carrying out relevant serological investigations, hospital blood banks have played an increasing role in collaboration with the HTC and clinicians in initiatives outside their laboratories to improve the safety and effectiveness of transfusion practice. Such activities include providing data on the safety of transfusion practice e.g. the number of samples rejected by the blood bank because of poor labelling, and on the effectiveness of transfusion by comparing the blood usage of clinical teams for similar procedures to other clinical teams in the same hospital, region or nationally.

Retrospective or prospective audits of transfusion practice may be co-ordinated by the blood bank, and reported direct to clinicians, clinical teams and the HTC.

In some hospitals blood bank staff are 'empowered' to challenge blood orders which appear to be outside local guidelines. Such empowerment is facilitated by providing relevant blood count data, e.g. haemoglobin concentration for a red cell transfusion, to blood bank staff when requests for blood are entered into the blood bank IT system. [70] These 'out of blood bank' activities of hospital blood banks are often facilitated by transfusion nurses, and senior and junior medical staff involved in transfusion medicine. In some centres, the 'out of blood bank' transfusion team might also include staff carrying out near patient haemostasis testing, intra-operative cell salvage, and training of clinical staff in safe transfusion practice, the appropriate use of blood, and measures for the avoidance of blood. These latter activities are increasingly being employed in some hospitals, and are being described as 'patient blood management', which will be described in detail in the next section on 'Emerging Interfaces'.

2.3. Emerging Transfusion Chain (Patient Driven)

The Institute of Medicine (IOM) report identified six aims for health care in the United States. [71] Health care should be safe, effective, patient-centred, timely, efficient, and equitable. Since its publication over a decade ago, the emphasis on safety and patient-centred care has been growing.

For example, more and more hospitals are considering implementing a patient-centred blood management programme (PBM). PBM is a patient-centred and patient-driven initiative that focuses on an evidence-based, multidisciplinary approach to optimizing the care of patients who might need transfusion. As described in a recently published report on best practices, a PBM programme needs a clearly defined structure and resources allocated to manage it and monitor its effectiveness. [72] To be successful, these programmes require collaboration among different specialties, each treating the patient as a member of the healthcare team.

This results in multiple interfaces between the patient and various medical and surgical specialists and ancillary staff (Figure 4). In most institutions, the HTC (or a similar committee) offers a perfect opportunity to bring all stakeholders on board to initiate a PBM programme. [73] PBM programmes are aimed at treating the reason for transfusion and avoiding transfusion in the first place, if possible. Several strategies can be employed to achieve that goal.

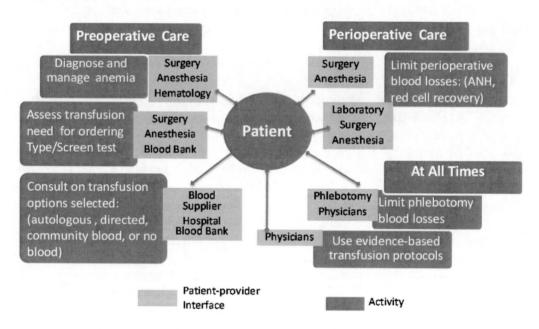

Figure 4. Emerging interfaces: multidisciplinary Patient-Centred Blood Management.

2.3.1. PBM - Pre-Operative

Elective surgical patients can be enrolled into a PBM programme when they visit a clinic for their pre-operative evaluation (see Annex 1, Table 1 – C1a & 1b). In a typical PBM programme, patients undergo medical evaluation by an anaesthetist. A part of that evaluation includes screening for anaemia. Where the haemoglobin concentration is low, the patient is treated by the clinical team using an agreed algorithm for anaemia management or referred to a haematologist for evaluation and correction of anaemia before the surgery is scheduled.

To ensure that the blood bank will have compatible blood available should the patient need a transfusion for surgery, a blood sample for type and screen (T&S) testing is drawn on all patients who are scheduled to undergo surgical procedures that have a reasonable likelihood of requiring a transfusion. [74] A second sample to verify the ABO type is drawn when the patient is admitted to the hospital. Informed consent is obtained after the patient is informed of risks and benefits of transfusion as well as alternatives to receiving allogeneic blood in accordance with the local accrediting and legal requirements as is described earlier in the chapter. This process provides an added benefit; it helps to identify patients who do not wish to receive transfusions so alternate strategies can be planned in advance. These patients are asked to sign an informed refusal to transfusion. Some patients may use options such as autologous or directed blood donation (see Annex 1, Table 1 – C2). They are referred to the local blood supplier or the hospital blood bank for obtaining additional information and scheduling the requested type of blood donations. Regardless of the option the patient selects, the blood bank is alerted to the special needs to ensure that the patients are transfused (or not transfused) according to their wishes. While it is convenient and quite effective to initiate the PBM in the outpatient setting, the full benefit of the programme can be realized only if the inpatient components of the programme, e.g. minimizing phlebotomy blood losses and use of autologous blood and auto-transfusion techniques, are also completed, which can be a much more complex and challenging task.

2.3.2. PBM – Peri-Operative

In the hospital setting, care is typically provided by a team of experts. As a result, patient and providers have to navigate multiple interfaces to ensure that optimal care is delivered. Minimizing blood losses due to phlebotomy is an important part of any PBM programme. Since diagnostic testing can contribute to anaemia among the hospitalised patients, only the tests that are medically justified and necessary should be ordered and the volume of blood sample collected should be reduced to the minimum needed for testing (see Annex 1, Table 1 – C1c). [75]

If transfusion is needed, exposure to allogeneic blood can be prevented by the use of autologous blood and implementing auto-transfusion techniques, such as acute normovolaemic haemodilution (ANH) or intra- or post-operative red cell recovery (see Annex 1, Table 1 – C1e). The use of targeted blood component therapy aided by point-of-care testing (POCT) can also help reduce the exposure to allogeneic blood. Instead of transfusing red cells, plasma, cryoprecipitate, and platelets all at the same time to control the bleeding, POCT can identify the specific component(s) that would be most effective in controlling the bleeding (see Annex 1, Table 1 – C1d). POCT also offers other advantages, such as a smaller blood volume requirement and rapid turn-around times. PBM programmes are applicable to both surgical and non-surgical patients. Strategies such as limiting blood losses through phlebotomy and use of evidence-based practice guidelines for red cells, platelet, and plasma transfusions should be adhered to for all patients and regularly monitored by appropriate committees, e.g. HTC for all services (see Table 1 – C1f). [73] Finally, modern healthcare, which includes transfusion practice in the context of this chapter, needs to adapt to new evidence about optimal patient care. For example, blood suppliers are responding to a better understanding of serious complications of transfusion and taking measures to minimise the risk of TRALI and bacterial contamination of platelets. However, it may sometimes be difficult to know how to respond to new data. For example, the controversy about 'stored' versus 'fresh' blood has been reignited by the finding of poorer clinical outcomes associated with 'older' blood in some observational studies. These studies have been the subject of critical reviews which have also pointed out the need for higher quality studies [76, 77], and several randomised controlled trials are underway. In addition, these reviews have also raised valid concerns about the effect of a radically shortened shelf-life on the blood supply which is taken for granted in the advanced and emerging transfusion chains.

Conclusion

This chapter has outlined the multiple current and emerging clinical interfaces in the transfusion chain between the blood supplier, the hospital blood bank, the clinician and the patient, and how they may be influenced to maintain and where necessary improve the quality of care and patient safety.

The clinical interfaces in hospitals and other settings where blood is used require engagement, co-operation and co-ordination by staff and with patients to ensure the safe and appropriate use of blood and alternatives to blood. There is also the interface between the blood supplier and hospitals connecting the supply chain which starts with blood donors.

The clinical interfaces are different depending on the setting. For example, the supply and safety of blood are the main concerns in the transfusion chain in developing countries ('traditional transfusion chain'), whereas avoidance of transfusion errors resulting in wrong blood transfusions and the inappropriate use of blood are the major issues in developed countries ('advanced transfusion chain').

At the level of the 'traditional' and certainly the 'advanced' transfusion chains, it would be expected that there would be a hospital transfusion policy, an active HTC, a quality management system to provide traceability of blood and haemovigilance, guidelines for safe and appropriate use of blood, and education, training and continuous professional development.

The emphasis of modern transfusion practice is on further reducing blood use through PBM programmes involving initiatives such as the robust implementation of evidence-based transfusion triggers, cell salvage, pre-operative anaemia management, and point-of care haemostasis testing ('emerging transfusion chain').

Whatever the setting, constructive engagement by those involved at the interfaces between the blood supplier, the hospital blood bank, the clinician and the patient are essential to ensure patient safety, an efficient blood bank service, and the best use of the finite blood supply. This engagement requires good communication in daily operational settings, and opportunities for the exchange of information and to address concerns such as at meetings of the HTC. Increasingly it is being recognised that further opportunities for discussion are required at the different interfaces, for example between blood supplier and hospital blood bank, hospital blood bank and clinical teams and clinicians with patient groups. Higher level discussions at regional or national level may be useful for setting strategy and agreeing initiatives for improving transfusion practice. All these discussions are facilitated by the sharing of data about transfusion practice. The availability and quality of such data is improving with the use of IT and the linking of IT systems within hospitals and between hospitals and blood services. Centralisation of hospital transfusion services and the integration of blood services with hospital transfusion services are likely to be significant enablers for better transfusion services in the future.

4. Final Recommendations

These final recommendations on key drivers for good transfusion practice for each type of transfusion service we have considered in this chapter, i.e. 'traditional', 'advanced' and 'emerging', are based on the content of this chapter and the supporting information provided in the references.

Traditional Transfusion Chain (supply driven):

1. Development and endorsement of policies for blood transfusion at both national and individual hospital level integrated in national and hospital health care policies;
2. Establishment of operational HTCs with clear terms of reference and membership;
3. Development of a working relationship with the supplier of blood and blood components;
4. Development of integrated quality management systems for transfusion by both blood suppliers and hospitals, to include the traceability of blood and haemovigilance;
5. Institution of education (teaching and training) with continuous professional development for all the many staff involved in blood transfusion;
6. Development and implementation of national and local guidelines for blood transfusion practice and a system for regular review;

Advanced Transfusion Chain (demand driven):

1. Further development and implementation of the above recommendations;
2. Provision of specialist scientific and clinical advice by blood suppliers advice and regular consultation between blood suppliers and hospital blood banks to strengthen the hospital blood bank-blood supplier interface;
3. Development and implementation of patient-oriented evidence-based blood transfusion practice including documented informed consent;

Emerging Transfusion Chain (patient driven):

1. Further development and implementation of the above recommendations;
2. Development of an integrated patient-centred blood management programme;
3. Creation of policies aimed at including the patient as a member of the healthcare team;
4. Development of a national and hospital transfusion epidemiology programme to better understand how blood is being used and how practice may be improved.

References

[1] Knowles, S; Cohen, H. (eds). On behalf of the Serious Hazards of Transfusion (SHOT) Steering Group. *The 2010 Annual SHOT Report, 2011* [online]. Available from: *URL: www.shotuk.org*

[2] US Food and Drug Administration. Fatalities Reported to FDA Following Blood Collection and Transfusion: Annual Summary for Fiscal Year 2010 [online]. Available from: *URL:http://www.fda.gov/BiologicsBloodVaccines*

[3]   Murphy MF; Stanworth SJ; Yazer M. Transfusion practice and safety: current status and possibilities for improvement. *Vox Sang*, 2011 100, 46-59.

[4]   UK Blood Transfusion & Tissue Transplantation Services. UK Blood Safety and Quality Regulations [online]. Available from: *URL: www.transfusionguidelines.org.uk*

[5]   Australian Commission on Safety and Quality in Health Care. *National Safety and Quality Health service Standards*, Sydney: ACSQHC; 2011.

[6]   Joint Commission on Accreditation of Healthcare Organizations.. Available from: *URL: www.jointcommission.org*

[7]   Hebert, PC; McDonald, BJ; Tinmouth, A. An overview of transfusion practices in peri-operative and critical care. *Transfus Alterna Transfus Me*, 2005 6,15-22.

[8]   Orlov D, Farrell RO, McCluskey SA, et al. The clinical utility of an index of oxygenation for guiding red blood cell transfusion in cardiac surgery. *Transfusion*, 2009 49, 682-688.

[9]   Carson JL, Terrin ML, Barton FB, et al. A pilot randomized trial comparing symptomatic against hemoglobin-level-driven red blood cell transfusion following hip fracture. *Transfusion*, 2003 38, 522-529.

[10]   Tinmouth AT, Freedman, J. Prophylactic platelet transfusions: which dose is the best dose? A review of the literature. *Transfus Med Rev*, 2003 17, 189-193.

[11]   World Health Organisation. Global database on Blood safety [online]. [cited 2009 Aug 3] Available from: *URL: http://www.who.int/bloodsafety/GDBS_Report_2001-2002.pdf*

[12]   Napier A, Chapman JF, Kelsey FP, et al. Guidelines on the clinical use of leukocyte – depleted blood components. *Transfus Med*, 1998 8, 59-71.

[13]   Rebulla P. Revisitation of the clinical indications for the transfusion of platelet concentrates. *Rev Clin Exp Hematol*, 2001 5, 288-310.

[14]   Hui CH, Williams I, Davis K. Clinical audits of the use of fresh-frozen plasma and platelets in a tertiary teaching hospital and the impact of a new transfusion request form. *Internal Medicine Journal*, 2005 35, 283-288.

[15]   Yeh CJ, Wu CF, Hsu WT, Hsieh LL, Lin SF, Liu TC. Transfusion audit of fresh frozen plasma in Southern Taiwan. *Vox Sang*, 2006 91, 270-74.

[16]   Maegele M. Frequency, risk stratification and therapeutic management of acute post-traumatic coagulopathy. *Vox Sang*, 2009 97, 39-49.

[17]   Grayson AD, Jackson M, Desmond MJ. Monitoring blood transfusion in patients undergoing coronary artery bypass grafting: an audit methodology. *Vox Sang*, 2003 85, 96-101.

[18]   *The clinical use of Blood*. WHO revised interactive edition (CD-ROM), 2005. Geneva, CH.

[19]   Expert Work Group. Guidelines for Red blood cell and Plasma transfusion for adults and children. *Can Med Ass J*, 1997 156 (11th Supplement).

[20]   Eindhoven GB, Diercks RL, Richardson FJ, et al. Adjusted transfusion triggers improve transfusion practice in orthopedic surgery. *Transfus Med*, 2005 15, 13-18.

[21]   Rosencher N, Kerkkamp HEM, Macheras G, et al. Orthopedic Surgery Haemoglobin Europe Overview (OSTHEO): Blood management in elective knee and hip arthroplasty.*Transfusion*, 2003 4, 459-469.

[22]   Rennie D. Informed consent by "Well-nigh abject" adults. *N Engl J Med*, 1990 302, 917-918.

[23] Drane JF. Competence to give an informed consent: A model for making a clinical assessment *JAMA,* 1984 252, 925-27.

[24] Ingelfinger FJ. Informed but uneducated consent. *N Engl J Med*, 1972 287, 465-66.

[25] Holland PV. Informed consent for Transfusion recipients: How much is enough?. In: Smit Sibinga CTh, Snyder EL, editors. *Triggers factors in Transfusion Medicine.* Dordrecht, Netherlands: Kluwer Academic Publishers; 1996; 17-24.

[26] Rock G, Berger R, Filion D, et al. Documenting a transfusion: How well is it done? *Transfusion,* 2007 47, 568-572.

[27] Holland PR, Schmidt, PJ. *Standards for Blood banks and transfusion services.* 12th edition. Arlington (VA). American Association of Blood Banks; 1987

[28] Krever H. Commission report: Commission of inquiry on the blood systems in Canada. *Final Report 1-3 Ottawa: Public works and Government Services Canada;* 1997, 11.

[29] Saxena S, Ramer L, Shalman IA. A Comprehensive assessment programme to improve blood administering practices using the FOCUS- PDCA MODEL. *Transfusion,* 2004 44, 1350-1356.

[30] Stowell CP. Informed consent for patients: Blood transfusion and Cellular therapies. In: Stowell CP, and Sazama K, eds. *Informed Consent in Blood Transfusion and Cellular Therapies: Patients, Donors, and Research Subjects.* Bethesda MD USA: AABB Press; 2007; 59-112.

[31] *Development of quality systems to improve the clinical use of blood.* Report on a WHO Regional Workshop. Groningen, The Netherlands. 2001 Oct 29-31.

[32] World Health Organisation. *Universal access to safe blood transfusion.* [cited 2009 Aug 3] Available from: *URL:http://www.who.int/bloodsafety/Publications/Universal AccesstoSafeBT.pdf*

[33] Larsson C, Saltredts S, Pahlen S, Andolf E. Estimation of blood loss after cesarean section has a low validity and a tendency to exaggeration. *Acta Obstet Gyn,* 2006 85, 14448-14452.

[34] Hughes K, Chang CY, Sedrak J, Torres A. (2007) A clinically practical way to estimate surgical blood loss. *Dermatol Online J* [Online serial], 13 (17).

[35] Gardner AJS, Dudley HAF. The measuring of blood loss at operation. *Brit. J. Anaesth*, 1962 34, 653-656.

[36] Dzik WH. New Technology for Transfusion safety. An analysis of surgical blood use in United States Hospitals with application of the Maximal Blood Order Schedule. *Transfusion,* 1979 19, 268-278.

[37] Guerin S, Collins C, Kapoor H, McClean I, Collins D. Blood transfusion requirement prediction in patients undergoing primary total hip and knee arthroplasty. *Transfus Med,* 2007 17, 37–43.

[38] Nuttal GA, Santrach PJ, Oliver WC, et al. A prospective randomized trial of the surgical blood order equation for ordering red blood cells for total hip arthroplasty. *Transfusion,* 1996 38, 828-833.

[39] Australian Society of Blood Transfusion. *Special edition on Guidelines for Autologous Blood collection.* 2002 April; Volume 9. No.2.

[40] Newman JH, Bowers M, Murphy J. The Clinical Advantages of Autologous *Transfusion*, JBJS (Br) 1997 79-B, 630-632 .

[41] Friedman, BA; Oberman, HA; Chadwick, AR. The maximal surgical blood order schedule and blood use in the United States. *Transfusion,* 1976 16, 380-387.

[42] Nuttall GA, Santrach PJ, Oliver WC, et al. Possible guidelines on preoperative autologous blood donation before total hip arthroplasty. *Mayo Clinic Proc*, 2000 75, 10-17.

[43] Dzik WH. Emily Cooley Lecture 2002: Transfusion safety in the Hospital. *Transfusion*, 2003 43, 1190.

[44] Linden JV, Wagner K, Voytovich AE, Sheehan J. Transfusion errors in New York State: an analysis of 10 years' experience. *Transfusion*, 2000 40, 1207-1213.

[45] Butch SH. Comparison of seven years of occurrence reports (abstract). *Transfusion*, 2000 40(Suppl 1), 159-S

[46] Lumadue JA, Boyd JS, Ness PM. Adherence to a strict specimen-labeling policy decreases the incidence of erroneous blood grouping of blood bank specimens. *Transfusion*, 1997 37, 1169-1172.

[47] Dzik WH, Murphy MF, Andreu G, et al. The Biomedical Excellence for Safer Transfusion (BEST) Working Party of the International Society for Blood Transfusion An international study of the performance of sample collection from patients. *Vox Sang*, 2003 85, 40–47.

[48] Murphy MF, Stearn BE, Dzik WH. Current performance of patient sample collection in the UK. *Transfus Med*, 2004 14, 113–121.

[49] Universal access to safe blood transfusion. Available from *URL:http://www.who.int /bloodsafety/Publications/UniversalAccesstoSafeBT.pdf*

[50] ResolutionWHA28.72. *Utilization and supply of human blood and blood products.* Twenty-eighth World Health Assembly, Geneva, World Health Organization, 1975.

[51] Kajja I, Bimenya GS, Sibinga CS. Blood request form at a University teaching hospital: evaluating design and clinician compliance. *Int J Health Sci*, 2008 1, 69-73.

[52] Armstrong B, Hardwick J, Raman L, Smart E, Wilkinson R. Introduction to blood transfusion technology. *ISBT science series*, 2008 3, 197-215.

[53] Rossmann SN. Scientific Section Coordinating Committee. *Guidelines for the Labeling of Specimens for Compatibility Testing.* Bethesda, MD: AABB; 2002.

[54] Klein HG, Lipton KS. Noninfectious serious hazards of transfusion. *AABB Bulletin 2001-04.* Bethesda, MD: American Association of Blood Banks.

[55] Linden JV, Paul B, Dressler KP. A report of 104 transfusion errors in New York State. *Transfusion*, 1992 32, 601-606.

[56] Robillard P, Itaj NK, Corriveau P. ABO incompatible transfusions, acute and delayed hemolytic transfusion reactions in Quebec hemovigilance system—Year 2000 (abstract). *Transfusion*, 2002 42, 25s.

[57] Andreu G, Morel P, Forestier F, et al. Hemovigilance network in France: organization and analysis of immediate transfusion incident reports from to 1998. *Transfusion*, 2002 42, 1356-1364.

[58] Shulman IA, Saxena S, Ramer L. Assessing blood administering practices. *Arch Pathol Lab Med*, 1999 123, 595-598.

[59] Zimmermann RZ, Linhard CT, Weisbach V, Büscher M, Zingsem J, Eckstein R. An analysis of errors in blood component transfusion records with regard to quality improvement of data acquisition and to the performance of look back and trace back procedures. *Transfusion*, 1999 39, 351-356.

[60] Goldman, M; Rémy-Prince, S; Trépanier, A; Décary F. Autologous donation error rates in Canada. *Transfusion.* 1997 37, 523-527.

[61] Donahue JG, Munoz A, Ness PM, et al. The declining risk of post transfusion Hepatitis c infection. *N Engl J Med,* 1992 327, 367-373.

[62] Department of Health. Better Blood Transfusion. HSC 2007/001. London: HMSO [online]. Available from: URL: *http://www.transfusionguidelines. org.uk/docs/pdfs /nbtc_bbt_hsc_07.pdf*

[63] Saxena S, Shulman IA. (2006). *The Transfusion Committee: Putting Patient Safety First* AABB Press, Bethesda, MD.

[64] Haspel RL, Uhl L. How do I audit hospital blood product utilization? *Transfusion,* 2012 52, 227-230.

[65] Dzik S. Use of a computer-assisted system for blood utilization review. *Transfusion,* 2007 47, 142S-144S.

[66] Gann P. Blood Safety Act [online]. Available from: *URL: http://www.mbc.ca.gov /publications/blood_transfusions.html*

[67] Advisory Committee on the Safety of Blood, Tissues and Organs. Patient Consent for Blood Transfusion [online]. Available from: *URL: http://www.dh.gov.uk/en /Publicationsandstatistics/Publications/PublicationsPolicyAndGuidance/DH_130716?s sSourceSiteId=ab*

[68] Davis RE, Vincent CA, Murphy MF. Blood transfusion safety: the potential role of the patient. *Transfus Med Rev,* 2011 25, 12-23.

[69] Aubuchon JP, Linauts S, Vaughan M, Wagner J, Delaney M, Nester T. Evolution in a centralized transfusion service. *Transfusion,* 2011 51, 2750-2757.

[70] Murphy MF. Reducing blood use: how we did it. *Transfusion,* 2007 47, 149S – 151S.

[71] Institute of Medicine of the National Academies. Crossing the quality chasm: a new health system for the 21st century/Committee on Quality Health Care in America, Institute of Medicine [online]. Availalble from; *URL: http://www.nap.edu/openbook. php?record_id=10027&page=R2*

[72] *Best Practices for a Patient Blood Management Program* (draft). April 2012 AABB Press, Bethesda, MD, USA download from *http://www.aabb.org/resources/bct/pbm /Documents/best-practices-pbm.pdf*

[73] AuBuchon JP, Puca K, Saxena S, et al., eds. *Getting started in blood management.* Bethesda, MD: AABB, 2011. download from *http://www.aabb.org/Pages/Product. aspx?Product_Id=1903&class=DOWNLOADS*

[74] Saxena S, Nelson JM, Osby M, Shah M, Kempf R, Shulman IR. Ensuring timely completion of type and screen testing and the verification of ABO/Rh status for elective surgical patients. *Arch Pathol Lab Med,* 2007 131, 576–581.

[75] Saxena S, Belzberg H, Chogyoji M, Wilcox S, Shulman IA. Reducing phlebotomy losses by streamlining laboratory test ordering in a surgical intensive care unit. *Lab Med,* 2003 34, 728-732.

[76] Dzik W. Fresh blood for everyone? Balancing availability and quality of stored RBCs. *Transfus Med,* 2008 18, 260-265.

[77] Glynn SA. The red blood cell storage lesion: a method to the madness. *Transfusion,* 2010 50, 1164-1169.

Annex 1

Table 1. Clinical Interfaces in Patient Safety and Quality Management

	Type of activities	Current interactions	Measures to assess outcomes	Interventions to improve outcomes	Evidence for effectiveness of interventions
A. Traditional interfaces (supply driven)					
1. Clinician and patient	Information about the risks and benefits of transfusion, alternatives to transfusion and measures for blood avoidance Obtaining and documenting consent	Decision to transfuse Documentation in medical record	Audits of documentation – Diagnosis, intervention and expectation, order	Education of clinicians, nurses and patients Development of information leaflets Development of in-hospital quality system; Introduction of informed consent	Change in professional behaviour and practice Improved documentation.
2. Clinician/ward and Hospital Blood Bank	Request for blood components ABO/Rh/alloantibodies Xmatch	Request for blood made to blood bank and blood sample provided	Audit of sample labelling and adequate provision of clinical information on paper requests Percentage completed forms	Refusal by hospital blood bank to accept poorly labelled samples or requests with inadequate clinical information	Improved practice of ordering and sample labelling, fewer 'wrong blood in tube' events, and better information of the reason for transfusion to facilitate audit
3a. Hospital Blood Bank and Blood Supplier	• Request for supply of blood and blood components • Request for advice	Ad hoc/daily requests for blood and blood components	Audit of requests and stock	Introduction of hospital blood stock management	Improved blood stock management Reduced clinical shortages
3b. Blood supplier and Hospital Blood Bank	• Supply of standard and special blood components and products for transfusion • (Scientific) advice about serological problems and the investigation and management of adverse events • Advice about regulatory issues and quality management • Other services e.g. stem cells, tissues, therapeutic apheresis	Almost daily and ad hoc (emergency) supplies of blood and blood components Regular shortages in the supplies	Audit of request and supply of blood and blood components	Introduction of clinical consultation Epidemiology of blood consumption	Improved supply; Reduced shortages Reduced emergency requests and supplies

	Type of activities	Current interactions	Measures to assess outcomes	Interventions to improve outcomes	Evidence for effectiveness of interventions
4. Hospital Blood Bank and clinician	Advice about: • Safe transfusion practice • Appropriate use of blood and blood avoidance • Use of alternatives to transfusion • Investigation and management of adverse events • Provision of blood in emergencies	Ad hoc advice, and draw attention to local and national guidelines for good practice	Local, regional and national audits of the safety of the transfusion process, the usage/epidemiology of blood and alternatives to blood, blood wastage, and the timeliness of provision of blood in emergencies	Development of hospital transfusion quality system and management Development of hemovigilance system; Feedback of results of audits, and educational events	Improved practice as assessed by repeat audits Reduced transfusion related morbidity and mortality
5. HTC* and clinical teams	Guidelines for: • Safe transfusion practice • Appropriate use of blood and blood avoidance • Use of alternatives to transfusion • Management of adverse events Monitoring of practice and feedback to clinical teams (and possibly to individual clinicians)	Ad hoc or absent	Existence of functioning/active HTC Guidelines Documentation	Creation of HTC with appropriate Terms of Reference Introduction of evidence-based hospital transfusion practice	Regular HTC reports Presence of clinical standards and guidelines Improved hospital transfusion practice
6. Blood supplier and HTC*	Provision of data on: • Quality of blood components • New developments and services Feedback on blood supplier's services	Commonly absent or ad hoc	Regular reports from blood supplier e.g. time to expiry of supplied blood components, data on quality monitoring of blood components, time to deliver diagnostic and reference serology services Satisfaction surveys of clinical prescribers and users	Following creation of HTC: requests by HTC for better data, quality improvements, or further development of products or services Explore additional methods of feedback from clinical users	Compliance by the supplier with requests by HTC for improvements in services and components. Use of comparative data of transfusion practice with other hospitals to support HTC's efforts to improve the safety and effectiveness of transfusion practice Improved satisfaction with the supplier's services and components

Table 1. (Continued)

	Type of activities	Current interactions	Measures to assess outcomes	Interventions to improve outcomes	Evidence for effectiveness of interventions
B. Advanced interfaces (demand driven)					
1. HTC* and clinical teams	Guidelines for: • Safe transfusion practice • Appropriate use of blood and blood avoidance • Use of alternatives to transfusion • Management of adverse events Monitoring of practice and feedback to clinical teams (and possibly to individual clinicians)	Distribution of local and national guidelines by hard copy, email or intranet Local (and possibly regional and national) audits Investigation of incidents of poor practice	Local audits of practice of the safety of the transfusion process and blood usage and participation in national audits Follow up audits	Feedback of results from audits, and educational events Educational events and revision and reissue of guidelines	Reducing number of 'wrong blood' events, 'near misses' and inappropriate use of blood As above
2. Clinician and patient	Information about the risks and benefits of alternatives to transfusion and measures for blood avoidance Obtaining and documenting consent	Issue of patient information leaflets and discussion with individual patients Documentation in medical records	Audits of documentation of provision of information and consent. Patient satisfaction surveys As above	Distribution of local guidelines and educational events As above	Improved documentation of provision of information and consent Improved patient satisfaction Improved documentation of consent
3. Clinician and Hospital Blood Bank	Request for • Blood components • ABO/Rh/alloantibodies • Xmatch	Request for blood made to blood bank and blood sample provided	Audit of sample labelling and adequate provision of clinical information on paper requests	Refusal by hospital blood bank to accept poorly labelled samples or requests with inadequate clinical information Electronic systems for blood requesting, patient identification and sample collection	Improved practice of sample labelling, fewer 'wrong blood in tube' events, and better information of the reason for transfusion to facilitate audit
4. Hospital Blood Bank and clinician	Advice about: • Safe transfusion practice • Appropriate use of blood and blood avoidance • Use of alternatives to transfusion • Investigation and management of adverse events • Provision of blood in emergencies	Ad hoc advice, and draw attention to local and national guidelines for good practice	Local, regional and national audits of the safety of the transfusion process, the usage of blood and alternatives to blood, blood wastage, and the timeliness of provision of blood in emergencies	Feedback of results of audits, and educational events	Improved practice as assessed by repeat audits

	Type of activities	Current interactions	Measures to assess outcomes	Interventions to improve outcomes	Evidence for effectiveness of interventions
5. Blood Supplier and Hospital Blood Bank	• Supply of standard and special blood components for transfusion • Scientific advice about serological problems and the investigation and management of adverse events • Advice about regulatory issues and quality management • Other services e.g. stem cells, tissues, therapeutic apheresis	Regular (up to several times/day) interaction for blood ordering, requests for special investigations and blood components, and advice	Monitoring of timely supply of blood components and other services Blood components meeting required quality standards Timely investigation of serological and diagnostic problems Provision of high quality scientific and clinical advice	Requests by hospitals or regulatory bodies for improved quality of blood components or other services Forums for discussion between blood suppliers and representatives of blood banks	Documented improvements in the quality of blood components and other services provided by the blood supplier
6. Blood Supplier and HTC (and Hospital Blood Bank)	Provision of data on: • Quality of blood components • New developments and services • Blood usage and blood wastage in comparison with other similar hospitals Feedback on blood supplier's services	Provision of intermittent data on the quality of blood components, and other services, and any new developments. Ideally, provision of comparative data of blood usage and blood wastage with other similar hospitals Feedback from the HTC on the supplier's products and services	Regular reports from blood supplier e.g. time to expiry of supplied blood components, data on quality monitoring of blood components, time to deliver diagnostic and reference serology services Satisfaction surveys of clinical users	Requests by HTC for better data, quality improvements, or further development of components or services Explore additional methods of feedback from clinical users	Compliance by the supplier with requests by HTC for improvements in services and components. Use of comparative data of transfusion practice with other hospitals to support HTC's efforts to improve the safety and effectiveness of transfusion practice Improved satisfaction with the supplier's services and products
C. Emerging interfaces (Patient-centered & Patient-driven Blood Management Programme)					
1. Multidisciplinary collaboration among key departments and patient	Develop and implement the following components of a PBM program, as appropriate	Not applicable (NA)	Monitor compliance with different components of the PBM program (see below)	Engage "opinion leaders" Involve HTC early in the development of the programme Provide lectures, presentations at departmental meetings	PBM programme is fully implemented

Table 1. (Continued)

	Type of activities	Current interactions	Measures to assess outcomes	Interventions to improve outcomes	Evidence for effectiveness of interventions
a) HTC*, surgery/anaesthesia, and haematology services	Establishing a Pre-operative Anaemia Management Clinic	NA	Monitor compliance with pre-operative anaemia evaluation protocols	Develop standardised protocols for anaemia evaluation and management Provide timely feedback on non-compliance	Pre-operative patients are evaluated for anaemia and managed appropriately
b) HTC*, Hospital Blood Bank, surgery/obstetric/anaesthesiase rvices	Ensuring type and screen (T&S) evaluations on all qualifying elective surgery and obstetric patients	NA	Monitor compliance with pre-op T&S ordering protocol	Develop and disseminate a list of surgical procedures that qualify for pre-op T&S testing Provide timely feedback on non-compliance	T&S test is ordered on all patients scheduled to have qualifying surgeries
c) Laboratory and various clinical services	Minimising blood losses through phlebotomy	NA	Review diagnostic test utilisation patterns	Use smaller blood collection tubes Redesign test ordering requisition and on-line screens to reflect evidence-based ordering guidelines Educate physicians and house staff about appropriate test utilisation	Diagnostic tests are ordered only when considered medically necessary Standing orders for tests are discontinued
d) Laboratory and surgery /obstetric/anaesthesia services	Implementing point-care testing (POCT) aided transfusion therapy in the operating rooms	NA	Review POCT usage and its impact on blood ordering	Benchmark blood usage among various services and share at leadership and departmental meetings	Blood components are ordered based on patient's clinical condition and POCT results

Type of activities	Current interactions	Measures to assess outcomes	Interventions to improve outcomes	Evidence for effectiveness of interventions
e) HTC, Hospital Blood Bank, and surgery/obstetric/anaesthesia services				
Limiting peri-operative blood loss through ANH** and red cell recovery programmes	NA	Monitor the extent of utilisation of ANH** and red cell recovery programmes among surgical patients	Develop guidelines for the use of ANH** and red cell recovery procedure in accordance with the published standards Collaborate with surgeons, obstetricians and anaesthetists to implement ANH and red cell recovery programmes	ANH** and red cell recovery programmes are fully implemented
f) HTC*				
Ensuring reasonable and justifiable blood utilisation practices	See under B.1	Review blood usage for both over- and under-utilisation of blood Review transfusion orders, by physician and by service	Develop evidence-based blood utilisation guidelines Redesign transfusion ordering requisition and on-line screens to reflect evidence-based ordering guidelines Provide timely feedback to physicians and service chiefs	Usage of blood products is appropriate and improving
2. Blood Supplier to patient				
Advice about: • Autologous donation • Directed donation	Provision of information on the autologous and directed donation options to patients who are planning to have surgery or may need blood in the future because of their underlying medical condition	HTC monitors the use of autologous and directed blood. in the hospital	• Providing guidance to physicians on ordering autologous and directed donations	A documented declining trend in the use of autologous and directed blood (except for patients with special needs)

Table 1. (Continued)

Type of activities	Current interactions	Measures to assess outcomes	Interventions to improve outcomes	Evidence for effectiveness of interventions
• Volunteer or Community blood supply	Provision of information on the option to receive blood from the community blood supply to patients who are planning to have surgery or may need blood in the future because of their underlying medical condition	HTC monitors the use of volunteer blood supply in the hospital	• Educating physicians on safety of the community blood supply	A shift towards ~100% use of the community blood (except for patients with special needs)

* Hospital Transfusion Committee.
** Acute Normovolaemic Haemodilution.

In: Quality Management in Transfusion Medicine
Editor: Cees Th. Smit Sibinga

ISBN: 978-1-62618-665-1
© 2013 Nova Science Publishers, Inc.

Chapter X

Quality Management at the Societal Interface

Ton A. P. M. Los†,[1],* Sarah Mutegombwa[2],† and Che Lin Kit[3],‡
[1]APM Los Consultancy, Groningen, The Netherlands
[2]Uganda Red Cross Society, Kampala, Uganda
[3]Chief Executive Hong Kong Red Cross Blood
Transfusion Service, Kowloon, Hong Kong

Abstract

The first section of this chapter comments on the very beginning of the blood transfusion chain i.e. the general population as it is before motivational efforts reach individual people who may potentially register for blood donation. In this section mainly external outcome indicators are used in assessing the quality of an intervention (e.g., campaign, PR, advertisement, messages). Measurement of outcome of motivational efforts will always be a bottle neck in the quality chain because interventions cannot be organized without external interfering factors.

It should be encouraging to learn that of the most important factor in society, i.e. religion, no negative or donation preventing attitude can be expected since all defined world religions accept blood donation as an act of helping humanity.

Second section discusses the possible quality assessment methods and measures to assess the quality of donor handling, planning, approach and donation sessions with emphasis on measurement of performance and outcome indicators through (donor) satisfaction surveys.

Final section discusses the various aspects of quality assessment in the hospital and patient surrounding and their interaction with the blood establishment leaving finally

* Ton A.P.M. Los†, MscMedSoc: APM Los Consultancy. P.O. Box 1089, 9701 BB, Groningen, Netherlands. Tel: +31-6-51677443; E-mail: apmlos@hotmail.com and info@ apmlosconsultancy.org.http://www. apmlosconsultancy.org.
† Sarah Mutegombwa: Uganda Red Cross Society. P.O. Box 494 Kampala, Uganda. Tel: +256-772-366121; E-mail: smutegombwa@redcrossug.org and mutegombwa@yahoo.co.uk.
‡ Che Kit Lin, MD: Chief Executive Hong Kong Red Cross Blood Transfusion Service. 15 King's Park Rise, Kowloon, Hong Kong. PRC: Tel: +852-27101301; E-mail: cklin@ha.org.hk.

room for social science application in diverse forms of measurement of client and organisational satisfaction with the related performance.

Keywords: Quality Management, Blood Donors, Donor Motivation, Patient Care, General population, Altruistic characteristics, Communication, Public relations (PR), Intervention, Demographic information, KAP assessment, PR tools

1. General Population

1.1. Introduction

Since 1900, blood transfusion therapy has become an increasingly important factor in health care. Two major discoveries were responsible for this development: First the discovery of the blood groups (ABO) system by Karl Landsteiner in the year 1900, and second in 1914, the use of Sodium citrate for anti-coagulation, invented by Albert Huestin. From that moment on as a basis for the application of blood transfusion therapy, there was a growing demand for human donor blood, implicating an appeal to the *altruistic characteristics* of the general population.

Altruism is a concept derived from the term 'alter' (L), which means 'the other'. Altruistic behaviour is behaviour which is unselfish, selfless. Altruism can be defined as "*doing something for the benefit of others at some cost to oneself*" [Wikipedia]. Altruistic behaviour in general and in diverse forms is found in all times and in all cultures. *Voluntary, non remunerated, blood donation* is in its essence a form of altruistic behaviour.

Since then, recruitment, mobilization (or using the preferred terminology: *motivation*) of volunteer blood donors in general was worldwide supported and organized by Red Cross and Red Crescent Societies, endorsing the principle of voluntarism and non-remuneration. In 1988 it was estimated that the Red Cross and Red Crescent Societies were responsible for the collection of one-third of the blood collected in the world [1] - result of the (enthusiastic) work of many local RC organisations and volunteer donor recruiters. It was initially in the field of '*welfare*'.

In that time the immediate result of 'recruitment' efforts counted as there was no long term policy, with systematic evaluation of the 'recruitment' efforts. Terms like quality or quality management were not (yet) applicable to these efforts.

The demand for human donor blood resulted worldwide in various approaches to meet the demand. Variation in approaches originated from social, organizational and political background and structure, and the level of economy and health care of the countries involved.

Although the principle of voluntary blood donation was and is (WHO statement) promoted worldwide, the reality shows us a different picture. Real voluntarism and non-remuneration is not always realised.

Remuneration in the form of food, facilities, and often but not always, under severe economic circumstances even payment for blood can be observed, for example in certain parts of East- and Western Europe, the United States, South America and the developing countries In 1976, the London social scientist Richard Titmuss in his book 'The Gift Relationship', described an applicable typology of blood donors / blood donation which is still up to date, covering the total range from complete and true non-remunerated voluntarism

(VNRBD) to professional and paid blood 'donation', with a number of in-between categories, like family credit or replacement donation, and fringe benefit donation. [Table 1] [2]

Let us consider the value of the following statements in terms of the ideal premises for blood transfusion emphasizing Titmuss's true voluntary donating donor type:

"The fundament of blood transfusion is the willingness of the community to share the blood", and "The willingness or motivation should be based on the concept of blood being a national resource to be shared by all".

The consequence of common agreement on the truth of these statements, is an accepted need for a *special educational approach* and mechanisms of continuous appeal of all groups in the society in order to achieve *general acceptance in the society.*

All efforts that have the ultimate goal to care for and to safeguard continuity, self-sufficiency and sustainability of the donor base and the related policy measures, could be reduced to the common denominator: 'donor management'.

Thus, specific educational research and mechanisms to reach the community are important aspects of 'donor management'.

We feel that such a comprehensive and fundamental approach on donor management is not yet generally accepted and applied worldwide. It can not be denied that donor management is still largely situated in a primarily good willing but rather amateurish corner.

It is certainly not our intention to question the integrity and dedication of staff and employees involved in the field of donor recruitment and/or donor management. The term amateurish should therefore not be regarded as unfavourable, but rather as a synonym for unsystematic, unscientific, and subject to insufficient evaluation.

Of course there has been abundance of scientific research on aspects of blood donation and donor management.

However, no doubt until the 1980s there has been a one-sided attention on the motivation of *becoming and being a blood donor.* In the literature on blood donation until the 90s of the previous century we find the majority of articles on this specific subject.

Over the last decades attention has shifted to donor retention and reasons for deferral.

Also donor satisfaction and the measurement of this aspect of blood donation became a topic of interest and study. This can be seen as a modest start of thinking in terms of *quality performance* of blood establishment personnel and blood establishment environment.

Table 1. R.M. Titmuss typology of donors

| Typology of donors –
Paid Donors
Professional Donors
Paid Induced Voluntary Donor
Responsibility Fee Donor
Family Credit Donor
Captive Voluntary Donor
Fringe Benefit Voluntary Donor
Voluntary Community Donor (VNRBD) | 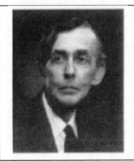 |

1.2. Recognition of the Notion of Quality

Since the notion of quality, quality systems and quality management was recognized in the non profit sector in the 90s of the previous century, and introduced as core topics in transfusion medicine, the organisations and institutions that were concerned with transfusion medicine in all its aspects, had to recognise and implement related policy measures, showing their concern and commitment to this new approach.

In this book the various aspects of transfusion medicine following the complete chain from approach to the general population, the source of the donors, the motivated donor and finally the patient are covered. There is a difference between the various aspects regarding the moment that attention to quality and quality systems was introduced for that specific topic. In general the more technical aspects were covered first and later on the attention became apparent for the societal and social aspects of blood transfusion and especially to the society interface, the approach to the information, motivation of the *general population*, the mobilisation and motivation to *become* blood donor and the aspects of the *donation process* from welcome/entrance to farewell of the donor. This paragraph covers the quality aspects of approach to the general population until registration as donor. The activities within this approach could be seen as preparation before the actual blood collection process starts. Recent publications consider donor recruitment (motivation) practices also as an objective of Quality Management of Blood Collection [3, 4]. This implies that all efforts (activities) should be judged against a background of quality management, quality processes, quality management processes, and using quality indicators. This paragraph wants to discuss whether this is feasible and to what extend.

1.3. Reaching the General Population: Quality of Communication and PR

When talking about quality of communication and public relations (PR), there must be a possibility to define the necessary characteristics of communication and PR and then to assess the quality of communication and PR. The starting point is always the population itself. About which population are we talking? Do we mean the complete world population in all its diversity or do we restrict us to the population in a small village in the rural area of North Siberia? Probably neither of the two. But then the question arises: which population are we aiming at? It can be the diverse population of an entire country or just a part of it such as the student population in the age of 18-25 years with their specific habits and language. These few examples make already clear that there cannot be such thing as 'the only correct or adequate way of communicating' or the only 'right' way of applying PR mechanisms.

So our first conclusion should be that the same variety that we notice in populations, parts of the world, countries, towns, villages, specific groups, students, Muslims, Catholics, etc., etc. can be found in adequate ways of communicating and applying PR. So there is not one right way in communicating. Each population / target group deserves and demands its own approach. Then the difficult question arises: How do we know that our chosen way of communicating is the most efficient way? In other words or *quality* terms: How do we assess the quality of our approach? In this sense we use the term quality as an indicator for the efficiency and effectiveness of our communication and PR method and tools. Quality indicators can be defined as measurable, objective indicators of the efficiency of the key segments of a system. [5] Measuring the efficiency and effectiveness of our communication and PR method and tools means knowledge about or insight in the situation *before and after* the intervention (PR method and Tool). This is called evaluation. What was the effect of our intervention and did it achieve the expected outcome? The effect of an intervention can be described in terms of outcome (number of donations, increase in number of donors, etc.) or any other important change that was planned. Measurement needs data about the old and new situation. Here we refer to outcome indicators. [5]

Before being able to design communication methods and PR tools it is of utmost importance to have insight in the characteristics of the focused population or part of the population (= target group). It starts with 'simple' demographics and ends with complex assessment of socio-cultural characteristics through Knowledge Attitudes and Practices (KAP) assessments or surveys (see par. 1.3.9).

1.3.1. Relevance of Demographic Information

Donor management should be approached in a professional, systematic and scientific way. The fundamental approach of donor management should be extensive, and should be based on good scientific documentation, monitoring and evaluation. Fundamental in this approach is a good notion and insight in the *characteristics and composition of the population* from which the (potential) donors should be mobilized and selected. These characteristics differ from place to place and from country to country.

1.3.2. Characteristics of the General Population

Basic information is needed on demographic characteristics of the general population from which the donor population should be mobilized. Important questions are: What data do we need? The availability of data and how should the data be collected?

In many countries there are population registries on different levels (country, department, city, etc.). From these registries the basic information on population demographics should be available. However, it should be realized that registration by census has yet to be implemented in many countries, so this basic information is often missing or incomplete.

For a basic demographic description of the general population the following data could suffice: Number of inhabitants, gender, age, domicile. However, the availability of additional data (religion; education; marital status, profession, etc.) could give more possibilities for gaining insight in and knowledge of the general population, the source of our prospective and potential donors. Another source could be the availability of data on postal code level (regional level) regarding the composition of household, consumptive behaviour, educational level, lifestyle, etc. through surveys among the general population by commercial organisations and bureaus for marketing research.

Then as a part of the communication methods and PR tools it comes to design, choice and evaluation of the quality of the used *message*. With what kind of message (written, audible, visible, etc.) do we approach our (target) population or target group?

1.3.3. Defining and Selection of Target Groups

Fundamental in this approach is a good notion and insight in the characteristics and composition of the population from which the (potential) donors should be mobilized and selected, their characteristics, and in further paragraphs the composition of the existing donor population: Characteristics of first-time donors, donor selection, the period donors are 'active' (length of the 'donor career'), the characteristics of resigned donors, the reason for resignation and deferral.

An example of target groups in the community is given in the following differentiation and selection criteria:

- Youth < 18 years; schools and > 18 years colleges, universities
- School curricula
- Vocational training
- Sports and recreation
- Clubs
- Religion, politics and cultural life
- Vocational practice; commerce, industry, institutions, government and private
- Family
- Aged people

1.3.4. Application of PR and Advertisement in Transfusion Medicine

Application of PR and advertisement starts with a good organization including a meticulous planning based on a clear and focused objective/expected outcome, adequate action, prepared mechanism for evaluation, all supported through an adequate budget. Hasty, *ad hoc* and poorly prepared actions should be avoided as well as lack of insight into the target group and inaccessible messages.

The effect of advertisement depends on objective of the presentation, the message, means used, timing, utilizing actualities, frequency of presentation; one time or repetitive, and visibility.

PR and advertisement for blood donation may include: Appeal on personal feelings and emotions, use of appropriate allusions and metaphors, appeal to public spirit – *blood is a national resource, of all of us, for all of us* – appealing to sense of responsibility; honesty, notion of value and possible risks for the recipient.

Some additional aspects to take into account are local style, simple, understandable, clear and repetitive messages, manners, habits of target group, identification and visibility, respect and appreciation, and a simple, expressive and strong logo.

Examples for presentation public transport, illuminated advertisement, posters at public locations, information to new citizens, community authorities, religion / politics / cultural life, information through driver licence-school, collection of drivers license, regional / local media (e.g., radio / television), internet, social media, mobile telephones.

Advertisements through announcements and messages should have the following points of attention: type of publication, area of distribution, circulation in relation to target group, interest of target group, culture, sports, recreation, hobby, business, vocation, religion, one time or repetitive, position in the publication. In practice and especially in developing countries all these aspects of PR and related activities can be carried out in the blood establishment environment through personnel. However, when sufficient funds are available, an option could be to delegate the activities to external commercial firms preferably with ISO certification to guarantee the necessary quality level and consistency of performance. This is called *outsourcing* and forms an adequate alternative. These commercial firms should apply external quality indicators to be able to monitor their performance and outcome.

1.3.5. Quality of Messages

Messages as tools for communication and PR should be fit for use (to the point, simple and understandable) and completely adapted to the goal of the planned intervention and the target population (target group).

The goal and final effect is not so difficult to define since all (society focused) efforts in transfusion medicine aim at realizing a safe and sustainable donor base with largely regular donors (outcome indicator). The goal can be to reach the general population in its totality to promote voluntary blood donation as an act of humanity and social solidarity. Or the goal can be to reach a selected target group for example college and university students. Messages should be understood by the population or target group and make use of the language and metaphors used and understood.

First and fundamental in this approach is a good notion and insight in the characteristics and composition of the population from which the (potential) donors should be mobilized and selected. Second, good knowledge of the way people perceive the given information is needed, since the comprehension of the information provided and the message given is of paramount importance for the appropriate action to be triggered.

Both aspects mentioned are of equal importance and are complementary, because before we can study the community we should have sufficient insight in the characteristics of the community. The message should fit each target group in a tailor-made fashion and should be given by adequate information materials.

Research on the characteristics of the community should provide us with sufficient information on the demographic composition of the different target groups. A relative under-representation of certain groups can be signalized through comparison of the existing donor population with the general population. Thus, special attention may be given to under-represented categories of potential donors identified. Adequate information about the population should result in proper adjustment of the message to the categories of interest. Additional information on the level of education, and professional status of the population could be helpful to make the message suit properly.

Some important aspects of donor motivation and mobilization could be summarized as follows:

- Emphasis on personal responsibility to support and to contribute.
- Blood donation should be voluntary but not without engagement.
- Adequate information and enlightenment should be given, and the very important final point: the language used should be simple, clear and metaphorical.
- Repetitive use of short and appealing slogans has proven their efficacy in many advertisements campaign.

A critical note regarding the aspects of PR and messages so far as the measurement of the effect is always after the intervention has taken place. In the most of the cases it will be an outcome indicator. The problem with these interventions and proposed effect is always and contrary with 'controlled experiments', that it can *never* be proven that *only* the intervention has resulted in the outcome or effect. There may be always societal circumstances that also influence the outcome, for example the influence of mass media, disasters. There is no control group! In other words: a planned and effectuated increase of number of donors can also be the side-effect of simultaneous events which happen in the society and are not under control.

1.3.6. Definition and Selection of Low Risk Groups

Fundamental criterion for this selection is privacy protection and confidentiality. For the procurement of the blood supply, the donor needs to meet international criteria of health for the selection. This includes the information in relation to risk factors and other confidential information. The medical profession has the responsibility to protect the privacy of the volunteer donor and to support evaluation of deferral criteria, both temporary and permanent.

The information to the *general population* regarding reasons for *not* giving blood and the relation of these reasons with specific behaviour has only one purpose – to prevent contamination of patients with donor blood that contains infectious agents. This means that in terms of quality of information, the communication, PR and messages, there is only one standard – to aim at and focus on 100% safety and exclusion of the risk of contamination.

A critical remark should be that there does not exist such a thing as 'zero-risk'. And behaviour of people can never be controlled in total. So selection of target groups which have proven to be low risk never guarantees the ultimate safety that we focus on. To apply standards of quality management to the selection of absolute *safe* potential donors out of the population to prevent risk of contamination will always face difficulties and probably will be not possible in its entire scope.

1.3.7. Information (Materials, Channels, News and Social Media)

A great variety of measures can be taken to motivate and mobilize persons to become a blood donor. The measures vary from well-designed educational programmes for young people at schools, to the use of mass media.

Regular publications in the newspapers can show the actual situation of the blood supply (stock) and the actual need (shortage) if present. This may have a shock effect. This may instantly motivate people to become blood donor. However, it is important to investigate what the real effect of (the) programme(s) is on the long run. A programme may sound very appropriate; the results can be seen on short term. However, there may be little or no insight in the effects (efficacy) of the measures on the long run.

It seems sometimes relatively easy to recruit first-time donors, especially with hard marketing techniques. However, the (long term) problem is how to retain them and guarantee continuity of blood donation. There should be long-term planning and adequate monitoring and evaluation of the measures taken.

There is often *ad hoc* and direct visibility of donor 'recruitment' programmes. However, the efficacy of these measures taken on the long run is not known. There is a need for more insight in 'long-term' effects and efficacy of given information materials and / or information methods used in reaching the community and target groups. In other words there is a need for adequate scientific monitoring and evaluation of measures taken to reach the general population. One efficient way of monitoring is through KAP survey, and assessment through permanent monitoring (questioning) and management of the collected data.

National guidelines should be developed based on the results of the KAP survey among other sources. A critical remark should be made here: The results of any KAP assessment should be seen as seeds to be sowed in fertile ground to be able to grow up to mature flowers, plants, trees, etc. If there is no fertile ground available or the ground is not prepared and dry, the seeds are bound to die and will never become of any value. This implies the existence of a basic structure of health care, a network of organisations which together form the platform that uses the results of the KAP survey and any other source of information to build up and improve the National guidelines on motivation and retention strategies.

First of all there is a need for this ground structure. A second remark relates to the expected impact of any sustained Public Awareness Campaign (PAC) based on the results of a KAP study. The effect will definitely be an ultimate increase of public awareness through the PAC.

Premises and restrictions are to be noticed regarding the necessary (local, regional) donor handling capacity. There should definitely be enough realistic opportunity to donate when the PAC is launched. In the design of PAC this donor handling capacity should be taken into account, and preferably result in a decision and choice between:1

1   low profile information to prepare to donate;
2   pro-active motivate and mobilize.

In other words; a certain amount of control over the generated effect of a PAC should be realized.

1.3.8. Assessment of Knowledge, Attitude and Practice (KAP) Regarding Blood Donation and Transfusion

Characteristics of the population and the various parts (groups – target groups) can be described in terms of number, gender, population density, age, and furthermore the socio-cultural characteristics that have an immense variety in origin: clubs, religion, education, free time, sport etc., etc. An adequate way to sample this socio-cultural information is through a KAP survey with besides the questions about the specific topic of the KAP survey, additional extended questions about socio cultural background and more extended demographic data.

1.3.9. General Introduction to KAP Studies

Knowledge, Attitudes and Practices (KAP) studies are highly focused evaluations that measure the actual situation regarding human knowledge, attitudes and practices in response to a specific subject e.g., voluntary blood donation. KAP studies have been widely used and valued around the world for at least forty years in several sectors under which public health. KAP studies tell us what people know about certain things, how they feel, and how they behave. Each KAP study is unique to a particular setting and designed for a specific issue.

- Knowledge possessed by a community refers to their understanding of that topic
- Attitude refers to their feelings toward the subject, as well as any preconceived ideas they may have towards it.
- Practice refers to the ways in which they demonstrate the knowledge and attitudes through actions and initiatives.

Understanding these three dimensions will allow a project to track changes over time, and may enable the project to tailor activities to the needs of that community. The specific topics of a KAP survey can be extended with demographic and socio-cultural questions. KAP studies preferably should be conducted twice, preferably to the same target population, both pre- and post-intervention, in order to measure impact of planned interventions.

1.3.9.1. KAP Research Protocol

A research protocol is a document that describes the methodology how a research study is designed, administered and analysed. The basic elements of a KAP study include:

a. Domain Identification

The domain is the subject for which the KAP study will be conducted, for example promotion of voluntary blood donation (VNRBD). More specifically, the domain would be the knowledge, attitudes and practices of a community in regard to VNRBD.

b. Identification of the Target Population

The first step in conducting a KAP study is the selection of the target group and the sample to which the survey will be given. The division of the population into smaller categories is typically desirable, as different groups in a community have varying educational, cultural and socio-economic backgrounds and therefore will likely have different levels of KAP.

c. Determination of Sampling Methods

A standard method for conducting the survey should be decided upon in advance, and should be consistent for each category to ensure that differences in the result are independent of the sampling method and depend solely on the characteristics of the population in question. KAP sampling methods typically use a *questionnaire* through interviews (in-person, phone, or mail), and finally can be a self-administered questionnaire completed by the target group persons.

Usually the design of questionnaires follows the standard operating procedures (SOP) of social science and can guarantee a certain level of quality. The method used for collecting the data through questionnaires followed the steps from design, distribution of hard copy questionnaires to the target group, collecting the completed questionnaires and entering the data manually, followed by description and analysis.

With the introduction of internet and e-mail a new way of collecting the data emerged through on-line questioning i.e., completing the questionnaires on-line at the personal computer (or in the future mobile telephones and i-pads, etc.) followed by central storage of the data in an external computer system (server) which prepares the data for description and analysis.

This method guarantees an increase of the quality of the data and related analysis, because human errors at the distribution, collection and data entry side are minimised.

Furthermore this method is extremely cost saving and therefore very interesting and useful for developing countries with modest budgets. The only disadvantage may be the high computer illiteracy, low availability of computers and low on-line access for various target groups.

However, the target group of young students (18-25 yr.) which is often a preferred group to be approached for surveying reasons for donation and investigating possibilities for motivating them to register as a blood donor, has by its origin of student registration extreme good access to internet and e-mail possibilities.

So the only bottleneck (computer access) seems to disappear. Inducing a good response can provide data of high quality and related analysis. [6]

d. Analysis and Reporting

KAP studies are very much like a standard social survey, although they are much more focused and limited in scope. KAP studies are also uniquely tailored to a specific location, project, or problem. Therefore they collect the least amount of information to determine whether KAP have changed from one time period to another. After collection, the data are analysed to determine the KAP level of the target group. The results / answers from the questionnaires are coded and entered in a spread-sheet (data base) or generated through on-line surveying.

In large populations software (programmes) like SAS, SPSS, Excel or other standard databases can be used to enter data, describe, analyse and present KAP data. Knowledge questions, which often have more than one component to a 'correct' answer, must be analysed differently from those in the Attitudes section, which must in turn be analysed differently from those in the Practices section.

Reporting of findings is typically done in the presentation of descriptive statistics in table format for each section (knowledge, attitudes, and practices). A KAP report should include an introduction, study design, findings, analysis and conclusions. Format and distribution depend upon the terms of reference of the study as defined by the commissioning agency. Most KAP reports contain detailed frequency data and histograms with attributes of the surveyed population, with clear tracking of pre/post intervention knowledge, attitudes and practices over time. To measure the effect of interventions it is therefore recommended to repeat a similar KAP study over a certain period of time.

1.3.10. Evaluation of Donor Management Activities through Application of Social Science Methods

The KAP studies and related protocol described in the previous paragraph follow their own Quality Management rules, quality assessment and guarantee according to the scientific standards of the social sciences and do not need a discussion in this book. We kindly refer to the literature on social science and methodology.

Some aspects of the attitude of the general population, however, towards blood donation are interesting to describe and one of the most important aspects is in general the reluctance in the various societies and cultures to give blood and general reasons for not donating.

1.3.11. Consciousness, Beliefs, Habits, Fears and Restrictions for Giving Blood

All over the world, blood is donated by only a minority of a country's population. The motivation of donors and non-donors has been surveyed many times. The American scientist R. M. Oswalt, who did extensive research on donor motivation, wondered in 1977 [7] whether it would still be necessary to do research on the motivation of donors and non-donors. He suggested that additional surveys of blood donor and non-donor motivations are not likely to produce any significant new information since essentially the same information has been forthcoming for the last 20 years or so. The findings of Oswalt were completed and confirmed by Boe and Ponder [8], and Piliavin. [9]

Reasons for *not* giving blood [10]:

- Medical ineligibility
- Medical (poor?) excuses

- Fear (fainting, needle, pain, sight of blood, infections [AIDS])
- Time constraints
- Inconvenience of opportunity
- Apathy

Most important reasons *for not* donating blood, described in the literature, seem to be 2-fold. First, it seems to be related to personal perception of the blood supply system and blood donation. This is influenced by misinformation, lack or paucity of information, misunderstanding, fear, and poor image. Second, non-donation seems to be related to several practical circumstances: infrastructure, time, distance, socio-cultural background, level of economy, and health status.

Reasons for not giving blood have always been largely dependent on cultural background of a population and socio-economic characteristics of a society. Also, the various religions and philosophies of life play an important role in determining public perception. This implies that the willingness of people to donate blood for their fellow human beings on a voluntary and non-remunerated basis could negatively be affected by various recent developments in society. Examples are – substantial change in the administration of the society (splitting up of the Soviet Union in multiple sections and later self-supporting countries), multi-media attention to scandals in the blood transfusion practice (e.g., France, Germany, Canada, Ireland), and the still apparent and increasing practice of payment for blood donation (e.g., Asia, Africa, other economy restricted countries). Therefore it could still be important to determine in detail the (contemporary) reasons why people do not give blood, and to continue research on the public perception of blood transfusion, blood donation and prejudices regarding giving blood, to guarantee safety and self-sufficiency of the blood supply. As already discussed, social surveys (KAP) among the general population could reveal a great part of the contemporary public perception of blood transfusion, donating blood, and reasons for not donating blood.

Based on such surveys (circumstantial evidence), up-to-date strategies for informing and motivating the general population about the need for donor blood should be designed and implemented. Personal communication with students from China and personal experience in Africa revealed the following reasons for not donating:

- Fear for loss of virility (China);
- Fear for loss of personal identity (China);
- Rumour that given blood is sold to hospitals (Uganda);
- Shortage of blood for own health (Uganda);
- Experience that family members have no access to given blood (Uganda);
- Rumour that Voodoo practices are related to donated blood (Zambia).

The willingness of people to give blood could be influenced by bringing about changes in the peoples' perception of the blood supply system and blood donation, and bringing about changes in the practical circumstances. When investigating possibilities to influence the willingness to donate blood, three main questions could be asked:

- What are the *perceptions* of the target population in a specific environment: country, region, domestic/working environment?

- Which specific *practical circumstances* could prevent people from giving blood?
- How can perceptions and circumstances be *changed* in order to promote blood donation?

Answers to the previous questions can be obtained through research, mainly focused on the reasons for *not* giving blood. Hence, this research should be carried out on samples of the *general population*. However, large research projects amongst the general population (surveys, polls, etc.) are relatively expensive and very often have a low response, which makes generalization of the results difficult and of insufficient quality. When there is a shortage of funds, other ways of achieving the goal of collecting substantial information from the general population regarding aspects of blood transfusion and blood donation should be investigated.

One of the possible ways is making use of the need for practical training of college or university students in the field of social sciences. These students can do field work (interviewing, etc.) of a survey amongst samples of the population (or subgroups, like students) under supervision of a senior social scientist.

Another way of obtaining information is to discuss aspects of blood transfusion and blood donation with high school students and have teachers in the classroom register the opinions of the students. This can also be done with short structured questionnaires. The basic principle of 'low-budget' surveys is making use of existing networks (schools, universities) and expertise.

Blood centres can benefit from the survey results, and simultaneously offer the opportunity to a university, i.e. students, to practice their skills. The studies in general are designed following the instructions (protocols or SOPs) from the relevant literature on methodology in social sciences. This approach has also the advantage of capacity building; educating people to help their own country to build up the necessary critical mass of knowledge to build up their own country instead of staying depended of external help.

- First, a literature search on the subject should be carried out for the various attention points.
- Next the attention points should be discussed with a few members of the target population to get a complete impression of the problem (e.g., why they are not donating blood).
- On the basis of these findings, a short half-structured (focused) questionnaire can be designed with 'structured' questions (with answer categories yes / no / do not know, etc.), and open questions to which the answers can be written down.

The questionnaires should be presented to a (sample) defined target group. The questionnaires can be completed personally (those who can read and write) or completed by field-workers (interviewers) when the questions are more complex or in case of illiteracy.

For more details on the various aspects of methodology the relevant literature in the social sciences should be consulted.

When the results are gathered, they should be recorded and thoroughly analyzed, and finally reported to the principals (blood centres, Government, etc.) with adequate advice and recommendations for policy, strategies, implementation and adjustment.

1.3.12. Information to General Population (Public), Media Possibilities (General), Peer Groups and Religious Groups (Specific)

One very important socio-cultural characteristic of world society is religion. Maybe it is the most important characteristic and at least very influential. Reasons for donating and not donating blood may have their origins in religious background. Therefore we pay attention to this characteristic in a separate paragraph.

Information on the (general and regional) religious principles of humanity in relation to blood donation and transfusion. Blood as the stream or elixir of life, the living tissue to be shared by those in health to the benefit of those in need. This paragraph gives an overview of the visions of various world religions on the donation of organs and tissue.

Here we consider blood donation as the donation of tissue.

'If you save one life, it is as though you save the world'.

The Talmud

An alphabetical overview of the positions and statements of various religions with regard to organ and tissue donation and transplantation. [11]

Summary of Statements of Various Theological Groups

AME and AME ZION (African Methodist Episcopal)

Organ and tissue donation is viewed as an act of neighborly love and charity by these denominations. They encourage all members to support donation as a way of helping others.

Amish

The Amish will consent to transplantation if they believe it is for the well-being of the transplant recipient. John Hostetler, a world-renowned authority on the Amish religion, wrote in his book, Amish Society, "*The Amish believe that since God created the human body, it is God who heals. However, nothing in the Amish understanding of the Bible forbids them from using modern medical services, including surgery, hospitalization, dental work, anesthesia, blood transfusions, or immunization.*"

Assembly of God

The answer to the question of organ donation, according to the General Council of the Assemblies of God, is rooted in one's understanding of the doctrine of resurrection, Article 13, "The Blessed Hope," in the council's Statement of Fundamental Truths. The council's response is as follows (Office of Public Relations, General Council of the Assemblies of God, November 2, 2005):

The apostle Paul makes it very clear that the mortal bodies we now have cannot inherit the kingdom of God (1 Corinthians 15:35-58; 2 Corinthians 5:1-10). The Bible also makes it clear that to be absent from this body is to be at home with the Lord (2 Corinthians 5:6-10).

When we go to be with the Lord to await the rapture and resurrection of those left alive until the coming of the Lord (1 Thessalonians 4:15), our bodies return to dust (Genesis 2:7, 3:19; 1 Corinthians 15:45-50). We have no more need of the fallen mortal bodies we now bear.

Donating our organs may give the gift of life to someone else long after we have gone home to be with the Lord. If the recipient is a Christian, the resource of the organ has the potential to facilitate continued Christian service and the living witness of a fellow believer here on earth. If the recipient is not a Christian, it may allow the individual additional time and opportunity to accept Christ.

A fascinating possibility is to imagine the impact if Christian donors were to stipulate that their donated organs be accompanied by a handwritten letter telling of the donor's life, testimony, and relationship with Christ.

The alternative is to keep our organs even in death. This also is a valid choice for the Christian. This was the practice for all until recent years when transplant procedures have proven viable. Ultimately, the question comes down to whether or not we view it right for our organs to be candidates for resource.

The realization that organ donations save lives and provide for a continuing witness of God's love and grace does not mean that failure to donate organs would be sinful. All of us should seek God's will for our choices in this matter. It should be discussed fully with one's entire family.

Many considering organ donation will have theological concerns and questions. If we donate our organs to others, will that have any effect on our resurrection? But we must also ask, "*Does God need any given molecule or atom from our bodies in order to resurrect us to life?*" The apostle Paul said, "*No.*" That which is perishable does not inherit the imperishable (1 Corinthians 15:49-50). The resurrection brings a new spiritual body.

Bahá'í
There is no prohibition in the Bahá'í Faith on organ donation. It is a matter left to the individual conscience (Office of Public Information, Bahá'í International Community, November 10, 2005).

Buddhism

Buddhists believe that organ and tissue donation is a matter of individual conscience, and they place high value on acts of compassion. The Rev. Gyomay Masao, president and founder of the Buddhist Temple of Chicago, said, "*We honor those people who donate their bodies and organs to the advancement of medical science and to saving lives.*" The importance of letting loved ones know your wishes is stressed.

There are no injunctions in Buddhism for or against organ donation. The death process of an individual is viewed as a very important time that should be treated with the greatest care and respect.

In some traditions, the moment of death is defined according to criteria which differ from those of modern Western medicine, and there are differing views as to the acceptability of organ transplantation. The needs and wishes of the dying person must not be compromised by the wish to save a life. Each decision will depend on individual circumstances.

Central to Buddhism is a wish to relieve suffering and there may be circumstances where organ donation may be seen as an act of generosity. Where it is truly the wish of the dying person, it would be seen in that light. If there is doubt as to the teachings within the particular tradition to which a person belongs, expert guidance should be sought from a senior teacher within the tradition concerned. When he discovered a monk sick and uncared for, the Buddha said to the other monks, "*Whoever would care for me, let him care for those who are sick.*"

Church of the Brethren

The Church of the Brethren commits itself and urges its congregations, institutions, and members to:

- Inform and educate themselves by taking advantage of resources within their region as to organ and tissue donation.
- Support and encourage individuals to be in discussion with clergy and family as to their wishes regarding the use of their organs and/or tissues for transplantation upon death.
- Encourage and support individuals to include within their advance medical directives instructions as to their wishes for organ and tissue donation. This may include the signing and carrying of a Universal Organ Donor Card.
- Support those living donors who, with prayerful consideration, make an organ or tissue gift, provided that such a gift does not deprive the donor of life itself nor the functional integrity of his or her body.
- Encourage our clergy to prepare themselves to respond to the special needs of family and friends at the time of organ and tissue procurement.

Catholicism

Roman Catholics view organ and tissue donation as an act of charity and love, as reported in the Catholic publication Origins in 1994.

Transplants are morally and ethically acceptable to the Vatican. According to Father Leroy Wickowski, Director of the Office of Health Affairs of the Archdiocese of Chicago, "*We encourage donation as an act of charity. It is something good that can result from tragedy and a way for families to find comfort by helping others.*" Pope John Paul II has stated, "*The Catholic Church would promote the fact that there is a need for organ donors and that Christians should accept this as a 'challenge to their generosity and fraternal love' so long as ethical principles are followed.*"

Health care institutions should encourage and provide the means whereby those who wish to do so may arrange for the donation of the organs and bodily tissues for the ethically legitimate purposes, so that they may be used for donation and research after death. The following is taken from the New York Organ Donor Network:6 In 1956, Pope Pius XII declared that: "*A person may will to dispose of his body and to destine it to ends that are useful, morally irreproachable and even noble, among them the desire to aid the sick and suffering....This decision should not be condemned but positively justified.*"

In August 2000, Pope John Paul II told attendees at the International Congress on Transplants in Rome: "*Transplants are a great step forward in science's service of man, and not a few people today owe their lives to an organ transplant. Increasingly, the technique of transplants has proven to be a valid means of attaining the primary goal of all medicine—the service of human life....There is a need to instill in people's hearts, especially in the hearts of the young, a genuine and deep appreciation of the need for brotherly love, a love that can find expression in the decision to become an organ donor.*"

In the Summer/Fall 2001 issue of On the Beat, a publication of the New York Organ Donor Network, His Eminence Edward Cardinal Egan, Archbishop of New York, wrote that, in thinking about the glorious gift of life God has given each of us, one of the greatest ways an individual can honor that gift is being an organ donor.

In his encyclical letter, Evangelium Vitae (On the Value and Inviolability of Human Life), His Holiness Pope John Paul II speaks of society's fascination with a 'culture of death'. He calls on Catholics and people of good faith everywhere to move from that culture towards a celebration and reflection of the glory of God in a culture of life. *"When asked to share my thoughts on the importance of organ donation for this publication, it was Evangelium Vitae that immediately came to mind. In thinking about the glorious gift of life God has given each of us, it would seem that one of the greatest ways an individual can honor that gift is by making a conscious decision to be an organ donor - a decision that enables another's life to continue—and in a very real and tangible way promotes a culture of life."*

Organ donation is, as His Holiness has stated, 'a genuine act of love'. The commitment of one person to give the gift of life to another person mirrors an essential foundation upon which the teachings of Christ and the theology of our Church are based. As Saint John tells us, *"For God so loved the world, that he gave His only begotten Son, that whosoever believeth in Him, should not perish but have everlasting life."* (John 3:16) By knowingly choosing the donations of one's bodily organs, one is acting as Christ would act—giving life to humanity.

The Catholic Church views organ donation as an act of charity. The Ethical and Religious Directives for Catholic Health Care Services, a set of principles that guide the healing mission of the Church, clearly explains the permissibility of organ donations. In Directive No. 30, we read: "The transplantation of organs from living donors is morally permissible when such a donation will not sacrifice or seriously impair any essential bodily function and the anticipated benefit to the recipient is proportionate to the harm to the donor. Similarly, Directives No. 63-66 treat organ donation as follows: Directive No. 63: *"Catholic health care institutions should encourage and provide the means whereby those who wish to do so may arrange for the donation of their organs and bodily tissue, for ethically legitimate purposes, so that they may be used for donation and research after death."* Directive No. 64: *"Such organs should not be removed until it has been medically determined that the patient has died. In order to prevent any conflict of interest, the physician who determines death should not be a member of the transplant team."*

The donation of organs in a morally acceptable manner, at the end of life, offers the gifts of health and life to those who are most vulnerable and who are at times without hope. It is one of the many pro-life positions an individual can choose in order to foster a culture that values life in our world.

As to what criteria constitute a 'morally acceptable manner', it is essential that organ transplantation occur in the context of love and respect for the dignity of the human person. There are, of course, parameters in determining when and how organs should be donated. It is the Church's position that transplanted organs never be offered for sale. They are to be given as a gift of love. Any procedure that commercializes or considers organs as items for exchange or trade is morally unacceptable. The decision as to who should have priority in regards to organ transplantation must be based solely on medical factors and not on such considerations as age, sex, religion, social standing or other similar standards.

In addition, it is of the utmost importance that informed consent by the donor and/or donor's legitimate representatives be had and that vital organs, those that occur singly in the body, are removed only after certain death (the complete and irreversible cessation of all brain activity) has occurred.

As Pope John Paul II observes in Evangelium Vitae, "*There is an everyday heroism, made up of gestures and sharing, big or small, which build up an authentic culture of life. A particularly praiseworthy example of such gestures is the donation of organs in a morally acceptable manner.*"

It is for the betterment of humanity, for the love of one's fellow human beings, that organ donation is undertaken. One of the most powerful ways for individuals to demonstrate love for their neighbor is by making an informed decision to be an organ donor.

Christianity

There is definite evidence for Christian support of organ donation.

The Lord demonstrated with his own life how, even in sorrow, love enables us to embrace the needs of others. We can choose to donate our organs to save the lives of many people. The decision to donate at the end of life is the beginning of healing for many others. Healing and saving life is a great gift. Jesus sent his 12 disciples out with the imperative to heal disease and illness: "*Heal the sick...freely ye have received, freely give.*" (Matthew 10:8)

Christian Church (Disciples of Christ)

The Christian Church encourages organ and tissue donation, stating that individuals were created for God's glory and for sharing of God's love. A 1985 resolution, adopted by the general assembly, encourages "*members of the Christian Church (Disciples of Christ) to enroll as organ donors and prayerfully support those who have received an organ transplant.*"

Christian Science

The Church of Christ, Scientist does not have a specific position regarding organ donation. According to the First Church of Christ Scientist in Boston, Christian Scientists normally rely on spiritual instead of medical means of healing. They are free, however, to choose whatever form of medical treatment they desire, including a transplant. The question of organ and tissue donation is an individual decision.

Church of the Nazarene

The Church of the Nazarene encourages members who do not object personally to support donor and recipient anatomical gifts through living wills and trusts. Further, the Church appeals for morally and ethically fair distribution of organs to those qualified to receive them (Manual, Church of the Nazarene, 1997-2001, paragraph 904.2).

Episcopal

The 70th General Convention of the Episcopal Church8 recommends and urges "all members of this Church to consider seriously the opportunity to donate organs after death that others may live, and that such decision be clearly stated to family, friends, church and attorney."

Evangelical Covenant Church

The following regarding the Evangelical Covenant Church is from the New York Organ Donor Network: 6 - A resolution passed at the Annual Meeting in 1982 encouraged members to sign and carry organ donor cards. The resolution also recommended '*that it becomes a policy with our pastors, teachers, and counselors to encourage awareness of organ donation in all our congregations.'*

Evangelical Lutheran Church in America
The Evangelical Lutheran Church in America:

- Regards the donation of deceased donor organs as an appropriate means of contributing to the health and well-being of the human family.
- Recognizes that the donation of renewable tissue (e.g., bone marrow) and live organs (e.g. kidney) can be an expression of sacrificial love for a neighbor in need.
- Encourages its members to consider the possibility of organ donation and to communicate their wishes to family members, physicians and health care institutions.
- Encourages those willing to donate to make the necessary familial and legal arrangements including the use of a signed donor card.
- Calls upon its pastors to acquaint themselves with the ethical and legal issues and clinical procedures involved in order that they may counsel persons and families considering the possibility of donation.
- Urges its pastors, congregations, synods, agencies and institutions to sponsor educational programs on organ donation.
- Calls upon government to establish public policies which will encourage voluntary donations, discourage coercive donation, assure the efficient, equitable distribution of human organs and tissues for transplants, and disallow both the sale and purchase of human organs.

Greek Orthodox

The Rev. Stanley S. Harakas, former professor of ethics at Holy Cross Greek Orthodox School of Theology, wrote the following about donation: *"In the case of organ transplants, the crucial ethical considerations are two-fold; the potential harm inflicted upon the donor and the need of the recipient."* Historically, the Orthodox Church has not objected to similar, though not identical, procedures, such as blood transfusions and skin grafts. In both cases, no radical threat to the life of the donor is perceived, and the lifesaving consequences for the recipient are substantial. Similar considerations affect the Orthodox Christian judgment of organ transplants. In no case should a person ignore or make light of the ethical implications of organ donation. Donating an organ whose loss will impair or threaten the life of the potential donor is never required and is never a moral obligation of any person. If the condition of health and the physical well-being of the donor permits, some transplants are not objectionable. Kidney transplants are a case in point. A healthy person may consent to donate a kidney knowing that his or her health is not thereby impaired.

The recipient of an organ transplant should be in otherwise good health, with the expectation of restoring to normal living in order to warrant the risk to the donor."

Gypsies (Roma)

Gypsies are a people of different ethnic groups without a formalized religion. They share common folk beliefs and tend to be opposed to organ donation. Their opposition is connected with their beliefs about the afterlife. Traditional belief contends that for 1 year after death the soul retraces its steps. Thus, the body must remain intact because the soul maintains its physical shape.

Hinduism

According to the Hindu Temple Society of North America, Hindus are not prohibited by religious law from donating their organs. This act is an individual's decision.

H. L. Trivedi, in Transplantation Proceedings, stated that "*Hindu mythology has stories in which the parts of the human body are used for the benefit of other humans and society. There is nothing in the Hindu religion indicating that parts of humans, dead or alive, cannot be used to alleviate the suffering of other humans.*"

The Swamis were universal in their approval of organ donation. They did not accept the concept sometimes heard in India that if one donated [his or her] eyes in this life, they would be blind in the next. Shri Mahant Krishan Nath Ji, based in Haryana, explained, "*If someone donates an organ willingly, then there is nothing wrong in that. And it is wrong to say that if you donate eyes in this birth, that in your next birth you would be born without eyes. We have the story of Baba Sheel Nath of Nath Sampradaya who transferred the sight of one of his eyes to that of a blind lady by his yogic powers. So our Nath Sampradaya has had such realized saints who even made people immortal. To them, eye donation was a very small thing.*"

Another source reports: "*Hindu methodology contains traditions in which human body parts were used for the benefit of other humans and society. There is nothing in the Hindu religion which would prevent living or cadaveric donation to alleviate suffering.*"

There are many references that support the concept of organ donation in Hindu scriptures. These include the following:

Daan is the original word in Sanskrit for donation meaning selfless giving. In the list of the 10 Niyamas (virtuous acts) *Daan* comes third.

Life after death is a strong belief of Hindus and is an ongoing process of rebirth. The law of Karma decides which way the soul will go in the next life. The Bhagavad Gita describes the mortal body and the immortal soul in a simple way like the relationship of clothes to a body:

> "vasamsi jirnani yatha vihaya navani grhnati naro 'parani tatha sarirani vihaya jirnany anyani samyati navandi dehi." ("As a person puts on new garments giving up the old ones the soul similarly accepts new material bodies giving up the old and useless ones.")
>
> Bhagavad Gita Chapter 2:22

Scientific and medical treatises (Charaka and Sushruta Samhita) form an important part of the Vedas. Sage Charaka deals with internal medicine while Sage Sushruta includes features of organ and limb transplants.

Independent Conservative Evangelical

Generally, Evangelical Christians have no opposition to organ and tissue donation. Each church is autonomous and leaves the decision to donate up to the individual.

Islams

Based on the principles and the foregoing attributes of a Muslim, the majority of Islamic legal scholars have concluded that transplantation of organs as treatment for otherwise lethal end stage organ failure is a good thing. Donation by living donors and by cadaveric donors is not only permitted but encouraged.

Organ donation should be considered as an expression of the believer's altruism and Islam encourages the virtuous qualities which are supportive of organ donation: generosity, duty, charity, co-operation, etc. Accordingly, the Islamic Code of Medical Ethics stresses that human life is sacred and it must be preserved by all possible means. It is permissible within the Shariat to remove the organ from one person and transplant it into another person's body in order to save the life of that person on the condition that such a procedure does in no way violate the dignity of the person from whose body the organ was removed.

One of the basic aims of the Muslim faith is the saving of life: This is a fundamental aim of the Shariah and muslims believe that Allah greatly rewards those who save others from death.

Violating the human body, whether living or dead, is normally forbidden in Islam. The Shariah, however, waives this prohibition in a number of instances: firstly in cases of necessity; and secondly in saving another person's life. It is this Islamic legal maxim al-darurat tubih al-mahzurat (necessities overrule prohibition) that has great relevance to organ donation.

UK Transplant also gives this summary of the lifesaving Fatwa (a religious edict): The Muslim Law (Shariah) Council of Great Britain resolved that:

- The medical profession is the proper authority to define signs of death;
- Current medical knowledge considers brain stem death to be a proper definition of death;
- The council accepts brain stem death as constituting the end of life for the purpose of organ transplantation;
- The council supports organ transplantation as a means of alleviating pain or saving life on the basis of the rules of the Shariah;
- Muslims may carry donor cards;
- The next of kin of a dead person, in the absence of a donor card or an expressed wish to donate their organs, may give permission to obtain organs from the body to save other people's lives;
- Organ donation must be given freely without reward;
- Trading in organs is prohibited.

Muslim scholars of the most prestigious academies are unanimous in declaring that organ donation is an act of merit and in certain circumstances can be an obligation.

These institutes all call upon Muslims to donate organs for transplantation:

- The Shariah Academy of the Organisation of Islamic Conference (representing all Muslim countries).
- The Grand Ulema Council of Saudi Arabia.
- The Iranian Religious Authority.
- The Al-Azhar Academy of Egypt.

Gatrad and Sheikh15 write this about the Fatwa in 1995 by the Muslim Law Council in support of organ donation: "Organ transplantation is now encouraged in many Arab Muslim countries, and considered by some as a 'perpetual' charitable act."

Jehovah's Witnesses

Jehovah's Witnesses do not believe that the Bible comments directly on organ transplants; hence: decisions made regarding cornea, kidney, or other tissue transplants must be made by the individual. The same is true regarding bone transplants.

Jehovah's Witnesses are often assumed to be opposed to donation because of their belief against blood transfusion. However, this merely means that all blood must be removed from the organs and tissues before being transplanted. (Office of Public Information for Jehovah's Witnesses, October 20, 2005.)

Judaism

According to Solomon, three Jewish principles govern the treatment of the body after death: respect and dignity to a cadaver, not benefiting from a corpse, and immediate burial.

Rabbi Elliott N. Dorff writes that saving a life through organ donation supercedes the rules concerning treatment of a dead body. Transplantation does not desecrate a body or show lack of respect for the dead, and any delay in burial to facilitate organ donation is respectful of the decedent. Organ donation saves lives and honors the deceased.

The Conservative Movement's Committee on Jewish Laws and Standards has stated that organ donations after death represent not only an act of kindness, but are also a "commanded obligation" which saves human lives. Refusal to participate in organ donation violates the commandment: "Do not stand idly by your neighbor's blood (Leviticus 19:16) which directs we use any resource possible to save a life.

UK Transplant reports: In principle Judaism sanctions and encourages organ donation in order to save lives (*pikuach nefesh*).

This principle can sometimes override the strong objections to any unnecessary interference with the body after death, and the requirement for immediate burial of the complete body.

It is understandable that there will be worries about organ donation. At a time of stress and grief, linked to sudden unexpected illness and death, reaching a decision about donation can be difficult for a family. It is at this time that halachic guidance is so important.

Judaism insists that no organ may be removed from a donor until death—as defined in Jewish law - has definitely occurred. This can cause problems concerning heart, lung and similar transplants where time is of the essence. Judaism insists that honor and respect are due to the dead (kavod hamet). After donation, the avoidance of unnecessary further interference with the body, and the need for immediate interment, are again of prime concern.

Lutheran Missouri Synod

The Lutheran Church-Missouri Synod encourages organ donation as an act of Christian love, but this choice is entirely up to the individual and/or his or her family, and should not be a cause of guilt or regret no matter what decision is made. The Bible has nothing specific to say regarding this issue. Therefore, it is a matter of Christian freedom and personal (or family) discretion.

In 1981, the Synod adopted the following resolution: To Encourage Donation of Kidneys and Other Organs Resolution 8-05: *Whereas, we accept and believe that our Lord Jesus came to give life and to give it abundantly* (John 10:10); and

Whereas, through advances in medical science we are aware that at the time of death some of our organs can be transplanted to alleviate pain and suffering of afflicted human beings (see Galatians 6:10); and

Whereas, our heavenly Father has created us so that we can adequately and safely live with one kidney and can express our love and relive the unnecessary prolonged suffering of our relative"; and

Whereas, we have an opportunity to help others out of love for Christ, through the donation of organs; therefore be it Resolved, that our pastors, teachers, and Directors of Christian Education be encouraged to inform the members of The Lutheran Church-Missouri Synod of the opportunity to sign a Universal Donor Card (which is to authorize the use of our needed organs at the time of death in order to relieve the suffering of individuals requiring organ transplants); and be it further

Resolved, that we encourage family members to become living kidney donors; and be it further

Resolved, that the programme committees of pastors and teachers conferences be encouraged to include 'organ and tissue transplants' as a topic on their agendas; and be it finally

Resolved, that the Board of Social Ministry and World Relief seek ways to implement this program so that the entire Synod may join in this opportunity to express Christian concern.

Mennonite

Mennonites have no formal position on donation but are not opposed to it. They believe the decision to donate is up to the individual and/or his or her family.

Moravians

The Moravian Church has made no statement addressing organ and tissue donation or transplantation. Robert E. Sawyer, president, Provincial Elders Conference, Moravian Church of America, Southern Province, states, "*There is nothing in our doctrine or policy that would prevent a Moravian pastor from assisting a family in making a decision to donate or not to donate an organ.*" It is, therefore, a matter of individual choice.

Mormon (Church of Jesus Christ of Latter-Day Saints)

The donation of organs and tissues is a selfless act that often results in great benefit to individuals with medical conditions. The decision to will or donate one's own body organs or tissues for medical purposes, or the decisions to authorize the transplant of organs or tissue from a deceased family member, is made by the individual or the deceased member's family.

The decision to receive a donated organ should be made after receiving competent medical counsel and confirmation through prayer.

Pentecostals

Pentecostals believe that the decision to donate should be left up to the individual.

Presbyterians

Therefore, be it resolved that the Presbyterian Church (US) recognize the life-giving benefits of organ and tissue donation, and thereby encourage all Christians to become organ and tissue donors as a part of their ministry to others in the name of Christ, who gave life that we might have life in its fullness;

Whereas selfless consideration for the health and welfare of our fellows is at the heart of Christian ethic; and

Whereas organ and tissue donation is a life-giving act since transplantation of organs and tissues is scientifically proven to save the lives of persons with terminal disease and improve the quality of life for the blind, the deaf, and the crippled; and

Whereas organ donation may be perceived as a positive outcome of a seemingly senseless death and is for maintaining the dignity of the deceased; is conducted with respect and with the highest consideration for maintaining the dignity of the deceased and his or her family; and

Whereas moral leaders the world over recognize organ and tissue donation as a[n] expression of humanitarian ideals in giving life to another; and

Whereas thousands of people who could benefit from organ and tissue donation continue to suffer and die due to lack of consent for donation due primarily, to poor public awareness and lack of an official direction for the church.

Protestantism

Because of the many different Protestant denominations, a generalized statement on their attitudes toward organ and tissue donation cannot be made. However, the denominations share a common belief in the New Testament. (Luke 6:38: *"Give to others and God will give to you"*) The Protestant faith respects individual conscience and a person's right to make decisions regarding his or her own body. In addition, it is generally not believed that resurrection involves making the physical body whole again.

In the Winter/Spring 2002 issue of On the Beat, a publication of the New York Organ Donor Network, the Rev. Dr. James A. Forbes Jr, senior minister, The Riverside Church of New York City, wrote:

Medical technology which has made organ and tissue transplantation possible opens up new opportunities for human beings to become partners with God in sustaining and extending the precious gift of life. The fact that we can donate an organ while we live without compromising our health should lead us to exclaim: *"I praise you, for I am fearfully and wonderfully made."* (Psalm 139:14 New Revised Standard Version) Even death cannot prevent us from making a magnanimous offering of new hope for those desperately clinging to life until an appropriate donor has been identified.

Some of the most touching moments of human compassion are associated with organ and tissue transplantation: a mother to a child, a sister to a brother, a neighbor to a neighbor, and stranger to a stranger. Dr. Wyatt T. Walker, Pastor of the Canaan Baptist Church of New York City and former Chief of Staff for Dr. Martin Luther King, Jr., loves to preach about such an event, which for him became a moment of revelation. He tells of an interview he saw on national TV following a fatal mass shooting at a school in Paducah, Kentucky. The reporter asked the mother of one of the slain students what her first thoughts were after being informed of the shootings. The mother said she rushed to the hospital hoping that her daughter had survived. "*And after you were told that she had passed, what was your next thought?*" The mother said, "*I hoped that it would be possible for someone to receive the gift of life from her through an organ donation.*" The little girl was white. Interestingly, the best friend of the little white girl was a black girl. They called each other 'my twin sister.' It turns out that the little girl's heart was donated to a black man. When the mother was finally able to visit the gentleman who had received her daughter's heart, she had one request: "*May I place my ear on your chest so that I can hear the heart of my wonderful daughter?*" Perhaps heaven was also monitoring that episode of sublime human love.

As wonderful as such moments are, some persons are still not sure if offering an organ is compatible with the demands of their faith. Is it pleasing to God to give part of oneself in this way? Shouldn't we strive at any cost to keep intact all of the parts of the body God gave us? Will we be less whole if a part of us is missing in the 'great getting up morning'? Is it mutilation of the flesh to allow someone to take one kidney when the Lord gave us two?

It may be surprising to some to learn that with only a few exceptions all of the major religions affirm and celebrate the godliness of organ and tissue transplantation. Words like caring, sharing, compassion, and sacrifice are at the heart of true religion. The cross, a central Christian symbol, is about Jesus giving himself for the salvation of the world. John 3:16 says, "*God so loved the world that God gave his only son...*" With this understanding, becoming a donor takes on sacramental meaning. Organ and tissue donation is considered to be the ultimate humanitarian act of benevolence.

As a Protestant minister, I think of the following perspectives as I respond to questions regarding organ and tissue donation:

1   Each person of faith needs to order his or her behavior to confirm to a spirit-guided and biblically nurtured conscience. "*Whatsoever is not of faith is sin.*" (Romans 14:23) It is helpful for members of our congregations to discuss the issue with their leaders and to form a solid sense of what is appropriate. Theological discussions in our communities of faith tend to lead to a strong encouragement of organ and tissue donation.

2   One should not expect proof text from the Bible on this issue. Transplantation was not even a possibility at the time the gospels were being written. There were many things Jesus did not address directly. It is the Holy Spirit who leads us into the ways of enlightenment on matters which have surfaced in our time. The spirit of generosity and sacrifice are encouraged in all seasons. Our bodies are the temples of the Holy Spirit. Holy deeds of generosity are to be commended.

3   The opportunity to donate organs and tissue may be one of the most effective ways to counteract the pervasive selfishness of these modern times. The golden rule urges us to think and act from the perspective of what we would desire of others if we were similarly situated.

4   Christian commitment calls us to show respect for the sanctity of the body. A loving sacrificial offering of the gift of life is a holy honoring of our flesh and blood. To be able to live as good stewards of our bodies, then to extend the lives of others reveals something of the nature of our heavenly parent and our Lord, Jesus Christ.

5   Romans 8:28 reminds us that in everything God is at work to bring good out of whatever happens. It is not appropriate to claim that God wills all the tragic events, which result in the death of any of us. Nevertheless, in such tragic circumstances, there is the good of organ and tissue donation, which upstages the evil, which has occurred.

Finally, so much of life is lived as if our own individual well-being is of ultimate significance. Before God, each life is precious and deserving of respect and care. But we are not only individuals before God. We are a family bound by love and mutual care. Organ and tissue donation gives dramatic witness to our interconnectedness. The first citizens of our nation, Native Americans, understood this [interconnectedness]. Perhaps we will be willing to sign a donor card and make an organ and tissue donation when we recover the spirit of Chief Seattle who inspired Ted Perry to write:

This we know. All things are connected Like the blood Which unites one family... Whatever befalls the earth, Befalls the sons and daughters of the earth. Man did not weave the web of life; He is merely a strand in it. Whatever he does to the web, He does to himself.

Salvation Army
The Salvation Army finds organ donation and transplantation acceptable.

Seventh-Day Adventist Church
The Seventh-day Adventist Church does not have an official statement on organ donation. However, the church does have a statement on the care of the dying, which includes the following excerpts:

1   God's plan is for people to be nourished within a family and a faith community.
2   Decisions about human life are best made within the context of healthy family relationships after considering medical advice (Genesis 2:18; Mark 10:6-9; Exodus 20:12; Ephesians 5-6). When a dying person is unable to give consent or express preferences regarding medical intervention, such decisions should be made by someone chosen by the dying person. If no one has been chosen, someone close to the dying person should make the determination.
3   Christian love is practical and responsible (Romans 13:8-10; 1 Corinthians 13; James 1:27, 2:14-17). Such love does not deny faith nor obligate us to offer or to accept medical interventions whose burdens outweigh the probable benefits. For example, when medical care merely preserves bodily functions, without hope of returning a patient to mental awareness, it is futile and may, in good conscience, be withheld or withdrawn. Similarly, life-extending medical treatments may be omitted or stopped if they only add to the patient's suffering or needlessly prolong the process of dying.

Additionally, Loma Linda University Medical Center, a Seventh-day Adventist institution, described as 'integrating health, science and Christian faith' and specializes in organ transplantation. Loma Linda's Transplant Institute provides adult and pediatric heart, kidney, liver, and pancreas programs, and performed a combined total of 138 deceased and living donor transplants in 2005.

Shinto

In Shinto, the deceased's body is considered to be impure and dangerous, and thus quite powerful. "*In folk belief context, injuring a dead body is a serious crime,*" according to E. Namihira in his article, "*Shinto Concept Concerning the Dead Human Body.*" "To this day it is difficult to obtain consent from bereaved families for organ donation or dissection for medical education or pathological anatomy... the Japanese regard them all in the sense of injuring a dead body." Families are often concerned that they not injure the itai, the relationship between the dead person and the bereaved people.

Sikhs

The Sikh philosophy and teachings place great emphasis on the importance of giving and putting others before oneself:

> "Where self exists, there is no God Where God exists, there is no self."
> Guru Nanak, Guru Granth Sahib

The Sikh faith stresses the importance of performing noble deeds. There are many examples of selfless giving and sacrifice in Sikh teachings by the 10 Gurus and other Sikhs.

> "The dead sustain their bond with the living through virtuous deeds."
> Guru Nanak, Guru Granth Sahib

> "The Sikh religion teaches that life continues after death in the soul, and not the physical body. The last act of giving and helping others through organ donation is both consistent with and in the spirit of Sikh teachings."
> Dr. Indarjit Singh OBE, Director of the Network of Sikh Organisations UK

> "The true servants of God are those who serve Him through helping others."
> Guru Nanak, Guru Granth Sahib

Sikhs believe life after death is a continuous cycle of rebirth but the physical body is not needed in this cycle—a person's soul is [the] real essence.

> "In my family we all carry donor cards and would encourage all Sikhs to do so"
> Dr. Indarjit Singh OBE, Director, Network of Sikh Organisations UK

Southern Baptist Convention

The Southern Baptist Convention (SBC) has no official position on organ donation. Such decisions are a matter of personal conscience, writes Dr. Steve Lemke, provost of the New Orleans Baptist Theological Seminary and fellow of the Research Institute of The Ethics and Religious Liberty Commission (January 20, 2006). Dr. Lemke further writes: However, the SBC did pass a nonbinding resolution in its 1988 convention that endorsed organ donation in certain situations. Citing the positive, lifesaving contribution of organ donation, the resolution encouraged *"physicians to request organ donation in appropriate circumstances."* The resolution denied that the bodily resurrection required the wholeness of the body at death, and praised the selflessness, stewardship, and compassion, and alleviation of suffering associated with organ donation.

The resolution also recognized the validity of living wills and organ donation cards, and the right of next-of-kin to make organ donation decisions in some circumstances and as allowed by statute. The SBC resolution on organ donation emphasizes that such action be life-affirming; for that reason the convention does not condone euthanasia, infanticide, abortion, or harvesting of fetal tissue for procurement of organs.

While Southern Baptists entrust the ultimate decision about organ donation to individual conscience, biblical principles such as the sanctity of human life, sacrificial and selfless Christ-like love, and the compassionate alleviation of suffering would appear to justify organ donation.

Society of Friends (Quakers)

Organ and tissue donation is believed to be an individual decision. The Society of Friends does not have an official position on donation.

Unitarian Universalist

Organ and tissue donation is widely supported by Unitarian Universalists. They view it as an act of love and selfless giving, according to the Unitarian Universalist Association, or UUA (Erika Nonken, public information assistant, UUA, October 26, 2005). The UUA has no official position on organ and tissue donation. It is up to each person to decide what is appropriate for [him or her].

Unitarian Universalist are free to make their own decisions about their bodies and their end-of-life arrangements. There are no spiritual or theological beliefs in Unitarian Universalism that would prevent an individual from choosing to donate [his or her] organs, as Unitarian Universalism is a creedless religion.

One of the principles of Unitarian Universalism is respect for the interdependent web of all existence of which we are a part. This principle often encourages Unitarian Universalists to choose have their organs donated after their death, and to otherwise use their bodies, lives, and deaths to help others whenever possible.

United Church of Christ

"United Church of Christ people, churches, and agencies are extremely and overwhelmingly supportive of organ sharing," writes the Rev. Jay Lintner, director, Washington Office of the United Church of Christ Office for Church in Society. He adds: The General Synod has never spoken to this issue because, in general, the Synod speaks on more controversial issues, and there is no controversy about organ sharing, just as there is no controversy about blood donation in the denomination.

While the General Synod has never spoken about blood donation, blood donation rooms have been set up at several General Synods.

Similarly, any organized effort to get the General Synod delegates or individual churches to sign organ donation cards would meet with generally positive responses.

United Methodist Church

The United Methodist Church issued a policy statement regarding organ and tissue donation. It states, "The United Methodist Church recognizes the life-giving benefits of organ and tissue donation, and thereby encourages all Christians to become organ and tissue donors by signing and carrying cards or driver's licenses, attesting to their commitment of such organs upon their death, to those in need, as a part of their ministry to others in the name of Christ, who gave his life that we might have life in its fullness."

A 1992 resolution states, "Donation is to be encouraged, assuming appropriate safeguards against hastening death and determination of death by reliable criteria." The resolution further states, "Pastoral-care persons should be willing to explore these options as a normal part of conversation with patients and their families."

"We are pro-organ donation," said the Rev. Blaine Bluebaugh of the Graham United Methodist Church in Falls Church, Virginia. "It's a major thing for us. It's one of our official days in the calendar. We just believe in it. God has given us the ability to do this, and we should share."

The United Methodists, as with several religions, believe that organ and tissue donation is an act of charity and that preserving life takes precedence over any beliefs that govern the treatment of the dead.

2. Donors

2.1. Introduction

Blood donation is an act of a person accepting to voluntarily give blood which will eventually be used for transfusion. Blood transfusion is a therapy so significant in the restoration of human life, as underscored by WHO in its manual on voluntary blood donation 2010 *"Blood transfusion is a core service within the health care system and individuals who donate their blood provide a unique contribution to the health and survival of others"*. [12] Blood donation has evolved ever since Landsteiner's discovery of blood type ABO, which proved the reality of human blood transfusion and the compatibility of the blood groups. The blood is sourced from human beings, as the only avenue and over time blood donation has survived with contributions from family replacement, paid and voluntary non remunerated blood donors. The evolution of these categories / types of blood donors is directly linked to the developments of safety and quality of the blood supply because blood safety is greatly enhanced by quality of the blood and blood products. Therefore donor management entails practices of checks and balances to observe the blood supply chain while giving the voluntary blood donor not only the opportunity to save lives but also provide quality blood and blood products to the recipients.

The WHA (1975) recommended the screening of Transfusion Transmissible Infections (TTI's) including but not limited to HIV, Hepatitis B, Hepatitis C, and Syphilis. [13] These infections are life threatening, yet blood transfusion is crucial for saving life. It is on this basis that the 'Melbourne Declaration' was passed by the WHO Global Consultation committee 2009 arguing national governments to support the achievement of 100% voluntary non-remunerated blood donations 2020 as the safest and sustainable way to manage blood 7 programme. [14]

The safety of voluntary non-remunerated blood donor is associated with Titmuss's value of their altruism referred to earlier in this chapter [4]; he describes it as creating a social cohesion and social wealth. Relating this to the societal interface level, blood donors have a sense of social responsibility for their own community to serve others in need of blood through donation. Communities that donate blood are believed to own social wealth which its members enjoy through the social network as compared to those with limited number of blood donors which may suffer from blood shortages. At this point we do recognize the valuable input of the blood donors who have availed blood supplies for the general population without discrimination. The blood banking and transfusion services' interface with the population should bring blood donors on board as critical partners not a 'mere' supply of raw materials but as people with specific needs and devise means to keep them treasured for sufficient and sustainable blood services.

Sustainable blood services are founded on 'safe blood' programmes, which start with safe input that is generated from a low risk population seen through the processes while emphasizing quality till the final blood component is transfused into the beneficiary patient. The importance of mobilizing and motivating safe blood donors who are the voluntary non-remunerated is strongly emphasized and all blood services are urged to aim at achieving 100% voluntary donation of blood and blood components.

2.2. Planning

This is a core function in quality management at the societal interface. Knowledge of the present situation of your blood donor motivation and retention programme (what it is) and the vision (where it should be) considerations is made to pave way and move the steps and strides to reach the desired destination of having enough and safe blood donors. The decision to walk, jump and run is therefore accelerated by the instituted plan of action that will be embraced in terms of time and resources committed to facilitate the process of donor motivation.

The resources required for this process are internal and external both material and human that inform the planning on how to acquire and dispense the resources. Though emphasis is mainly concentrated on the internal resources, this should be done comprehensively with due consideration to give adequate time allowing the delivery of the external resources which you may not have control over. Planning for blood service requires establishing a base line upon which the estimates of the need for blood are based in order to plan for the motivation and retention of blood donors that will provide adequate and safe blood supplies. Comprehensive planning focuses on a national strategic approach rather than a single product approach to understand the supply needs and factors that affect its availability and scarcity as affected by the seasons, disease out break and disasters. Contingency planning is critical in quality risk management which assists in the implementation, maintenance and continuously improves a quality management system [15] where all risks that could occur are identified, and plan for solutions in case they occur for instance a case of vaso vagal reactions that are found to deter both male and females from giving blood and therefore necessitate a coping plan prepared in advance to psychologically prepare blood donors for adverse reaction because of their effect on donor retention. [16]

Dedicated resources in terms of staff motivation coupled with proper and continued training together with the finances to support motivation and retention activities is at the corner stone of a quality programme. The staff should have the right knowledge and skills on the policies and strategies enhanced through education (teaching and training) to implement the standard operating procedures. Schedules for education of staff should be determined within the quality plan for example at entry of every staff, on rotation to perform a new task and after evaluation of performing a given task that shows noncompliance to the systems.

Blood establishments should also forecast and plan for achieving a set standard that will eventually form the basis for accreditation or certification by the authorized and recognized bodies such as AABB, ISO, AfSBT and others. These quality plans should include compatibility from vein to vein; right from donor identification, education, motivation, selection, blood collection, testing, processing and distribution. It should also include definition and specifications of component such as whole blood frozen, fresh plasma (FFP), platelet concentrate and process specifications. Identification of the necessary indicators as well as inspection/verification points along the donor management process should also be addressed as early as quality planning.

2.3. Approach

The method of addressing quality at societal interface requires instituting quality systems in the blood establishments that involve organizational policies on blood donor management that will stipulate the identification of the right staff for this kind of job, and train them to effectively perform their functions. Establishing quality standards that staff will observe in the processes of donor identification, motivation, selection, blood collection and donor care. Documentation is cross cutting at every stage in these procedures and processes, which involves development and utilization of standard operating procedures and efficient donor records system. Periodical assessment to validate procedures, equipment, materials, software and the monitoring and evaluation of all activities related to donors and donations. [12] These are all aimed at giving the precious blood donor quality service and care to maintain high levels of motivated and satisfied donors that will be loyal to the blood donor programme, which is a good thing to share with others in the society and motivating for them to become blood donors.

Identification of potential blood donors requires good knowledge of the target audience to design approaches to reach the population with the right messages in the right language catering for the specific group interest. Considerations should be made in terms of age, level of education, marital status, culture, occupation, gender, religion, medical history and seasons for a good understanding of risk, fears, myths and misconceptions surrounding blood donation and expectations of the blood donation procedure that may impact on their attitudes towards blood donation. This can be obtained through simple and less costly research such as reviewing existing records, knowledge, attitudes and practice (KAP) studies to facilitate the development of approaches and information to address the needs in order to respond to the call for voluntary regular blood donation. The World Health Organization/ International Federation of Red Cross and Red Crescent Societies produced basic guiding questions to include in these studies. [12] Embracing these guidelines is expected to result into evaluation and developing new strategies for donor motivation and retention.

The outcome of donor motivation and retention as a process is a critical control point (CCP). The outcome becomes a critical input for other processes which rely on the quality of the input, e.g,, the testing and processing. Hence observation of quality standards at this stage is not an end in itself but affects the entire chain of the blood service from vein-to-vein. This justifies the importance of quality donor management which requires the enhancement of forward and backward linkages that necessitate continuous improvement. This can be informed by Deming cycle an iterative four-step management method for the control and continuous improvement of processes and products. [17] The improvement cycle operates on the principle of Plan-Do-Check-Act. It involves planning where objectives and processes required to produce results are established, followed by implementing the plan, study actual results and instituting corrective actions in case of differences in plan and actual results. It is an iterative process that recommends a continuous feedback loop for identification of processes that needs improvement. Though this was explained in the business processes to improve customer satisfaction it can as well be applied in donor management which also focuses on quality for donor satisfaction. In this case a quality donor management system must be put in place entailing quality plans that are monitored within this system, stipulating a decision point (forum) to ensure that incidences are corrected and prevented from re-occurring referred to as corrective action and preventive action (CAPA). [18] This approach will help in learning from experience and continuously improve the quality of the donor motivation and retention processes.

2.4. Communication

The process of communication is regarded as sharing information, thoughts and feelings between people through speaking, writing, pictures or body language. Effective communication requires that content is received and understood by the receiver in the same way it was intended, so as to achieve the goal of creating a common perception, changing behaviours and acquiring information. [19]

Quality communication in blood donor management is intended to create awareness on the need for blood for people to develop a positive attitude towards blood donation. Needs, desires, fears and aspirations should be assessed in order to develop messages that address the cultural constraints, social and psychological fears. [12] Quality communication considers communication gaps and failures in order to bridge the gaps between awareness and the actual act of blood donation.

In order to overcome the barriers to communication, the target audience's age, sex, culture and intellectual abilities to comprehend the message and translate it into action, must be identified and handled through the communication strategy. Equally important are the receptivity, emotional state, the time of communication and the body language of the donor motivation staff. This staff should be very observant and an active listener to the feedback from the recipients of the message in order to know whether they understood the message and are able to acquire knowledge, change their attitude and respond positively to blood donation. The medium of communication will greatly influence the message reception and should be designed to suit the audience's characteristics and needs.

The medium can include:

- Print Media (magazines, newspapers, leaflets, fliers, posters, brochures);
- Broad cast media (Television, radio);
- Digital media (websites, blogs, online forums).

These and many more can be utilized to communicate to the target audience. The donor management team should build confidence in the public media and feed them with facts on blood donor motivation because the general public trusts the media for being 'professional' and a 'reliable' source of information. The public media is also obliged and committed to transmit information at any cost because they are accountable to the public. Therefore media will always feed the general public and the blood donors with information. So if the blood donor management staff creates a vacuum they risk the media to misinform the public on blood donation. The blood donor services should therefore harness the skills of their staff because of their 'front line' role as public relations 'gurus' to handle the media since they are a friend and a foe. The donor motivation staff should always plan and document whatever they are to communicate to the general public and the media as well as their fellow staff to whom they hand over donors after motivation do donate. This is aimed at efficient donor care from 'welcome' to 'please return again'

All communication materials must be transcribed in local languages, designed and tested for their suitability to a given target audience before they can be used for donor education. They should provide in simple and understandable language the detail on the importance of blood donation, safety of the blood donor and recipient, quality processes and procedures in blood donor management, assure confidentiality and emphasize voluntary blood donation. [20] Use of appropriate metaphors and icons could certainly contribute to good understanding. Periodical reviews of the communication strategies are recommended to accommodate the changes in the population tastes and preferences, up coming diseases, infections, advancement in communication applications to suit blood donor life style.

The communication strategy design should institute provisions for receipt of general public and blood donors feedback (complement or otherwise) about the service and mechanisms to respond as part of the continuous improvement process.

2.5. Donor Service

Blood donors are important resources that are input (raw materials) in the blood donor motivation and mobilization process, not only valued for the one donation they can give in a single time but for the many other functions such as advocacy and motivation of other potential blood donors. This can be attained through suitable blood donor handling giving donors the most pleasant experience every time they interface with the blood establishment. Share this wonderful experience with peers and motivate them as donors (donor motivates donor).

Good Manufacturing Practice (GMP) calls for having the right input, into the right processes to achieve the right output. Thus the identification of the 'right' blood donors in this context is a crucial step. The potential blood donors should be mobilized from low risks populations that have low risks of infections such as HIV, Hepatitis B, Hepatitis C, Syphilis,

Chagas and others, which can be transmitted through blood transfusion commonly known as Transfusion Transmissible Infections (TTIs). The recommended category of safe donors is the voluntary non-remunerated blood donors as compared to paid or family/replacement blood donors. [12]

At the reception of the potential blood donors a well prepared donor information package should be delivered in consideration of the socio-demographic characteristics such as age, gender, marital status, literacy levels in countries where there are major disparities, and recent travel information especially to disease endemic areas. The information package should contain the right message for the right target group at the right time and place. Such messages should be motivational, educative and informative to the potential donor to make an informed decision and encourage self exclusion.

2.6. Donation Sessions

Quality management under blood donor management focuses on the motivation, selection, collection, documentation, care, satisfaction and retention of blood donors [21] National blood transfusion services (NBTS), National Red Cross /Crescent blood centres, Community Hospital blood banks and other blood establishments involved in blood donor motivation and screening of blood for transfusion have guiding policies for organizing and handling blood donation sessions for the collection of either whole blood or its components in fixed premises and mobile blood collection teams aimed at quality assurance of the collection. These policies are regulated by authorities or reputable bodies such as the WHO, FDA, EDQM, ShFDA, PAHO, AfSBT, AABB and other regulatory bodies the world over by setting standards to ensure systematic ways in which donors are identified, blood is collected, tested and transfused and have donor vigilance and haemovigilance procedures for adverse reactions or unexpected outcomes by epidemiologically following up donors and recipients.

To ensure efficacy, safety and efficiency in the mentioned processes there is need to educate (teach and train) personnel that will handle the different stages guided by the standard operating procedures (SOPs). These are initially developed by the actual people that handle the specific tasks in a way of describing the procedures step by step in a logical flow with due attention to critical processes that determine decision making. The SOPs are an integral part of the organizational policies, strategies and guidelines which are endorsed and approved by governance of the institution. The policies, strategies and guidelines should have in built systems and strategies on donor motivation, eligibility, retention and assessment of the post donation period, incident and accidents to blood donors, customer satisfaction, complaint handling. Donor vigilance and management should review these systems regularly.

The procedures entail venue selection in consideration of the health and safety factors, accessibility and other measures to minimize the risk of contamination to the blood. Potential donors at this stage also require information on the characteristics of blood and its components, the blood tests, risky behaviours. The donor should provide bio data, provide information on the health status, medical history and informed consent to donate blood. They should be encouraged to voluntarily donate and be assured of the confidentiality on any given information. The procedure (session layout), time expected to take, and assurance on a positive outcome of the donation exercise from donor identification, medical examination, haemoglobin determination, venepuncture, observation /refreshment until the donor is seen out of the donation site. A donor should receive a pleasant experience given by the blood collection staff through paying attention (listening) to the donors, motivating them, appreciating and recognizing their precious contribution to save lives.

The blood should be collected in a clean environment, using sterile equipment and materials free from any contamination, due attention should be paid to any leakages, expiry date and the blood collected in a closed system, to minimize infections of the blood and the donor. While collecting the blood, proper mixing of the blood with the anticoagulant and weighing for the right amount of blood to be collected to avoid imbalances in the solutions. After collection the tubing is sealed off not to allow cross contamination and the samples are separated and packed as a ready material (input) for the testing and processing.

The packaging of the collected blood should be in the right containers with regulated temperatures and transported using the right means as a quality control measure to ensure that the final product will not be affected.

3. Hospitals and Patient Care

3.1. Introduction

Blood transfusion is a key part of modern health care and transfusion medicine is a multi-disciplinary service. It encompasses donor recruitment, blood collection, manufacturing, distribution, laboratory investigation and patient care activities. Transfusion therapy has made possible many treatments that were previously unattainable. However, there are also inherent problems such as transfusion reactions, blood group incompatibility and transmission of diseases. Moreover, the public continues to demand for safety and quality for blood and blood products up to international standard.

All activities in a transfusion service, from the collection of blood to its infusion, are interrelated. Problem in one area of service may affect the final outcome of the recipient. To ensure quality service and maximum safety for blood donors and recipients, all the critical points in the transfusion service have to be identified and mechanisms established to control them. It is important that a safe and sound hospital transfusion procedure is in place and complied by the staff involved in the handling, use and administration of blood and blood components. It is also imperative for hospitals to set up peer review mechanisms to monitor and audit transfusion practices to keep pace with current developments.

3.2. National Strategies

blood products provided for clinical use by the national blood programme are safe, adequate to meet demand, effective and produced consistently to the appropriate standards. Hospitals having blood transfusion activities are required to develop their own internal procedures in line with the national guidelines that define the basic standard for hospital blood transfusion procedures. [22] The purposes are to ensure safe, effective and timely blood transfusion to patients; and to minimise any chance of error throughout the transfusion process. Internal procedures drawn up on blood transfusion apply to all relevant staff involved in the particular steps of the blood transfusion process irrespective of their professional disciplines. Hospitals may adopt internal procedures with more stringent requirements. However, they must be practicable in order to facilitate the smooth operation of the blood transfusion process. Blood is a scarce human resource and essential for the care of many patients. When used correctly, it saves lives and improves health. However, blood transfusion carries a potential risk of acute or delayed complications and transfusion transmitted infections and should be prescribed only to treat conditions associated with significant morbidity or mortality that cannot be prevented or managed effectively by other means. Ensuring blood safety and clinical effectiveness requires investment – both human and financial. The national health programme should develop policies and strategies to reduce the need for transfusion, minimize unnecessary transfusions and ensure the safe and appropriate use of blood and blood products. [23] These strategies should include:

- Prevention, early diagnosis and effective treatment of conditions that could result in the need for transfusion;
- Use of good surgical and anaesthetic techniques, pharmaceuticals and medical devices to reduce blood loss;
- Availability and use of simple alternatives for volume replacement, including intravenous replacement fluids (crystalloids and colloids);
- Appropriate prescribing of blood and blood products in accordance with national guidelines;
- Safe pre-transfusion procedures;
- Safe administration of blood and blood products;.
- While responsibility for the decision to transfuse ultimately rests with individual clinicians, consistently effective clinical transfusion practice cannot be achieved unless the following are in place;:
- A well organized, nationally coordinated blood transfusion service to ensure the availability of, and access to, safe blood and blood components;
- National blood policy and plan incorporating the clinical use of blood, with appropriate supportive regulations;
- National committee on the clinical use of blood within the national blood programme;
- Availability of intravenous replacement fluids, and medical devices and pharmaceuticals to reduce blood loss;
- Quality system for the BTS, hospital blood banks and all clinical departments involved in transfusion, including:
  o Standard operating procedures
  o Documentation of requests for blood, blood sampling, the administration of blood and monitoring the transfused patient
  o Systems to monitor adverse events and errors related to transfusion
  o Clinical audit

The national committee on the clinical use of blood should work to ensure the effective implementation of the guidelines. Transfusion guidelines should represent a consensus by clinical specialists, the BTS, pharmacists and professional bodies on the most effective treatments for specific conditions. They should be practical, comprehensive and relevant to local conditions. They should include:

- Clinical and laboratory indications for the use of blood, blood products and alternatives to transfusion;
- Information on available blood products and alternatives to transfusion: dosage, storage conditions, risk of transfusion-transmissible infection, means of administration, contraindications and precautions;
- Standard blood request form to provide full information about the patient and the need for transfusion;
- Blood ordering schedule, as a guide to the number of units of blood and blood products that should normally be requested for each type of operation, with guidance on its adaptation by each hospital;
- Instructions for the development of standard operating procedures at hospital level.

3.3. Communication with Hospital and Tuning/Adjusting Demand and Supply

There should be regular and open communication between the Blood Service and client hospitals on the inventory level of blood and components in both the Blood Service and client hospitals. In many countries, this can be achieved through IT system which enables real time checking on the inventory situation including expiration of products. The system can also serve the function of transacting blood request and supply. [24]

Blood Service should establish written blood supply agreement with user hospitals. In addition to the blood supply quotas serve as the baseline for adjusting stock replenishment, the agreement should define clearly the respective responsibilities of both parties such as:

- The Blood Service has manufactured Blood in compliance with legal and professional requirements;
- The Blood Service has tested and confirmed that all products supplied are non-reactive to various assays for HBV, HCV, HIV-1+2, HTLV-I and syphilis;
- The Blood Service shall use its reasonable endeavours to maintain permanent records of all donors and their blood distribution history;
- The Blood Service Supplier shall provide blood and blood components to Client according to the actual number requested by the Client's need and Supplier's availability;
- The Client has established blood bank facilities to take custody of the blood received and to perform the necessary pre-transfusion tests;
- The Client has established documentation to track destination of each blood unit received;
- The Client shall provide requirement forecast to Supplier annually;
- The Client shall agree to return blood to the Blood Service on request and provide evidence on its suitability for re-issue if necessary;
- The Client shall maintain records of transfusion or disposal of blood in accordance with legal and professional requirements;

- The Client shall provide monthly Blood utilization statistics to the Blood Service, assist in product recall, recipient look back and notification as and when required by the Blood Service.

Based on the activities and utilization records, the regular blood supply quotas for stock replenishment should be agreed for each type of products and blood groups. An example is provided below:

Product type	Mon				Tue				Wed				Thur				Fri				Sat			
	O+	A+	B+	AB+	O+	A+	B+	AB+	O+	A+	B+	AB+	O+	A+	B+	AB+	O+	A+	B+	AB+	O+	A+	B+	AB+
WB/RBC (excluding LRBF)	150	90	70	20	150	100	95	30	150	100	95	30	150	130	130	50	200	130	130	50				
WB ≤ 5day	Nil																							
Pl. Conc.	50				50				50				50				50				50			
FFP	O+ 80 A+ 60 B+ 60 AB+ 40																							
Cryo	O+ 5 A+ 5 B+ 5 AB+ 5																							
Others:																								
c- E- Mi- RBC	2 x Group O (on replenishment basis)																							
O neg. WB/RBC	1				1				1				1				1				1			

Figure 1. Regular blood supply quotas for stock replenishment.

The above also serves as the baseline for adjusting the stock level should either party feels that it is necessary at any time or during an annual review of the agreement. In addition, to address fluctuation in inventory, the Blood Service and client hospital should have an agreement to the principle for replenishment of blood components in the event that the overall blood inventory is below optimal. An example is provided as follows:

Supplier's Inventory Grades[*]			
RBC	Platelets	FFP	Supplier's Commitment
I	I	I	Top up Client's stock as requested, provided that Client's RBC, Platelet and FFP stocks do not exceed 110%, 100% and 100% of agreed levels respectively.
II	II	II	Top up Client's RBC, platelet and FFP stocks to at least 90%, 70% and 70% of agreed levels respectively.
III			Top up Client's RBC stock to ≥70% of agreed level.
< III	< II	< II	Further reduce stock supply and handle difference by case requests.

[*]As determined at or before 8 am each morning.

Figure 2. Agreement for replenishment of blood components in the event that the overall blood inventory is below optimal.

3.3. Evaluating Clinical Use of Blood

A transfusion committee should be established in each hospital to implement the national policy and guidelines and monitor the use of blood and blood products at the local level. The committee should have authority within the hospital structure to determine hospital policy in relation to transfusion and resolve any identified problems. The main functions of a hospital transfusion committee include:

- Developing systems for the implementation of the national guidelines within the hospital;
- Liaison with the BTS to ensure the availability of required blood and blood products at all times;
- Liaison with the relevant department to ensure a reliable supply of intravenous replacement fluids and other alternatives to transfusion at all times;
- Developing a hospital blood ordering schedule;
- Developing hospital standard operating procedures for all steps in the transfusion process;
- Training all hospital staff involved in transfusion;
- Monitoring the usage of blood and blood vomponents within the hospital;
- Monitoring and investigation of severe adverse effects or errors associated with transfusion, taking any corrective and preventive action required and reporting through the haemovigilance system to the national committee on the clinical use of blood.

At national level, responsibility for monitoring and evaluation should be shared by the BTS, the national committee on the clinical use of blood and the department responsible for the supply of intravenous replacement fluids and other alternatives to transfusion. The monitoring system should cover:

- The safety, adequacy and reliability of the supply of blood, blood components and alternatives to transfusion;
- The traceability of all blood and blood products, from blood collection to transfusion;
- Compliance with the national guidelines on transfusion and the impact on prescribing practice;
- Differences in blood usage within hospitals and between similar hospitals at regional, provincial and district level;
- Haemovigilance – the monitoring, reporting and investigation of all adverse events related to transfusion.

3.3.1. Assessment of Quality of Service to Hospitals

Every blood service should develop an effective quality system. [25] This should provide a framework within which BTS activities are established, performed in a quality-focused way and continuously monitored to improve outcomes. It should also reflect the structure, needs and capabilities of the BTS, as well as the needs of the hospitals and patients that it serves.

Blood Service should closely monitor the product supply satisfaction for client hospitals. [26] It should also establish a mechanism to regularly assess the quality of its service provided to hospitals. A client committee chaired by a member elected among the client hospitals can provide a regular platform for clients to feedback comments and complaints. Blood Service should have also a formal mechanism to receive and follow up client complaints on product and services. The number of complaints should be monitored and analyzed for the purpose of identifying problem areas that need to be rectified. In addition, Blood Establishment should conduct survey, at least once a year, to assess clients' satisfaction on its services.

Acknowledgments

The summary of general religious views was originally compiled by Christine Gallagher, MAR, while the public education consultant/religious community liaison at Colorado Organ Recovery Systems. Some church position statements from various religious denominations were collected by the Rev. Charles H. Chandler, DMin, UNOS clergy consultant. We also thank the New York Organ Donor Network for the possibility to copy from its Web site.

References

[1]   Leikola, J. How much blood for the world? *Vox Sang*. 1988;54:1-5.
[2]   Titmuss, R. M. *The gift relationship: from human blood to social policy*. New York, NY, US. Vantage Books 1970.
[3]   Strengers, P. Quality management of the blood collection. *ISBT Sci. Ser*. 2012; 7:12-15
[4]   *Donor Management Manual 2010*: DOMAINE project. W. de Kort, Veldhuizen, I. (Eds). Nijmegen, the Netherlands, Domaine 2010. ISMN 978-90-815585-1-8, http://www.domaine-europe.eu
[5]   Vuk, T. Quality indicators: a tool for quality monitoring and improvement. *ISBT Sci. Ser*. 2012; 7:24-28
[6]   UniPark Enterprise Feedback Suite (EFS). GlobalPark AG Cologne. Germany 2011.
[7]   Oswalt, R. M. A review of blood donor motivation and recruitment. *Transfusion* 1977; 17:123-25
[8]   Boe, G. P., Ponder, L. D. Blood donors and non-donors: a review of the research. *Am. J. Med. Technol*. 1981;47:248-53.
[9]   Piliavin, J. A. Why they "give the gift of life to the unnamed strangers": A review of research on blood donors since Oswalt (1977). *Transfusion* 1990; 30:444-59.
[10] Piliavin, J. A. and Callero, P. L. *Giving blood: The development of an altruistic identity*. Baltimore, MD, US: Johns Hopkins University Press 1991
[11] UNOS corporate headquarters. Post Office Box 2484, Richmond, Virginia 23218 / updated *Organ and Tissue Donation: A Reference Guide for Clergy*. Cooper ML, Taylor GJ, eds. 4th ed. SEOPF/UNOS, Richmond, VA, US 2000.
[12] *Towards 100% Voluntary Blood Donation: A global framework for action*. Ms Jan Fordham and Dr Neelam Dhingra, editors. Blood Transfusion Safety, World Health Organization Geneva, CH 2010, ISBN 978 92 4 159969 6

[13] WHA28.72 Utilization and supply of human blood and blood products. 1975 *Handb. Res., Vol. I, 1.5.2.2; 8.2.4* Thirteenth plenary meeting, 29 May 1975.

[14] Melbourne Declaration

[15] Agoston, S. M. I., van Mourik, P. C., Strengers, P. F. Quality Risk Management: a valuable tool in implementing, maintaining and improving a quality management system. *Vox Sang, ISBT Science series*, 2011;6:52-55

[16] Veldhuizen, I., Atsma, F., van Dongen, A., de Kort, W. Adverse reactions, psychological factors, and their effect on donor retention in men and women. *Transfusion*, 2012;521871–1879. doi: 10.1111/j.1537-2995.2011.03551.x

[17] Deming, W. E., *The New Economics For Industry, Government and Education*. Cambridge: Massachusetts Institute of Technology Center for Advanced Engineering Study, 1993, Cambridge, MA, US

[18] Strengers, P. F. Key Elements of a blood transfusion quality management system, the tools and objectives. *Vox Sang, ISBT Science series*, 2011;6 (number 1):21-25,

[19] Barbara Brown. What is Effective communication? August 11, 2011. Downloaded September 27, 2012 www.livestrong.com

[20] WHO, Strategies for Safe Blood Transfusion, SEARO Publications on HIV/AIDS Downloaded April 26,2012 www.searo.who.int

[21] Mohammed, N., Moftah, F., Ezzat, S. Improve donor satisfaction National Blood Transfusion Service Cairo - Egypt, *Vox Sang*, 2011;101 (Supp. 1):127 -128.

[22] *Aide-Mémoire for Ministries of Health - Developing a National Blood System,* World Health Organization, Geneva, CH 2011.

[23] *Aide-Mémoire for National Health Programmes - The Clinical Use of Blood*, World Health Organization, Geneva, CH 2003.

[24] Guidelines for blood bank computing. Working party of the British Committee for Standards in Haematology Blood Transfusion Task Force, *Transfusion Medicine*, 2000;10:307-314

[25] *Aide-Mémoire for National Health Programmes - Quality Systems for Blood Safety*, World Health Organization, Geneva, CH 2002.

[26] *Standards for Blood Banks and Transfusion Services*, current Edition, AABB Press, Bethesda, MD, US

In: Quality Management in Transfusion Medicine
Editor: Cees Th. Smit Sibinga

ISBN: 978-1-62618-665-1
© 2013 Nova Science Publishers, Inc.

Chapter XI

Management of Blood Safety: Prevention and Precautions

Elizabeth M. Dax,[1,*] Alan Kitchen,[2,†]
Kumanan Wilson[3,‡] and Henk W. Reesink[4,§]
[1]Associate Professor, The Dax Centre,
University of Melbourne, Victoria, Australia
[2]National Transfusion Microbiology Reference
Laboratory, NHS Blood and Transplant, London, UK
[3]Associate Professor at Ottawa Hospital, Ottawa, Canada
[4]Associate Professor at Academic Medical Center,
Amsterdam, The Netherlands

Abstract

Blood transfusion can transmit certain infections (e.g. HIV, viral hepatitis) with a high degree of certainty. These infections are termed transfusion transmissible infections or TTIs. Appropriate prevention measures such as selective questioning of donors, testing for the presence of infection in donations and assuring the integrity and quality of all processes and through all blood service procedures can avoid transmission; also with a high degree of certainty. The public, health care workers and recipients have assumed governments' stances of a "zero risk expectation" for transfusions' safeness. However, it is essential that transfusion services educate governments, users and recipients that zero

[*] Elizabeth M. Dax, AM; MD,BS; PhD, ARCPA; GAICD: Associate Professor, The Dax Centre, Kenneth Myer Building, at the University of Melbourne, Genetics Lane off Royal Parade, Parkville, 3052 Victoria, Australia. Tel: +61 409 022 052; E-mail: lizdax@gmail.com.
[†] Alan Kitchen, PhD: Head, National Transfusion Microbiology Reference Laboratory, NHS Blood and Transplant, Charcot Road, Colindale Avenue, London NW9 5BG, UK. Tel: +44-20-8957 2733; E-mail: alan.kitchen@nhsbt.nhs.uk.
[‡] Kumanan Wilson, MD, MSc, FRCP(C):Associate Professor at Ottawa Hospital, Civic Campus, 1053 Carling Av, Box 684, Ottawa ON K1Y 4E9, Canada. Tel: +1- 613-798-5555 ext 17921; E-mail: kwilson@ohri.ca.
[§] Henk W. Reesink, MD, PhD: Associate Professor at Academic Medical Center, PO Box 22660, 1100DD, Amsterdam, The Netherlands. Tel: +31-20-5669111; E-mail: h.w.reesink@amc. nl.

risk does not exist. All interventions involving the transfer of human material between humans have an element of risk. Transfusion services in countries with developed healthcare systems have developed intricate applications and frameworks to assure that transmission of infection and other risks are minimized such that the risk approaches few chances per hundreds of thousands to millions of transfusions. The framework relating to managing risk and ensuring quality and efficacy is known as a quality management system. Quality management is only in place when all procedures are documented and this documentation is used according to the quality cycle. Risk management procedures should be included as well as management of non-conformances. Central to measures for prevention and precaution, are the testing programmes that have been established and blood centres' abilities to minimise any risk of transfusion transmissible infection and maximise the quality of their outputs and volumes of products. Achieving the degree of quality management necessary to assure the safety and efficacy of blood and blood products for transfusion is a laborious, stepwise journey that, in the long run, is cost saving but above all ensures the well being of the recipients of transfused products.

Keywords: Quality, Precaution, Prevention, Laboratory testing, Testing requirements, Risk management, Essential training, Efficacy, Cost effectiveness

I. Introducton

Quality Management is the mechanism that transfusion services world-wide, have embraced to assure the precautions against, and prevention of, risks associated with transfusion of blood and/or blood products. Not only is risk reduction achieved but cost effectiveness of services been achieved. This is particularly true of laboratory testing where donations are screened for Transfusion Transmissible Infections (TTI) in order to eliminate donations that may transmit infection. The need to use more costly, more sophisticated tests to continually reduce risk of transmission, has added to costs and the need for training and installation of more complicated equipment. Quality management systems assure cost effectiveness where risk and costs are expected to be minimised.

1.1. Considerations around Abilities to Test and the Importance of Prevalence

1.1.1. Skills and Infrastructure (Including Laboratory Structures)

The infrastructure surrounding preparation of blood for transfusion is wide and varied. At one end of the scale of blood service infrastructure, there are fully equipped centralized blood facilities. They have cultivated donor pools of largely, repeat donors, they produce blood and a variety of products that are all screened to identify donations that may transmit infectious agents, and these are stored before use and distributed according to the needs of associated medical systems. Uses of product range from transfusion and plasma product preparation to preparation and use of plasma fractions. The functions of laboratories in these centralised services that may conduct hundreds or even thousands of tests per day, are streamlined. Much of the testing is automated and the hands-on testing tasks of the staff are minimal. A large proportion of staff time and effort is spent is in maintaining quality and procuring and analysing information in order to secure safety and efficacy.

At the other end of the scale are small hospital or health care centre services that engage replacement donors, may screen with rapid tests and transfuse only whole blood. [1] There may be no, or inadequate storage facilities and no area for quarantine. The major use of blood in these small services tends to be for anaemia, peri-partum haemorrhage or trauma. [2] The laboratories are often poorly set out, and any equipment may be poorly maintained. The staff may be poorly trained or never given the opportunity to retrain. They may have only scant knowledge of quality assurance mechanisms. Sometimes, staff members are rotated and then not trained thoroughly for blood service functions and maintaining their quality. Testing may utilise rapid tests that change with the purchasing decisions of procurement offices removed from the laboratories or even removed from a health care facility altogether.

Then there are a range of services with varying degrees of development, wide-ranging proficiency of staff, varying and possibly unstable budgets, various levels of supervision and training. Thus, there are wide ranges in the quality of services. The range and development of human immunodeficiency virus (HIV) testing laboratories in China may be illustrative. [3]

It is necessary that *all* transfusion services (leaving aside the arguments made in favour of centralisation) assure quality management of each of their services in order to assure the safety of their products. Governments must be involved in insisting upon or regulating the quality of *all* blood services and in providing the necessary resources to assure safety. Training programmes should be designed to assure that all services benefit. In short, it is the ultimate responsibility of governments and authorities to prevent transfusion transmission and support precautions against transfusion risks. The responsibility includes obligation to budget for and fund, not only the transfusion services themselves but the necessary requirements for maintaining quality through audited quality management systems.

1.1.1.1. Understanding Process

As in all industries where outputs are achieved, there are processes concerned with the manufacture of transfusion products. That is, there are a defined series of steps that lead to specific outputs. In industry, a process involves taking raw reagents and pursuing a regulated series of manufacturing steps that result in transforming reagents into a consistently well-manufactured product. However, this is not strictly how processes operate in blood services. Rather, processes relate to delivering a service from one point to another. A schematic representation is shown in Figure 1.

Examples of processes in blood services include –

- screening donors for their suitability to donate,
- testing a donation for transfusion transmissible infections or
- transporting blood from the production facility to another where it will be used.

The steps in a process that may apply to numbers of areas of the service are termed procedures. Procedures are accomplished through a series of individual tasks (Figure 2). Examples of procedures include preparing donation samples for testing, assuring the identity of the sample with associated prepared blood components, maintaining the cleanliness of a service's laboratory, and waste disposal.

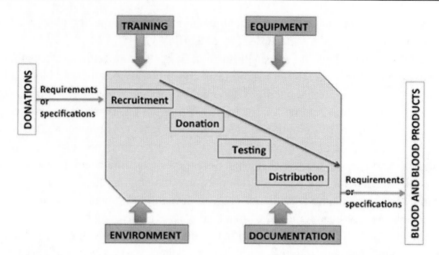

Figure 1. Process in blood transfusion services. Donations are collected and through a series of steps, blood and/or blood products are produced. There are a series of supports (e.g. training) to the process that contribute, and are essential to it.

1.1.2. Testing, Quality Principles and Approaches

How Much Testing?

All blood donations are expected to have been tested for the presence of relevant TTI.

WHO has produced guidelines for testing for TTI in blood donations. [4] The guidelines state that all donations must be tested for "the BIG four" – human immunodeficiency virus (HIV), hepatitis C (HCV), hepatitis B (HBV) and Syphilis. Other TTI should be tested for, according to prevalence and risk (Table 1).

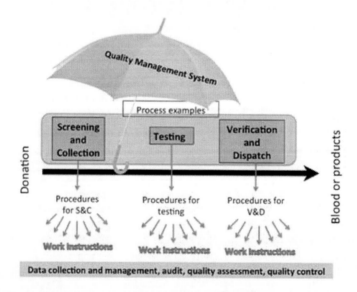

Figure 2. Quality Management Systems are vital to the prevention and precautions taken for managing risk. In each transfusion service the quality of each step in the entire process is assured through understanding the operation of every step. Documentation and the implementation of the documents' instructions and recording devices assure consistency and efficiency.

What Tests?

Blood screening for TTI has been accomplished with immunoassays and more recently with nucleic acid amplification tests (NAT). Immunoassays rely on the detection of antibody-antigen interactions (indirect detection of the virus or infective agent). Immunoassays detecting viral epitopes (e.g., HIV p24 antigen) are also used (direct detection).

NAT are designed to detect specific nucleic acid sequences of the target virus (direct detection of the virus). The mechanisms of these tests' operation are readily available on the internet or in testing literature. [5]

2. Prevention, Precautions and Quality

2.1. Prevention

2.1.1. Prevention of Transmission – Background

Clearly, the key way to avoid transmission of TTI is to secure donations that do not contain infectious agents. Prevention of transmission depends on a large number of influences. [6] If there are lesser numbers of blood services and of larger size (the so-called centralized services), that generate high quality of management within the services, prevention of TTI transmission may be higher than in areas where there are a larger number of small services with less attention paid to quality management.

The prevalence and incidence of infection in the community and in donors, the transmissibility of a TTI, the mode of transmission of an infection outside blood services [7], the tests and testing available, effective reagent procurement, government policy and guidelines, the state of the health services in general, regulation, and education, all play a part in the risk of transmission. [8]

To maximize the quality of blood available for transfusion, integrated strategies are necessary. WHO recommends [4]:

- Well-organized services, nationally coordinated supplying necessary blood and coordinated to meet needs
- Collection of blood from voluntary, non-remunerated donors at low risk of harboring TTIs
- Quality managed services with quality assurance mechanisms in place
- Screening of donations for infections, always for HIV, Hepatitis B and C and syphilis and for other infections according to prevalence and/or incidence
- Judicious use of blood and products.

There needs to be national policies, regulation and financial services in place to foster blood safety. Quality management of services cannot be achieved without authorities recognizing the absolute need and support for its development and maintenance.

Table 1. Transfusion transmissible infections (TTI) that must always be tested for (row 1) and others that may be tested for depending on their prevalence or threat. Usual modes of testing are listed in the column to the right

TTI	When to test	How to test
HIV, HBV, HCV, Syphilis serology	Every donation, always	Ab and or Ag; ChIA, EIA, Rapid-EIA, PA
HIV, HCV, HBV nucleic acid	Depends on incidence, transmissibility, budget, regulations	Multiplex or individual NAT; pooled or individual donation testing
Malaria, Chagas disease, HTLV serology	Depends on risk in donor population	ChIA, IA
CMV serology	Transfusion to immune-incompetent individuals	IA, Antigenic titres
WNV nucleic acid	Depends on risk in donor population e.g., during epidemics	IA, NAT

Abbreviations: HIV, Human immunodeficiency virus; HBV, hepatitis B virus; HCV, hepatitis C virus; HTLV, human T-cell lymphotropic virus; CMV, cytomegalovirus; WNV, West Nile virus; Ab, antibody; Ag, antigen; EIA, Enzyme immunoassay; ChIA, chemi-luminescence IA; PA, particle agglutination assay; NAT, nucleic acid amplification assay.

2.1.2. Public Health

Public health systems have an important role in management of blood safety. [9] The public health system is of great importance in developing the evidence that can be used to formulate policy and guide prevention measures. Furthermore, it is the public health systems that need to maintain the vigilance for changes in epidemiology of infections and identify new and emerging infections. [10] In a number of African countries, political unrest has contributed to the downfall of blood safety. [11] In other areas change of climate may contribute to changes in prevalence or the incidence of infections, particularly vector-borne, that may affect blood safety. [12]

Often it is the public health services that are equipped to conduct the appropriate research and recommend useful courses of action. [13]

2.1.3. The Role of Policy and Regulation

The outcomes of lack of policy and regulation to blood safety are clear. Examples include investigations into and outcomes of reviews on blood safety in Canada and France. [14]

Countries without policy and regulation are all too common in those of low to medium human development indices. National systems are necessary for most effective prevention. [9] Such systems include a hierarchy of components (Figure 3).

2.2. Precaution

Managing the safety of the blood supply has presented unique challenges that have required a modification of the standard approach to assessing evidence to determine risk. As part of the health care system transfusion medicine is guided by principles of evidence-based medicine.

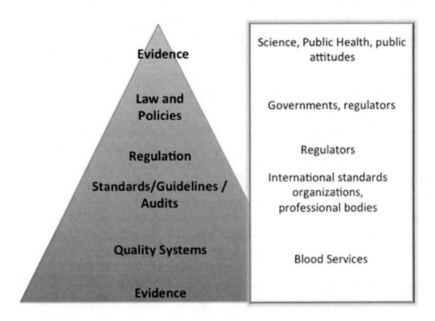

Figure 3. National components and players assure and support blood transfusion services, their quality systems and their management. They assure these are established and that they are coordinated.

These principles argue for high quality evidence of a high level of certainty to be present before the introduction of an intervention. Typically this has referred to health care interventions at an individual level, for example the introduction of a new treatment for a patient experiencing a myocardial infarction. Under the evidence-based medicine paradigm, such an intervention should ideally be supported by randomized controlled trial evidence with results suggesting a greater than 95% certainty that they did not occur by chance. [15]

Applying this approach to transfusion safety is problematic. At the time blood systems around the world were confronted by the twin threats of HIV and non-A non-B hepatitis (NA/NB hepatitis - now identified as HCV) the evidence-based approach to medicine was in its ascendency. This led some decision-makers to argue for high quality evidence of risk before introducing measures to protect the blood supply from the threats – in particular because the introduction of the measures had the potential to create harm in and of themselves by reducing the blood supply. [16] Unfortunately the decision to wait for definitive evidence, led to the preventable spread of the blood borne infections in the case of NA/NB hepatitis. [16]

This case is particularly illustrative of the dilemma facing policymakers in transfusion medicine at the time. NA/NB hepatitis was recognized as transfusion transmissible and as being caused by a blood borne pathogen. However the virus had not yet been identified and consequently there were no tests available to screen donors for NA/NB hepatitis. One approach utilised by some transfusion services was to screen donors using surrogate markers for NANB that included alanine-amino transferase (ALT) levels and/or HBV core antibody, serologically. Retrospective observational studies suggested that using specific cut-off levels of ALT in donors to defer donations could identify a substantial number of donors who were at risk of NA/NB hepatitis. [17]. A prospective study in the Netherlands showed a very high correlation of elevated ALT in donors and non-A/non-B hepatitis in recipients. [18]

However, it would also result in the deferral of donations from many individuals who did not harbour this virus and therefore waste their blood donation. [19] As well as reducing the blood supply this would also create substantial costs. In Canada, the decision to implement surrogate testing was deferred until the results of a randomized controlled trial were available. This trial confirmed the benefits of the test. [20] However, in the interim, thousands of individuals received blood from donors who could potentially have been deferred if the surrogate testing had been implemented. [18]

At the crux of the dilemma demonstrated by this example is that transfusion medicine lies at the interface of both health care delivery and public health. Blood borne infections (TTI) are a threat to the population and thus measures taken to protect against them are an essential component of public health/health protection activities. As such, these measures are governed by a different paradigm than evidence-based medicine but rather one governed by the precautionary principle. [21] Unlike other areas of medicine involving delivery of care to individuals, it is not sufficient to just prevent recognized harms but it is also necessary to prevent anticipated harms.

2.2.1. The Precautionary Principle

Transfusion medicine was not the only area confronted with the challenge of taking measures to protect against potential risks. The environmental sector has been addressing the possibility of managing theoretical catastrophic risks. In the process, emerging out of the environmental movement of the 1970's was the concept of the precautionary principle. [22] This principle argues that the absence of definitive evidence of harm does not need to exist for individuals to take action to protect against this harm. Because of the inherent ambiguity in this definition, there have been numerous different interpretations of the principle. [23] In general, strong formulations of the principle have argued that the primary consideration for taking precautionary action is the potential for a serious threat. The Wingspread Statement articulates a strong interpretation of the principle:

"When an activity raises threats of harm to human health or the environment, precautionary measures should be taken even if some cause and effect relationships are not fully established scientifically. In this context the proponent of an activity, rather than the public, should bear the burden of proof." [24]

Weaker interpretations allow for other considerations to enter into the decision-making process, for example the cost of the precautionary measure. The Rio Declaration on Environment and Development is illustrative of a weaker interpretation.

"*Where there are threats of serious or irreversible damage, lack of full scientific certainty shall not be used as a reason for postponing cost-effective measures to prevent environmental degradation.*" [25]

The numerous different interpretations have made the application of precaution problematic and have led to accusations of its being applied arbitrarily for other purposes, for example trade protectionism. Other criticisms of precaution include denying the public the benefits of new technology, arousing unnecessary fear, creating unnecessary costs and marginalizing the scientific risk assessment process. [26, 27]

The European Union, in an effort, to harmonize application of precaution put forth a guidance statement. [28] The key principles are as follows:

2.2.1.1. Specific Principles

Scientific Evaluation refers to a process through which the scientific evidence of what is known, and what is not or cannot be known is systematically evaluated.

Risk Evaluation refers to the calculation of the risks from the agent under study and the consequences of any actions under consideration as well as inaction.

Inclusive Participation refers to the deliberate representation of all interested parties in the evaluation processes.

2.2.1.2. General Principles

Proportionality means tailoring measures to the chosen level of protection. Risk can rarely be reduced to zero, but incomplete risk assessments may greatly reduce the range of options open to risk managers. A total ban may not be a proportional response to a potential risk in all cases. However, in certain cases, it is the sole possible response to a given risk.

Non-discrimination means that comparable situations should not be treated differently, and that different situations should not be treated in the same way, unless there are objective grounds for doing so.

Consistency means that measures should be of comparable scope and nature to those already taken in equivalent areas in which all scientific data are available.

Examining *costs and benefits* entails comparing the overall cost of action and lack of action, in both the short and long term. This is not simply an economic cost-benefit analysis: its scope is much broader, and includes non-economic considerations, such as the efficacy of possible options and their acceptability to the public.

Subject to review in the light of new scientific data, means measures based on the precautionary principle should be maintained so long as scientific information is incomplete or inconclusive, and the risk is still considered too high to be imposed on society, in view of chosen level of protection. Measures should be periodically reviewed in the light of scientific progress, and amended as necessary.

Assigning responsibility for producing scientific evidence is already a common consequence of these measures. [27]

2.2.2. Applying Precaution to Transfusion Medicine

While the precautionary principle originated in the environmental sector it has increasingly been used in public health [29], transfusion safety is illustrative on the application of precaution to a public health problem. [30] Perhaps most representative of the change in approach to safety that took place in transfusion medicine was the management of the risk of transfusion transmission of variant Creutzfeldt-Jakob disease (vCJD). Variant CJD represented the first major challenge related to infectious agents threatening the safety of the blood supply following hepatitis C and HIV. [31, 32] While, upon the initial recognition of the condition, no epidemiological evidence, including even case studies, existed to support potential transfusion transmission; biological models of risk suggested the possibility [33, 34] subsequent probable transfusion transmitted cases This was based on high prion concentration in tissues intimately linked with the blood system (lymphatics) and demonstration of peripheral transmission through an alternate route (oral). Blood systems around the world introduced measures to protect against this risk including deferring donations from individuals who had lived in areas where Bovine Spongiform Encephalopathy (BSE) was endemic and the institution of leukocyte reduction as a potential mechanism to reduce prion load in the blood. [32] Eventually, evidence presented itself warranting the precautionary measures including animal evidence and case reports of transfusion transmission of the prion. [35-39] Subsequent precautionary measures introduced to protect the safety of the blood supply have included donor deferral policies for Severe Acute Respiratory Syndrome (SARS) and for individuals with Chronic Fatigue Syndrome. [9, 40]

Managing vCJD illustrated a novel challenge to instituting specific precaution – the creation of one health risk by the introduction of a measure to protect against another health risk. In this instance the potential risk was the reduction in the blood supply that accompanied donor deferral policies. The broad reaching approaches and subsequent probable transfusion transmitted cases in the UK demonstrating at the very least a strong causal association. Another problem that precaution and the general movement towards risk aversion and minimal risk in blood supply added to, was increasing costs of transfusion services. The latter complementary component of a safer blood system means introducing measures to reduce residual risks to as low a level as possible. While cost-effectiveness ratios cannot be calculated for precautionary measures, because they deal with theoretical risks, the costs of residual risk removal are well above the cost-effectiveness ratios in other areas of medicine. While these traditionally range from $20 000 to $100 000/quality adjusted life year, the cost-effectiveness of nucleic acid amplification (NAT) testing for hepatitis C, hepatitis B and HIV are approximately $US 2,000,000/QALY. [41-43]

2.2.3. A Strategy for Applying Precaution to Transfusion Medicine

To reconcile the benefits of introducing precautionary measures with the potential harms a framework for applying precaution to transfusion medicine was published in the journal, Transfusion Medicine Reviews. [30] This framework is based on the response to the following questions:

These characteristics relate to the use of the following 5 questions:

1   Is the extent of the exposure large?
2   Is the consequence of the exposure serious?
3   Is the consequence of the exposure irreversible?
4   Is there a minimal cost associated with the removal of the exposure?
5   Is there a minimal negative health effect associated with removing the exposure?

The first three questions address how much evidence is necessary before a precautionary measure is instituted. The more affirmative the response to these questions the less evidence that is required to trigger precautionary action. The more likely the response to each of these questions is, "YES", the less evidence is needed by policymakers to trigger a precautionary action. Thus for exposures potentially involving a large amount of individuals, as would be the case in issues pertaining to a contaminated blood supply, where the exposure causes a serious condition which is irreversible, for example vCJD, then policy makers should not wait for high quality evidence and can act on lower levels of evidence with more uncertainty. The latter two questions address the extent of the precautionary measure that should be instituted. If there is a minimal cost associated with removal of the exposure and minimal health effect then a more aggressive measure can be introduced. In most instances, in transfusion medicine, the answer will be somewhere in between, removal of the exposure through a donor deferral policy will reduce supply and/or increase costs. In these instances a partial measure could be justified, as was done with vCJD and Canada's institution a donor deferral policy based on a 6 month's residence in affected areas. [34, 44]

As blood systems distance themselves from the tragedies associated with transfusion transmission of hepatitis C and HIV and countries prepare for a period of economic austerity, a new balance will need to be achieved between safety, maintaining and promoting quality management and costs. This will necessarily require revisiting how the precautionary principle has been put into operation.

2.3. Quality Management

2.3.1. Definitions of Quality, Safety and Risk

There are many definitions of quality but the most functional is perhaps "*that the product achieves fitness for purpose*". That is, whatever manoeuvre is performed should be aimed at achieving the expected outcome as effectively and efficiently as possible. If this definition is accepted, blood or blood products that are fit for purpose must be of the type and volume required for clinical requirements and uses and they must be 'low risk'. Low risk means that the chance of any adverse outcome in the recipient resulting from something present in the blood or products transfused is as low as possible; the product is of high integrity and is suitable for use in a given situation.

Safety again requires definition and is often perception related. It may be appropriate to invoke Hippocrates for this definition. His oath is, of course "*above all, do no harm*". The perception of safety in terms of necessary precaution, has been discussed but the risks that do remain are ever present (but low) in quality-managed facilities. They still may be substantial in some countries where their facilities are ill-equipped or poorly financed and transfusion outcomes are not followed up. Many blood services in countries with low to medium Human Development Indices are small, hospital-based, staffed by minimally trained people who have had little or no education in managing quality and risk. Once trained initially, staff may never be re-trained or have any ongoing training. Follow-up, once transfusion is conducted, may not occur. Thus, the outcome of their efforts may never be known to those preparing the blood. This situation cannot foster improvement in safety and quality.

Risk is also difficult to estimate and define. Risk depends very much on local factors, demand, facility and people, particularly human error. Where transfusion services are centralised, managing large numbers of donations and donors, preparing products and reserving plasma for fractionation, risks from infection or other laboratory managed risk-amelioration, are extremely low (risk of loss of safety either from the product's quality or post transfusion complication). Risk may be highest following transfusion of a product and often relates to human error (e.g. transfusing a unit of the wrong blood group) rather than the inherent quality of the product itself. Furthermore, there are post-transfusion complications to consider but these are discussed more fully elsewhere.

Often quality, safety and low risk are demanded as an absolute by funding bodies or by authorities. The definitions and achievement of these ideals are not absolute. They are not static but are the basis for improvement. Therefore, the generation of quality management starting small and building progressively should be the mantra. The building of a quality management system should follow an orderly process, applied over and over to every procedure carried out in the service (Figure 4). This approach is referred to as continual improvement.

Table 2. Issues preventing the universal implementation of Quality Management (QM) in Blood Services, world-wide. Training is the single, most essential element for prevention of and precaution against the risks involved in blood transfusion

Issue	Interim Solution	Risk to QM
Resources allocation	Training on how to maximise efficiency	High
Training of blood service staff in LDI ad MDI countries	Coordinate training efforts	High
Governmental control of resources and purchasing	Education on principles of quality management Education on effective and sustainable procurement	High
Decentralised services without oversight of quality	Establishing country-wide pyramidal training systems	High
Lack of sensitivity; identification and use of appropriate assays	Clear assay specifications developed and used to procure tests	Medium-High
Lack of service for equipment maintenance and repair	Funding, moving responsibility to providers of equipment with contracts	High to medium
Poor regulation of blood services and reagents	Education within governments	High

The greatest perceived risk for transfusion safety in the public mind in recent years has erroneously been the passage of TTI. However, the most common and ever-present risks stem from human error or inconsistency particularly in the cases of transfusing the wrong blood group or incorrect component's being transfused. The risk management of these threats depends upon the integrity in managing the quality and the checking mechanisms that assure that management of quality is in place from vein to vein.

Risk management procedures are encompassed in Quality Management Systems. Quality Management Systems are embodied in records of everything that is done, documentation, including changed procedures and the archives. They are living, growing and changing systems and, as has been cited, aimed at continual improvement. Major issues hindering the introduction of quality management are listed in Table 2.

By definition, a quality management system cannot be a set of written documents that sit on a shelf or in a cupboard that are brought out when a service is asked about the system or audited. The system is written, used, changed, used, and so on as the whole service improves. [Figure 4]

2.3.1.1. Principles of Quality Management

Attaining universal quality management in national blood services is best achieved within an orderly, nation-wide and stepwise system involving many groups. [45]

The principles of quality management are set out in a number of standards including ISO 9000. The ISO principles are summarised and slanted toward blood safety here:-

i   Customer focus: Blood services depend on their donors but also they must assure that the product is of quality and achieves the requirements for successful clinical outcomes. Not only does a blood service need to nurture a stable and 'safe' donor population but it needs to assure that the donors are rewarded for their donations in terms of appreciation and their careful medical management should it be necessary. Similarly the service needs to assure that the products fulfill users' needs.

ii Leadership: Blood service directors and managers assure and maintain unity of purpose within the service. They should create and maintain the internal environment in which people can become fully involved in achieving the service's objectives.

iii Involvement of people: People, at all levels, are the essence of a blood service and their full involvement and coordinated efforts enables their abilities to be used for the service's benefit and assuring effective outcomes.

iv Process approach: A desired result is achieved more efficiently when activities and related resources are managed as a process. This requires definition of the processes within a service as well as understanding an defining the procedures and tasks involved.

v   System approach to management: Identifying, understanding and managing interrelated processes as a system contributes to the organization's effectiveness and efficiency in achieving its objectives. Understanding processes by all staff members is an essential first step in establishing a quality management system.

vi *Continual improvement* of the organization's overall performance should be a permanent objective of the organization. All staff members must be dedicated to this aim (Figure 4).

vii Factual approach to decision making: Effective decisions are based on the analysis of data and information. It is therefore necessary and prudent for a blood service to maintain meticulous records. These records constitute the data that are used to inform improvements. The data are exclusive to a given service or services under the same auspices. They cannot be interchanged for use in facilities of unlike facilities or donor populations.

viii Mutually beneficial supplier relationships: A blood service should be assured that supplies are consistent and utilize suppliers that understand the needs of the service. Tight and specific contracts are essential. This is an area of difficulty for blood services where purchasing may be carried out by central [uninformed] purchasing offices.

2.3.1.2. Measures of Quality

Assessment of quality cannot be subjective. All measures of quality should be not only objective, but quantifiable. Audits of quality management systems provide objectivity.

The assessment of quality requires an understanding of:

- Process, procedures and tasks;
- The critical points i.e. points at which alterations in procedure will change the outcome of the process;
- How to assess when the requirements for quality are not met;
- How to use the documented system that assures the expected outcome consistently (i.e. ensuring the fitness for purpose).

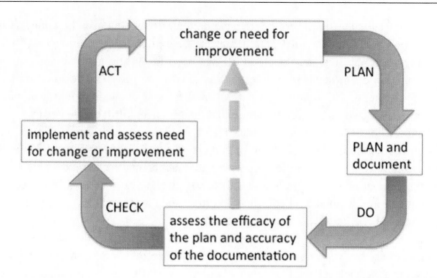

Figure 4. The cycle for achieving continuous improvement. The dynamics of planning (plan), following the plan (do), checking that the plan delivers the expected result or outcomes (check) and implementing the plan (act) affords the transfusion service a mechanism for managing risk and achieving efficiency.

Quality management systems assure that all understandings are in place and that all processes, procedures and tasks continue to proceed in a uniform manner. The assessment points should be built into the management system through audit, change procedure and corrective action. Examples of assessments include:

- That all test tubes in an assay contain sample. This may be done by simple inspection or there may be an indicator in the assay system that shows a sample has been added either by a colour change or by an indicator on a strip. The number of tubes with sample or other reagents added may be recorded as an indication of the assayist's skills; or lack thereof. This is an example of a task's verification.
- That an assay is performing consistently by assessing the variation (or lack of variation) in quality controls designed for that assay, over time. The variation in the quality control results within designated limits indicates the procedure is 'in control' over time. This is an example of verification of a procedure i.e. the testing procedure in this case.
- That all blood donations are assayed for TTIs with records in tact and any reactive donations quarantined. Any misplacement or omission may be recorded as a failure of process. This is an example of a process verification.
- That an audit of the documentation shows that the procedures are proceeding as documented. Non-conformances can be recorded with change procedures as a record of quality improvement. This is an example of verification of the integrity of documentation and is usually conducted through auditing.

A blood service creating the series of measures to verify that all procedures progress according to the documentation, should then construct a series of forms to be used to record the information. Regular review of these data offers opportunity to monitor the integrity of the quality management system, the skills of staff members and the performance of instruments and assays.

Perhaps the most important area for quality management as an implement for prevention of, and precaution against risk in blood service laboratories.

2.3.2. Laboratory Quality Management and Testing for TTI

Development and implementation of laboratory quality management systems varies greatly depending on geographic, national and educational conditions. Where resources and regulations are in place, compliance has assured that funding, resources and education (teaching and training) have been made available. However, in countries of lower human development indices often quality management systems are seen as a luxury or their necessity is not understood across sectors, and so the funds, resources and education are not made available. Furthermore, there may be limitations such as lack of power at least for some parts of a day or inadequate water supplies. Novel tests and other reagents, sometimes of poor quality, may be provided without warning when they are purchased without laboratory advice. In some cases reagents may not be available on occasions.

2.3.2.1. Tests for TTI and Their Uses

Both serological and molecular assays are now used in many in blood establishments to screen for the presence of a range of TTIs that may be present in blood donations. In any screening programme the first decision is to determine the infectious agents that need to be screened for. In addition to the main four infectious agents previously referred to, different countries may have different priorities according to the disease burden in the country and specifically in their donor population. Incident infectious diseases are of most concern and some countries may have to screen for a number of other infectious agents. Once the infectious agents of concern have been identified the appropriate specific screening target for each infectious agent must be identified. It is here that assay evaluation and validation is important, the particular assays selected for use must be properly evaluated as suitable for that purpose. However, modern screening assays, when performed correctly, perform at the high levels of sensitivity and specificity and their outcomes are generally reliable.

Once the appropriate assays have been selected the specific screening algorithm[1] to be used must be identified.

In general, screening algorithms should be simple and efficient, generating the final outcome as quickly and efficaciously as possible, but mindful of the circumstances of the screening programme. There are effectively two main blood screening algorithms in use today across the world.

The simplest algorithm is where the result of each screening test performed directly determines the fate of the donation; screen negative – issue, screen reactive – discard. However this approach is wasteful as it does not take into account the spurious and variable non-specific and false reactivity often seen when screening low risk populations.

The more commonly used screening algorithm requires the retesting, in duplicate, of any initially reactive donations with the final fate of the donation based on the repeat testing;

---

[1] A testing **STRATEGY** is a designated sequence in which tests (generically) are to be used (e.g. Test 1 EIA, Test 2 EIA) to achieve the result. An **ALGORITHM** is the way in which *specific* tests (i.e. by brand name and mechanism of action) are inserted into and used in a testing strategy.

screen negative – issue, screen reactive – repeat in duplicate and use the results to determine the donation's fate (Figure 5). If the screening assays used have been properly selected the outcomes are generally very reliable and a donation that screens negative for the infectious agents being screened for can be considered to be 'uninfected'.

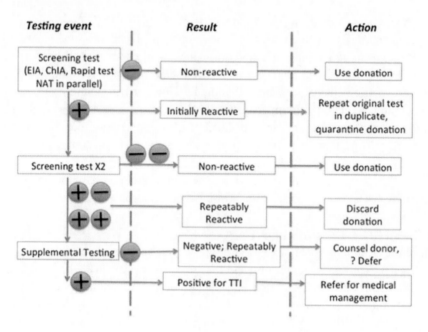

Figure 5. Testing strategy for Blood Services. The elements depicted in this schema are the broad components of all TTI testing strategies. Various steps may be modified or other steps inserted (e.g. NAT) according to the tests to be used for excluding the TTI in donations, determining those that contain TTI or for confirming the presence of a TTI.

However because sensitivity and specificity are somewhat mutually exclusive, a balance has to be found between them – potentially failing to detect and infectious donation against loosing too many donations owing to non-specific reactivity. In general, if high quality assays from the major international manufacturers are used, this balance between sensitivity and specificity can be achieved relatively easily, although the balance will always fall towards sensitivity with a (low) level of non-specific reactivity expected. Once the screening outcome has been obtained, and the donation fate determined, the status of any screen reactive donors must be determined. Confirmation of the screen reactivity obtained is critical to both providing the appropriate clinical care for the donor as well as properly understanding the actual level of infection in the donor population [and testing outcomes]. [4] These steps in the management of the donor are then conducted according to individual transfusion service's protocols. These protocols range from directing that the donor is referred for medical follow up or the donor, in some places, is not informed that their donation was found to react in one or more tests and no action is taken.

The true in-laboratory performance of the screening assays being used is important as there are differences between analytical and operational sensitivity. There are many factors that contribute to assay performance, including staff numbers and ability, the equipment available, its service and maintenance. However ongoing monitoring of performance is critical in maintaining the effectiveness of a screening programme. Initial and repeat reactive rates should be monitored and all outcomes related to the confirmatory results obtained. All information generated should be used continually to monitor the programme. Only then will a full picture of the situation be obtained and an effective and high quality screening programme be maintained.

Finally, and of varying relevance, the cost effectiveness of any proposed strategy should be evaluated fully. [46, 47]

Successful screening programmes
follow time-honoured and evidence-based principles.

2.3.3. Assessing the Efficacy of Testing

Validation of assays and algorithms in any laboratory is the most vital element of assessing testing efficacy. Although validation presents numbers of challenges, especially in small or poorly resourced blood services, it cannot be finessed. The performances of assays are often quoted in terms of sensitivity and specificity. These are important parameters and must be taken into consideration when contemplating which tests are to be used. These parameters should be assessed within the laboratory in which they are to be used wherever possible. From the perspective of understanding unnecessary loss of donations owing to poor specificity of the tests in use is most important to be aware of. It is difficult to assess this where specificity is high because a large number of samples is required and follow up testing needs to be available to identify true from false reactivity. If this is not practical, research in sufficient volume should be carried out in order to demonstrate the tests' integrity[2] (i.e., validated). Tests reported in peer-reviewed literature to deliver sensitivities and or specificities of less than 98% should be considered only with caution in a screening environment and data generated with local samples to support the test's integrity. However, the sensitivity and specificity will not offer a true picture of the test's performance in a given situation without considering the predictive values of their use. The positive and negative predictive values must be considered. Predictive values are the chance that a given result is correct. The broad calculation of predictive values is shown in Table 3. Predictive values can only be generated and used retrospectively from data obtained at a testing site, and even then only if proper confirmation is available. Information from other facilities, organisations or countries cannot be used unless the screening populations (demographics, risks and disease burden) and the laboratory systems are virtually identical. Understanding the predictive values of testing in any given facility, is essential to understanding and predicting risk and managing the appropriate precautions against risk.

In understanding laboratory-screening outcomes the prevalence and incidence of the infection in the donor population are relevant. If the prevalence and incidence are high it is likely that a higher proportion of donations will be reactive in a screening test. However, knowing the incidence of a give infection in the donor population is of greater value because it indicates the level of ongoing infection in the donor population and thus defines the specific risks to blood safety. The screen reactive donations are more likely to be from infected individuals where the prevalence of the target TTI in the donor population is high, and

---

[2] Integrity means that a test has been evaluated appropriately. It should be found to perform in line with its intended use. Appropriate validation means that the test is characterised and verified to meet evaluation performances in samples similar to those in which it will be used.

therefore the positive predictive value (or probability of a screen reactive result reflecting true infection) will be higher. If the prevalence and/or incidence is low it is more likely that reactive screening results are non-specific and the PPV will lower. However, donation screening assays should be selected on the basis of sensitivity first and specificity second, but assuring their performances are still high enough to minimise unnecessary wastage owing to non-specific reactivity.

Table 3. Calculation of predictive values of an assay. Predictive values are the chance of result's being correct. Calculating these parameters requires understanding of the assay's performance in terms of sensitivity and specificity but also the prevalence of the target in the population in which the assay is to be used. It may require that the sensitivity and specificity of an assay understood in the same population in which the predictive values are being assessed

Positive Predictive Value

$$\frac{\text{True Positive}}{\text{True Positive} + \text{False Positive}} \times 100\,\%$$

i.e.
$$\frac{\text{Prevalence}}{\text{Prevalence} + (100\text{-Specificty})} \times 100\,\%$$

Negative Predictive Value

$$\frac{\text{True Negative}}{\text{True Negative} + \text{False Negative}} \times 100\,\%$$

i.e.
$$\frac{(100 - \text{Prevalence})}{(100 - \text{Prevalence}) + (100\text{-Sensitivity})} \times 100\,\%$$

Therefore in populations at low risk of being infected with a TTI, it is expected that the NPV will always be high whereas the PPV should be low. It is most critical that a negative screening result is correct to assure a high probability that a donation does not contain the screening target. For accepting or rejecting donations this is the most relevant outcome of the testing or screening process. However, for donor management and care as well as testing programmes and their risks, further testing must be conducted wherever possible to determine the true status of donors once a reactive screening result has been obtained. It is only with knowledge of the true status of donors that the efficacy of testing and other related programmes may be assessed.

2.3.4. The Assays (Tests)

2.3.4.1. Immunoassays

Immunoassays are the backbone of BTS screening programmes.

The reduction of transfusion transmissible infections has been a long journey. The well-known and historic schema of Alter and Houghton [49] demonstrated the changes in risk over time during which major changes in blood screening were taking place (Figure 6). Since HIV antibody screening was introduced in 1985 the incidence of HIV transmission through blood transfusion, has been reduced to very low levels. Initially HIV immunoassays were based on antibody capture with crude viral lysate as the capture phase in the EIAs (1st generation assays). Subsequently, detection of antibody-antigen complexes was achieved. By today's standards these assays had inadequate sensitivity and poor specificity, but they set a pathway of assay development that has ultimately achieved unprecedented levels of assay performance. Subsequently with the use of recombinant and synthetic HIV proteins and peptides to capture antibody before detection of the antibody-antigen complex, assay were more specific as well as more sensitive (2nd generation assays). However, it was still very much a concern that donors in the very early phases of infection before antibodies developed (i.e., in the window period) would be missed and their blood transmit infections. There was a considerable pressure to reduce window periods. This could be done by introducing –

- more sensitive antibody assays
- detection of antigen
- direct detection of nucleic acid.

Third generation assays captured antibody from the sample with synthetic peptides on the solid phase. P24 antigen bound to a second anti-human IgG antibody was the used to 'sandwich' any captured sample antibody. TTI assays employing the sandwich technique are now most widely used and are highly specific as well as sensitive to all classes of antibody (IgM included). The HIV antibody window period was closed considerably compared with the antibody window period of the 2nd generation assays (2-3 weeks compared with 5-7 weeks).

The inclusion of HIV antigen detection in the 4th generation HIV serology assays ensured high sensitivity and specificity with added ability to identify infection even before an antibody response was developed in some cases of incidence infection. HIV antigen/antibody detecting, 4th generation assays from reputable international manufacturers now detect most of the identified types and subtypes.

Immunoassays for other TTI have paralleled the development of HIV assays. The ability to screen large numbers of samples with short time frames means immunoassays have become essential tools for maintaining blood safety. With detection systems that employ efficient detection of immunologic reactions, blood service screening can be fully automated with extremely high throughput. Operator input and this error is minimised with the use of these fully automated systems.

Information on blood safety and its quality management tends to focus on larger, well-resourced transfusion services. In reality, a large volume of testing of donations is carried out often using rapid tests, often in small hospital based facilities in developing countries. [1, 4, and introduction in 49] This is especially true of HIV screening. Whatever types of test are used, the quality assurance principles are essentially the same.

The major problems arise through lack of commitment by governments and competent authorities with the consequent lack resources including adequate budgets, lack of training and the constant rotation of staff or change of tests without laboratory consultation.

The message along with training about quality management systems and appropriate training needs to be filtered through to even the most basic facilities collecting and transfusing blood.

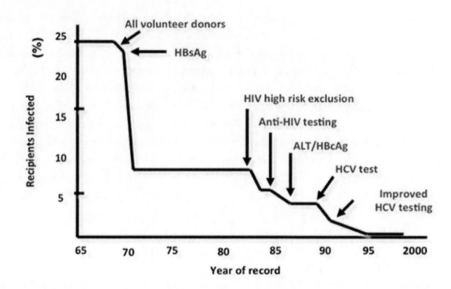

Figure 6. Reductions in transmission of TTI over time. Modified from Alter and Houghton [48].

Quality cannot be maintained with constant changes in staff or reagents that are beyond the control of [small] blood services.

This is essential for government departments and authorities to understand in the role of quality management.

Table 4. Estimates of Residual Risk for transmission of transfusion transmissible infections in 5 different countries after the implementation of antibody and nucleic acid testing for screening

	UK [54]	US [55]	Australia [56]	HK [57]	South Africa [58]
HIV	1 : 5.2m	1 : 2.14m	1 : 7.30m	1 : 10m	1: 0.48m
HCV	1 : 60m	1 : 1.94m	1 : 3.60m	1 : 50m	1:21.00m
HBV*	1 : 0.9m	1 : 0.25m	1 : 1.30m	1 : 0.001	1: 0.06m

2.3.4.2. Nucleic Acid Testing

The introduction of Nucleic Acid Testing (NAT) closed window periods beyond those of immunoassays but did not reduce the transmission of transfusion transmissible infections to zero. [50] The serological window periods are different from the molecular window periods. The window periods vary significantly between different infectious agents Thus, HCV detection with its longer serology window periods, is enhanced by the use of NAT, whereas the HIV NAT window periods that are not vastly different from the 4th generation tests' window periods have lesser yields. However these differences are also due to the biology of the viruses and virus/host interactions The odds against transmission are usually very high

(Table 4). However, the extremely low risk cannot be attributed to testing alone but testing with concomitant measures such as the introduction of quality management systems.

Introduction of nucleic acid testing should be made with an understanding of its efficacy (i.e., effectiveness and economic value) with particular reference to the incremental benefit of NAT over serological screening. Importantly the most sensitive serological screening must be used as the comparator, not the serological screening that simply happens to be in use in a particular blood establishment. If the cost effectiveness is to be determined the prevalence and incidences (particularly) of each TTI within the donor population should be understood.

Consideration of the efficacious use should take into account technical issues, for example –

- the incidence of each infection in the donor population
- predicted incremental pick-up rates as a result of implementing NAT
- costs and budgets
- whether testing is conducted in single donations or in pooled donations (for NAT). Multiplex testing for HIV and HCV may be implemented using minipools with sample numbers from 16-128 or even 500 donations [51] whereas the trend is towards small pool or single donation NAT.
- dilution may compromise analytical (dilutional) sensitivity but also presents challenges for staff in managing pools effectively. [52]
- the highly sophisticated automation and the need for very high sensitivity for HBV DNA detection has led (or is leading) to small pool or single donation testing for HIV and HCV RNA as well as HBV DNA
- Discriminatory/confirmation assays are necessary to decipher which TTI is present following multiplex testing presenting another challenge for the integrity of blood transfusion services' quality management systems.

2.3.5. Process Regulation

2.3.5.1. Quality Assurance

Quality Assurance may be defined as the procedures and steps that are taken to assure that procedures and tasks are undertaken in a specified, documented and uniform manner in order to achieve expected and consistent outcomes.

Thus, in the case of a blood service some examples of quality assurance would be –

- the quality of supplies being shown to meet specifications,
- checking that the batch testing by the manufacturer of tests was shown to be within set and specified limits,
- that training of staff is verified and documented as up-to-date
- reagents all shown to be within their 'use-by' dates and
- out-of-date reagents quarantined or discarded
- quality assessment and quality control procedures in place for all critical steps
- all procedures are properly documented including recording results etc.

After establishing quality management systems through analysis, full documentation and comprehensive training, quality assessment and quality control are the methods used to assure the integrity of processes, procedures and tasks. It is the information gleaned from the quality assurance procedures that will secure that risks are evidenced and documented. The evidence provides the grist for prevention and precaution against untoward events. Another most important implement of quality assurance is the audit process and procedures. Again, these quality measures are essential to the integrity of the testing process as well as all procedures in the blood transfusion service. The quality procedures for testing services are described below.

2.3.5.2. Quality Assessment

Quality assessment is the way in which an entire process is assessed to ensure the integrity of its outcome. For laboratory testing this is usually accomplished within laboratory networks. A designated laboratory or facility (e.g., a reference laboratory) conducts the exercise as demonstrated in Figure 7. This method has been in place for pathology laboratories since the late 1950s and has not been supplanted by any more useful methods.

2.3.5.3. Quality Control

Quality control is a method used to check that a task is performed correctly, that a reagent is of integrity and that equipment is operating as expected, as examples.

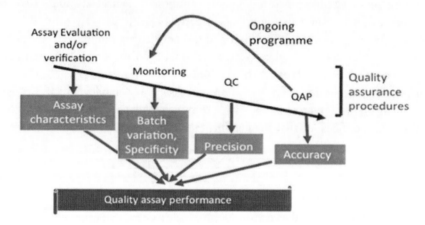

Figure 7. Quality Assurance mechanisms used to achieve performances for assays used in detecting TTI.

For the quality control of a laboratory test, a standard sample is made up in quantity sufficient for, say, a year's use and stored. It must be stable enough to give the same result over time. Quality controls are best prepared by a reference laboratory, using the correct raw materials and employing appropriate expertise.

In this way the controls are stable and give consistent results as long as they are appropriately stored. However, when no such products are available, quality controls can be prepared and used by *any* laboratory. There is no excuse for a laboratory's not using quality controls for assays. Training is the limiting factor.

2.3.6. Costs of Quality

The costs and cost effectiveness of implementing quality management and its quality assurance are difficult to specify (Figure 8).

For instance, the implementation costs in a small service will be proportionally greater than in a larger service.

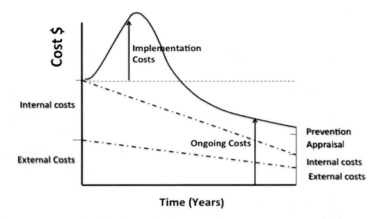

Figure 8. Relative costs of implementation and maintaining quality management systems. External costs include audit, contract costs, training and other costs paid outside the facility. Internal costs include staff salaries, reagent costs, costs of maintaining the environment etc. Implementation cost will vary according to the degree of quality management at the start of establishing a quality management system, training levels, the size of the service etc.

Costs of implemented quality systems will range between 8-25% of budget depending on where in the implementation process the service has reached, the sophistication of the service, the size of the service, the types of reagents and suppliers the service utilises, and so on. Larger costs include training fees, equipment maintenance, quality assessment, audit fees etc. If a transfusion service is necessary, if it is established, the costs of quality management must be included in its establishment and in planning the ongoing costs.

On the other side of the coin, there are savings to be made in utilising quality management. Trained staff members perform better and make fewer mistakes, reagents are suitable and ordered in the correct amounts and with their specified needs met (i.e. wastage is reduced), laboratory layout is more efficient and safer (therefore productivity is increased and running costs are reduced), results are reliable and repeat testing is avoided, as examples.

2.3.6.1. Effectiveness and Cost Effectiveness of the Measures

Blood Transfusion Service structures, size and resources vary greatly across the world. In western countries centralized systems that collect blood from a number of sites, process them centrally and distribute as necessary have proven to have reduced risks and operate more efficiently. [45]

However, the bulk of systems across the world in terms of facility and staff numbers, do not operate centralized systems. The sophistication and quality may vary widely. The support for establishing quality and cost effective procedures may be minimal or absent. [49] These systems are likely to be hospital based and very often receive no priority in the administration of the hospitals.

The solutions to problems in establishing quality management and quality assurance in the more peripheral systems rest on improving training throughout the entire system. If there is no national system issuing guidelines for transfusion services this requires establishment. Sometimes there are adequate resources but they are poorly used. Training resources require careful use and recognition that the establishment of national efficient systems takes considerable time and effort from numbers of trainers with various skills, working in coordination. [53]

Conclusion

TTI are the *perceived* major risk to the safety of blood and blood product transfusion. The major risks stem from poor practice because sufficient quality management and adequate quality assurance procedures are not in place. Governments in medium to low human index countries generally do not recognise the importance of blood safety principles and often even basic funds for establishing and maintaining quality management systems are not made available.

Human error is a critical factor in compromising transfusion safety. Countering human error is best accomplished by implementing comprehensive quality management systems. In the long run quality management, especially in laboratory services, is the mechanism to assure prevention and offer precaution against errors and risks. It is cost effective.

The 'take-home messages' of this Chapter are –

1   Quality Management Systems provide mechanisms for risk management in transfusion services where procedures and supply management have become increasingly complex.
2   Training often is the critical factor missing in achieving precaution against, and prevention of, risks of transfusion. Training should be continual until quality management is in place and being maintained.
3   If governments and authorities expect risk to be minimal, they need to acknowledge that quality management systems are integral to assuring transfusion safety and fund transfusion services accordingly.
4   Governments and authorities need to be convinced that quality management is cost effective.
5   Consistency of supply is not only necessary to quality management but is also cost effective.

References

[1]   Ala, F., Allain, J. P., Bates, I., et al. External aid to blood transfusion services in sub-Saharan Africa (SSA) – A need for reflection. *PLoS Med.* 2012;9: e1001309. doi:10.1371/journal.pmed.1001309
[2]   Allain, J. P. Volunteer safer than replacement donor blood: a myth revealed by evidence. *ISBT Science Series,* 2010;5:169-175
[3]   Jiang, Y., Qiu, M., Zhang, G., et al. Quality assurance in the HIV/AIDS laboratory network of China. *Intern. J. Epidemiology*, 2010;39, ii72–ii78
[4]   WHO Geneva, CH. (2009). Screening donated blood for transfusion-transmissible Infections: Recommendations.

[5] Chappel, R. J., Wilson, K. M., Dax, E. M. Immunoassays for the diagnosis of HIV: meeting future needs by enhancing the quality of testing. Review. *Future Microbiol.,* 2009;4:963-982.

[6] Choudhury, N. Can there be blood units of high and low quality? *Asian J. Transfus. Sci.,* 2009;3:1-2

[7] Frey, B. M., Schlenke, P. Safeguards in blood supply: a national and European challenge. *Transfus. Med. Hemother.,* 2010;37:109-110

[8] Gonçalez, T. T., Sabino, E. C., Schlumpf, K. S., Wright, D. J., Mendrone, A., et al. NHLBI Retrovirus Epidemiology Donor Study-II (REDS-II). International Component. Analysis of donor deferral at three blood centers in Brazil. *Transfusion,* 2012;52:870-879

[9] Wilson, K. The Kreever Commission – 10 years later. *CMJA* 2007;177: 1387-1389

[10] Hayes, E. B., Gubler, D. J. (2006). West Nile Virus: Epidemiology and Clinical Features of an Emerging Epidemic in the United States 181-194 - doi, 10.1146/annurev.med.57.121304.131418

[11] Appiah, B. Africa's road to blood ruin. *CMAJ* 2012;184:E 341-E342

[12] Bambrick, H. J., Woodruff, R. E., Hanigan, I. C. Climate change could threaten blood supply by altering the distribution of vector-borne disease: an Australian case-study. *Glob. Health Action.,* 2009;10:2 doi: 10.3402/gha.v2i0.2059.

[13] Attaullah, S., Khan, S., Khan, J. Trend of transfusion transmitted infections frequency in blood donors: provide a road map for its prevention ad control. *J. Transl. Med.,* 2012;10:20. doi: 10.1186/1479-5876-10-20

[14] Angelotta, C., McKoy, J. M., Fisher, M. J., et al. Legal, financial, and public health consequences of transfusion-transmitted hepatitis C virus in persons with haemophilia *Vox Sang.,* 2007;93:159–165

[15] Upshur, R. E. Are all evidence-based practices alike? Problems in the ranking of evidence. *CMAJ* 2003:169:672-673.

[16] Krever, H. Canada's rejection of surrogate testing. Commission of Inquiry on the Blood System in Canada. Final Report. Ottawa: *Canadian Government Publishing,* 1997:649-686.

[17] Aach, R. D., Szmuness, W., Mosley, J. W., et al. Serum alanine aminotransferase of donors in relation to the risk of non-A,non-B hepatitis in recipients: the transfusion-transmitted viruses study. *N Engl. J. Med.,* 1981;304: 989-994.

[18] Van der Poel, C. L., Reesink, H. W., Lelie, P. N., et al. Anti-hepatitis C antibodies and non-A, non-B post-transfusion hepatitis in The Netherlands. *Lancet* 1989*ii*;8658:297-298.

[19] Alter, H. J., Purcell, R. H., Holland, P. V., Alling, D. W., Koziol, D. E. Donor transaminase and recipient hepatitis. Impact on blood transfusion services. *JAMA,* 1981;246:630-634.

[20] Blajchman, M. A., Bull, S. B., Feinman, S. V. Post-transfusion hepatitis: impact of non-A, non-B hepatitis surrogate tests. Canadian Post-Transfusion Hepatitis Prevention Study Group. *Lancet* 1995;345:21-25.

[21] Krever, H. Commission of Inquiry on the Blood System in Canada. Final Report. Ottawa, Canada: *Canadian Government Publishing.* 1997.

[22] Foster, K. R., Vecchia, P., Repacholi, M. H. Risk management. Science and the precautionary principle. *Science,* 2000;288:979-981.

[23] Van der Zwaag, D. The precautionary principle in environmental law and policy: elusive rhetoric and first embraces. *J. Environmental. Law and Practice*, 1999i;8:355-375.

[24] Wingspread statement on the Precautionary Principle. Wingspread Conference, 1998. January 23-25 1998; Racine, Wisconsin.

[25] United Nations. Report of the United Nations Conference on Environment and Development, Rio Declaration on Environment and Development UN Doc A/CONF. 151/26 (Vol1) (Annex 1). New York: United Nations, 1992:31 ILM. 874.

[26] Wildavsky, A. Trial and error versus trial without error. In: J. Morris, Editor. *Rethinking risk and the Precautionary Principle.* (22-45). 2000, Oxford, UK: Butterworth-Heinemann.

[27] Morris, J. Defining the precautionary principle. In: Morris, J., editor. *Rethinking risk and the Precautionary Principle.* (1-21) 2000, Oxford, UK, Butterworth-Heinemann.

[28] EC Commission, Communication on the Precautionary Principle COM (2000) 1 (Brussels: 2 February 2000), online: Europe Gateway to the EU *http://europa.eu.int/comm/dgs/health_consumer/library/pub/pub07_en.pdf.*

[29] Goldstein, B. D. The precautionary principle also applies to public health actions. *Am. J. Public Health,* 2001;91:1358-1361.

[30] Wilson, K., Wilson, M., Hebert, P. C., Graham, I. The application of the precautionary principle to the blood system: the Canadian blood system's vCJD donor deferral policy. *Transfus. Med. Rev.,* 2003;17:89-94.

[31] Wilson, K., Ricketts, M. N. Transfusion transmission of vCJD: a crisis avoided? *Lancet,* 2004;364:477-479.

[32] Wilson, K., Ricketts, M. N. The success of precaution? Managing the risk of transfusion transmission of variant Creutzfeldt-Jakob disease. *Transfusion,* 2004;44:1475-1478.

[33] Cashman, N. *New Variant Creutzfeldt-Jakob Disease and the Canadian Blood Supply: Scientific Basis of Risk.* Laboratory Centres for Disease Control, Atlanta GA, US 1999.

[34] Wilson, K., Hebert, P. C., Laupacis, A.., et al. A policy analysis of major decisions relating to Creutzfeldt-Jakob disease and the blood supply. *CMAJ,* 2001;165:59-65.

[35] Houston, F., Foster, J. D., Chong, A., Hunter, N., Bostock, C. J. Transmission of BSE by blood transfusion in sheep. *Lancet,* 2000; 356: 999-1000.

[36] Llewelyn, C. A., Hewitt, P. E., Knight, R. S., et al. Possible transmission of variant Creutzfeldt-Jakob disease by blood transfusion. *Lancet,* 2004; 363(9407):417-421.

[37] Peden, A. H., Head, M. W., Ritchie, D. L., Bell, J. E., Ironside, J. W. Preclinical vCJD after blood transfusion in a PRNP codon 129 heterozygous patient. *Lancet,* 2004;364:527-529.

[38] Wroe, S. J., Pal, S., Siddique, D., Hyare, H., Macfarlane, R., Joiner, S., et al. Clinical presentation and pre-mortem diagnosis of variant Creutzfeldt-Jakob disease associated with blood transfusion: a case report. *Lancet,* 2006;368:2061-2067.

[39] Wilson, K., Ricketts, M. N. A third episode of transfusion-derived vCJD. *Lancet,* 2006;368:2037-2039.

[40] Wilson, K. A framework for applying the precautionary principle to transfusion safety. *Transfus. Med. Rev.,* 2011;25:177-183.

[41] Laupacis, A., Feeny, D., Detsky, A. S., Tugwell, P. X. How attractive does a new technology have to be to warrant adoption and utilization? Tentative guidelines for using clinical and economic evaluations. *CMAJ*, 1992;146:473-481.

[42] AuBuchon, J., Petz, L. Making decisions to improve transfusion safety. In: AuBuchon, J., Petz, L., Fink, A., (Eds), *Policy Alternatives in Transfusion Medicine.* 2001:184-226. Bethesda, MD, US: AABB Press.

[43] Van Hulst, M., de Wolf, J. T. M., Staginnus, U., Ruitenberg, E. J., Postma, M. J. Pharmaco-economics of blood transfusion safety: review of the available evidence. *Vox Sang.*, 2002;83:146-55.

[44] Wilson, K., Graham, I., Ricketts, M., Dornan, C., Laupacis, A., Hebert, P. Variant Creutzfeldt-Jakob disease and the Canadian blood system after the tainted blood tragedy. *Soc. Sci. Med.*, 2007;64:174-185.

[45] Kim, D. U. The quest for quality blood banking program in the new millennium the American way. *Int. J. Hematol.*, 2002;76 Suppl. 2:258-62.

[46] Barreto, A. M., Takei, K. E. C. S., Bellesa, M. A., et al. Cost-effective analysis of different algorithms for the diagnosis of hepatitis C virus infection. *Braz. J. Med. Biol. Res.*, 2008; 41:26-134

[47] Custer, B., Busch, M. P., Marfin, A. A., Petersen, L. R. The cost-effectiveness of screening the US blood supply for West Nile virus. *Ann. Intern. Med.*, 2005;143:486-492

[48] Alter, H. J., Houghton, M. Hepatitis C and eliminating post-transfusion hepatitis *Nat. Med.*, 2000;6:1082-1086

[49] Lara, A. M., Kandulu, J., Chisuwo, L., Kashoti, A., Mundy, C. Laboratory costs of a hospital-based blood transfusion service in Malawi. *J. Clin. Pathol.*, 2007;60:1117-1120

[50] Stramer, S. L., Glynn, S. A., Kleinman, S. H., et al. Detection of HIV-1 and HCV Infections among Antibody-Negative Blood Donors by Nucleic Acid–Amplification Testing. *N Engl. J. Med.*, 2004;351:760-768

[51] Ohnuma, H., Tanaka, T., Yoshikawa, A., et al. for the Japanese Red Cross NAT Screening research group. The first large-scale nucleic acid amplification testing (NAT) of donated blood using multiplex reagent for simultaneous detection of HBV, HCV, and HIV-1 and significance of NAT for HBV. *Microbiol. Immunol.*, 2001; 45:667-672

[52] Westreich, D. J., Hudgens, M. G., Fiscus, S. A., Pilcher, C. D. Optimizing screening for acute human immunodeficiency virus infection with pooled nucleic acid amplification tests. *J. Clin. Microbiol.*, 2008; 46:1785-1792

[53] Seitz, R., Heiden, M. Quality and safety in blood supply in 2010. *Transfus. Med. Hemother.*, 2012;37:112-117

In: Quality Management in Transfusion Medicine   ISBN: 978-1-62618-665-1
Editor: Cees Th. Smit Sibinga   © 2013 Nova Science Publishers, Inc.

Chapter XII

Health Economics of Technologies in Blood Transfusion within the Context of General HTAs

Marinus van Hulst,[1,] Maarten J. Postma[2,†]*
and Brian Custer[3,‡]
[1]Groningen Research Institute of Pharmacy (GRIP), University
of Groningen *and* Department of Clinical Pharmacy and
Toxicology, Martini Hospital, Groningen, The Netherlands
[2]Unit of PharmacoEpidemiology and PharmacoEconomics
(PE2), Department of Pharmacy, University of
Groningen, Groningen, The Netherlands
[3]Associate Investigator, Epidemiology and Health
Policy, Blood Systems Research Institute *and* Adjunct
Associate Professor, Laboratory Medicine, University of
California San Francisco, San Francisco, CA, US

Abstract

The demand for structured and generic health technology assessments (HTAs) is considered a pathway for achieving the combined goals of increasing quality of care and access to care, controlling expenses and achieving value for money. In the blood safety and transfusion medicine these evaluations are particularly relevant because of the high

[*] Marinus van Hulst, PharmD, PhD: Groningen Research Institute of Pharmacy (GRIP), University of Groningen and Department of Clinical Pharmacy and Toxicology, Martini Hospital. PO-BOX 30033, 9700 RN, Groningen, The Netherlands). Tel: +31-6-2909.6932; E-mail: hulstr@mzh.nl.
[†] Maarten J. Postma, PharmD, PhD: Professor, Unit of PharmacoEpidemiology and PharmacoEconomics (PE2), Department of Pharmacy, University of Groningen, Groningen, The Netherlands NL. Tel: +31-6-5121.2767; E-mail: postmamj51@googlemail.com.
[‡] Brian Custer, PhD, MPH: Associate Investigator, Epidemiology and Health Policy, Blood Systems Research Institute and Adjunct Associate Professor, Laboratory Medicine, University of California San Francisco, 270 Masonic Ave, San Francisco, CA, US. 94118. Telephone: 415 901 0756. E-mail: bcuster@bloodsystems.org.

costs of many interventions and the lack of consensus on priorities and acceptable risk transfusion recipients should bear. The value of HTA in the area of blood safety and transfusion medicine is understood, however, consistent application of HTA lags. The threshold willingness to pay for optimal safety in blood transfusion is expected to remain substantially higher than the threshold for medical therapies. The use of health economic methods in HTAs will increase in importance because of the presence of competing interventions in blood safety and transfusion. The recognition of the need to change the decision-making paradigm in transfusion safety coupled with need to make decisions with scarce resources will bring HTAs that include health economics to greater prominence.

Keywords: Health technology assessments, Health economics, Quality assurance, Safety, Cost-effectiveness

1. Introduction

Economic analyses are critical for quality improvement because these analyses identify the health gains that can be achieved and costs that are incurred for all activities or interventions that seek to improve healthcare. In the blood safety and transfusion medicine context this is particularly relevant because of the high costs of many interventions and the lack of consensus on priorities and acceptable risk transfusion recipients should bear. For example, the policy of the Dutch government has been to strive for optimal blood transfusion safety with a recognition that zero risk or a maximum risk avoidance policy is perceived as an unobtainable goal for medicinal products originating from a human sources. [1, 2] This viewpoint is shared by many others. [3, 4] Although the policy of optimal safety in transfusion medicine is expressed in every Ministerial Blood Supply Plan, implementation by the Dutch government of new technologies which improve the safety of blood and its components are mainly driven by availability of technology, merely suggesting that economics may not be within the set of evidence that defines optimality. In the last decades several health economic evaluations of blood transfusion safety strategies have been published either as papers in peer reviewed journals or reports. [5-7] The appropriate role that economic analysis should have in contributing to decision making and therefore managing the quality for blood transfusion safety strategies will continue to evolve.

Health care markets are becoming more and more complex and the number of stakeholders is generally increasing. This can be explained by increasing regional decision making with concomitant centralization, increasing privatization leading to more health care insurers with stakeholders' interest in new fields, and increasing recognition of the need to include health economics within the broader context of health technology assessment (HTA). National bodies such as NICE (National Institute of Clinical Excellence) in England, SMC (Scottish Medicines Consortium) and iQWIG (Institut für Qualität und Wirtschaftlichkeit im Gesundheitswesen) in Germany, and the Pharmacy Benefits Advisory Committee (PBAC) in Australia have now been in place for at least a decade. Purchasers in general (also including health care insurers, managed-care organizations, patient bodies and private clinics) are more concerned than ever about getting value for money, demanding increased evidence of proven added value even before granting market access, let alone reimbursement and widespread use of technologies. This also applies for local levels where considerations on evidence, costs and cost-effectiveness are becoming more relevant. Even before the recent economic crisis, decisions on reimbursement for drugs, diagnostics, and vaccines often required economic evidence in terms of cost-effectiveness in many European countries and other international settings. Notably, the approach on evidence, costs and cost-effectiveness stems from the area of drugs, which are relatively easy to control. However these expectations extend to all other areas in health care. These same trends apply to the disciplines of blood safety and transfusion medicine but not with the same level of formal guidelines. Importantly, new technologies for blood components and the need for prioritization among them are increasing the need of such assessments.

2. Consequences of Demanding HTAs

The demand for structured and generic health technology assessments (HTAs) is considered a pathway for achieving the combined goals of increasing quality of care and access to care, controlling expenses and achieving value for money. HTA uses evidence-based medicine techniques and is based on sets of guidelines for methodologies to be used, inclusive of health economics guidelines. [w101] As a result, the reimbursement environment is often stringent, both at the central as well as at the local health-care insurance and hospital levels. For instance, in the Netherlands, the implementation of technology assessment, inclusive of pharmacoeconomic analysis, has resulted in the denial of various new technologies for reimbursement. [w102] Further examples of some recent innovative therapies that have gone through HTA in Western countries include various new anti-thrombotic therapies, antimicrobial agents, psychotropic drugs and orphan drugs. [8-10]

Such stringent rules and procedures have various consequences. On the one hand, stringent rules and procedures hamper the dissemination of new technologies, in particular if this leads to denial for reimbursement (The Netherlands, Belgium, Sweden, et cetera) or negative guidance on use (NICE and SMC in the UK). On the other hand, denial for reimbursement of interventions which showed a negative balance between health gains achieved and resources used would enable resources to be used for more effective interventions with in the end more health gains achieved for the society. Furthermore, denial of such less cost-effective health care interventions may eventually stimulate the innovation of health care interventions with more added value to society.

Despite being stringent, procedures and the set of requirements it encompasses do provide suppliers of technologies with rather clear-cut pathways to follow for market access and reimbursement. Indeed, in many Western economies the pathways for manufacturers to get new drugs on the market is straightforward, generally including clear steps and decision criteria. Also, and most clearly at the central level, timelines generally exist in the technology assessment, reassuring that the evaluation will be finished within an adequate amount of time both regarding market access and reimbursement although clock-stops (extending this legislation timeline) are obviously more rule than exception.

In many Western economies such procedures exist for outpatient and inpatient drugs with processes and criteria and with specific requirements on how to report evidence with regard to some of the decision criteria (for example guidelines for pharmaco-economic analysis). In some areas, however, lags in this respect still exist and ample potentials for further development of rational procedures, criteria and requirements exist. This is the case for blood safety, derived products from donated blood (e.g. albumin, specific immunoglobulins, clotting factors) and transfusion medicine. [w103]

The value of HTA in the area of blood safety and transfusion medicine is understood, however, consistent application of HTA lags. The experiences gathered in assessing drug technologies are informative and the trend towards use of rational technologies in blood transfusion safety provides a new challenge for HTAs.

3. Structure of the Chapter

As mentioned earlier, this chapter specifically focuses on health investment decisions for technologies in blood safety and transfusion medicine within the scope of quality management, whereby it is acknowledged that such decisions can be expected at several levels (e.g., country, regional, and hospital). For uniformity reasons so that the health economic evidence base is robust, it is highly relevant to identify the set of procedures and criteria to develop a toolkit for decision making procedures on health investments in blood transfusion. Focus in this chapter will be on those aspects of HTA that primarily concern health economics. In the following sections we discuss and propose health-economic criteria for decision making related to investments in blood transfusion technologies as well as refer to processes and requirements. In addition, three aspects of HTA that remain particularly challenging for blood transfusion safety technologies will be developed in detail –

a) assessing and understanding uncertainty in the transfusion medicine context;
b) the role of modelling because of limited data from large blood recipient cohorts, and
c) appropriate thresholds for defining what is 'cost-effective'.

4. Criteria for Decision Making

In our current approach, we define criteria as various items to be considered within the whole toolkit to assess new blood transfusion technologies. The toolkit comprises the process of which steps to take in an assessment, who actually performs these (national or local level decision-makers and advisors), specific procedures and the consideration of methodological standards or even guidelines for conducting specific parts within the toolkit. Previously, the EUnetHTA Core Model for HTA was developed within an EU-project. [w104] The model employs 10 domains or criteria within the process that can be applied for assessing a new screening or diagnostic test. Next to issues on safety, effectiveness, ethics and organisation, these criteria involve costs and economic evaluation.

5. Health Economics Terminologies

The methodology of cost-effectiveness analysis (CEA) and health economics has been discussed in detail in recent review papers. [5, 11-13] The main study types used in economic evaluation are cost-effectiveness (CEA) and cost-utility analysis (CUA) in which the incremental net costs of a programme are related to the incremental health benefits.

CEAs measure health effects in physical units such as increments in life-years gained, infections averted, cases found, cases cured, etc. Cost-minimisation analysis (CMA) is a specific form of cost-effectiveness analysis whereby the health effects of the intervention and the current practice are equivalent (or are expected to be equivalent). In a CMA, the focus is on comparing only the costs of difference practices. Whereas, in CUA, the incremental life-years gained are adjusted for quality of life, to arrive to a common denominator known as a quality adjusted life-year (QALY). Both costs and effects may or may not be the same for different practices. For developing countries disability adjusted life-years (DALY) averted are often used as the burden of disease measure. DALYs are estimated by adding the years of life lost due to the disease and the adjusted years lived on with disease. While a different conceptualisation of effects exists between QALYs and DALYs for a CUA the same analysis approach is used. Costs are measured in monetary units. Cost-effectiveness or cost-utility ratios are expressed as net costs per unit of effect by comparing a new intervention with current practice or another competing intervention (incremental analysis). The primary result of a CEA or CUA is this incremental cost-effectiveness ratio (ICER).

The perspective of a health economic evaluation defines which costs are explicitly included or excluded from the evaluation, depending on the perspective different types of costs are considered. Generally, all health economic analyses include *direct* costs for medical care borne by the health system, community, families of patients, and patients themselves. Direct costs can either be *programme-related*, such as tests in a screening programme or can be *patient-related*, such as hospital, outpatient and community care. Health economic analyses performed from the health care providers' perspective tend to focus on direct costs only. The current consensus in health economics is that a more complete assessment of cost-effectiveness is achieved with the use of a societal perspective and therefore that all relevant costs and consequences for society should be considered, including productivity and leisure losses. [14] However, discussion remains whether loss of productivity caused by morbidity and mortality should be incorporated as *indirect* costs or as quality adjustments in cost-utility analysis [15-20], and how to exactly measure indirect costs using human capital or friction costing approaches. Patient-related costs – direct as well as indirect – may transfer to *benefits* if illnesses and related costs are averted, for example through screening or inactivation procedures of blood components. The basic conceptualisation in health economic analyses is to evaluate the net costs, i.e., programme costs and net patient-related benefits. Results for cost-effectiveness studies can also be plotted on the cost-effectiveness plane. For each intervention the incremental costs and incremental effects are plotted as Cartesian coordinates, depending on the quadrant an intervention falls in certain conclusions can be made about its value relative to its comparators. Even within the same quadrant, this provides a visual method for displaying results and also allows for classification of interventions as being dominant over or dominated by other interventions. From a health economic viewpoint any new programme with negative net cost (offering overall cost saving programmes) and non-negative health gains should be implemented since it is a dominant strategy. Positive net costs should be related to health gains such as life-years gained. To determine whether implementation is justified, the cost-to-health-gains (cost-effectiveness) ratio should be carefully considered and compared to acceptability thresholds, if available. The threshold for health economic acceptability that has been published is US$50,000 per QALY [21] and to this day continues to be considered a threshold defining cost-effectiveness in the US. According to WHO and World Bank guidelines, strategies that show a cost-effectiveness ratio below the per capita gross national income (GNI) of a country are regarded as cost-effective, whereas strategies with cost-effectiveness ratios above three times the per capita GNI are regarded as not cost-effective. [22, 23] Interventions with cost-effectiveness ratios between these two values would have to be considered on a context-specific basis. Thresholds of adopted blood safety and transfusion thresholds do not conform to these standards and will be discussed later in this chapter.

Another aspect of health economics is the expectation that analyses will discount future costs (and effects). Discounting is a method to adjust future costs and benefits to their present value (cost and benefits are weighted less the farther in the future they occur). In transfusion medicine, transmission of agents with the potential to establish long term chronic infections is particularly relevant. As viral infections often involve serious complications requiring complex health-care interventions occurring several years after infection, the concept of discounting of future costs is highly relevant. Examples of long-term complications are cirrhosis after years of chronic hepatitis or development of AIDS in the late stage of HIV-infection. Discounting is a method to adjust future costs and benefits to their present value (cost and benefits are less weighted the farther in the future they accrue). The discounting procedure applies two major principles. First, capital invested in a new technology could have been invested otherwise and may have gained interest. Second, there is a pure time preference with short-term benefits being preferred to future benefits because of uncertainty as to whether one will be able to benefit from the same monetary amount next year as one is now. The value of the discount rate should be chosen in accordance with marginal rates on investment and market interest rates. Many countries use average interest rates of long-term government bonds. [24] Often, discount rates are specified in the national guidelines for health economic research and vary between for example, 1.5% in the Netherlands, 3% in the US to 6% as previously used in the United Kingdom. [14] Discounting is common practice in health economics, although a fruitful field for discussions on exact numericals and methods used [17] this is beyond the scope of material presented here. The existing set of tools is adequate to apply to blood transfusion technologies. Sensitivity analysis is an important tool to investigate the outcomes obtained from health economic models. Whereas most parameters used in health economic models are derived from clinical trials or from retrospective data sources, others may be based on individual expert opinions. Often, few parameters are known with a high degree of undisputed accuracy. To estimate the effect of uncertain variables on the robustness of the model results, sensitivity analysis is performed.

Economic evaluation has become paramount in the last decades to help priority setting in health care; i.e., to spend health-care budgets optimally to ensure the highest health gains for limited resources. It is undertaken to inform health-care decision makers with the explicit goal to enhance rational decision making. Guidelines are used as explicit tools for designing, executing and judging economic evaluations. Health-economic/pharmaco-economic guidelines exist for various countries all over the world. [w101] Setting the methodological standards, most guidelines require the transparent presentation of cost-effectiveness planes, cost-effectiveness acceptability curves, value-of-information analysis, uncertainty analysis using both sensitivity and scenario analysis, and explicit probabilistic sensitivity analysis reporting averages, credibility intervals surrounding the cost-effectiveness estimates, international transferability and sometimes explicit thresholds for willingness-to-pay. [25-28]

6. Health Economics within the HTA-Context

Next, we will consider in more detail which tools, methodological standards and guidelines exist for assessing health economics of new technologies in blood transfusion.

Regarding tools to judge and structure health-economic parts of HTAs, guidelines for health-economic or pharmaco-economic evaluations can be extremely helpful. As an illustration, we list the Dutch guidelines for economic evaluation as presenting such a set of tools. This specific set of guidelines reflects one set of many possible sets of guidelines that are now available all over the world and that can be considered and compared at www.ispor.org. [w101] Generally, these sets of guidelines are quite comparable between countries and institutions (for example, the Dutch guidelines resemble the Belgian ones and those of the National Institute of Clinical Excellence [NICE] resemble those of the Scottish Medicines Consortium). Yet, notable differences exist, for example, where the first Dutch guideline prescribes the societal perspective, NICE generally recommends the third-party payer (NHS) perspective to be adopted. In particular, the Dutch guidelines consist of a set of 11 guidelines with several subheadings being specified. The table below consistently lists this set of items that can be applied to structuring or evaluating any HTA, inclusive those concerning blood transfusion technologies. These guidelines are used for assessing and evaluating files on drugs that are prepared by *the manufacturers* themselves, inclusive of pharmaco-economic analysis (generally outsourced to a consultancy specialized in this area, but under strict supervision of the company/manufacturer). Obviously, ideally the process of HTA should be a fruitful collaboration between authorities and the manufacturer. However, analyses and assessments are being performed primarily by independent bodies (NICE).

Some general aspects are reflected in this set of tools and therefore should all apply to economic analyses of blood transfusion technologies. [16] In particular, transparency in reporting is an important issue, as economic evaluations are often performed by (under the strict supervision of) the manufacturer. Also, effectiveness versus efficacy is important with the goal to analyse on population/real world level rather than on clinical trial level; i.e., a cost-effectiveness analysis is necessary and a cost-efficacy analysis is insufficient for real-world decision making. For donor screening tests this means the analysis should be one assessing clinical utility rather than analytical validity or clinical validity. A related issue is the desire to measure effects in 'hard endpoints' for morbidity and mortality rather than intermediate or surrogate endpoints (such as, blood pressure, albuminuria, HB1Ac and cholesterol levels) which may have been used in phase III clinical studies. This often requires the use of models, which is allowed according to the guidelines if adequately motivated. In practice, most economic evaluations HTAs involve some level of modelling to infer from efficacy to effectiveness and from intermediate to 'hard' endpoints.

7. Uncertainty in Health Economic Evaluations

The role of uncertainty analysis in health economics is different than its role in other medical research. The objective of health economics is to inform decision makers on the optimal allocation of scarce health care resources to maximise health gains. Decision makers always make a choice between mutually exclusive options. Even if decision makers chose not to implement a new technology, the decision is made to continue the current technology with the associated costs and consequences.

Therefore, traditional rules of inference do not apply to decisions on resource allocation in health care. [30, 31] Statistical tests, p-values and confidence intervals are less relevant in decision making. Maintaining current health care technology based on a statistical insignificant difference with a new technology also implies that a new intervention has a mean benefit which is no better than current practice. In health economics the role of uncertainty is to inform decision makers on the level of uncertainty surrounding the decision and if it is worthwhile to conduct additional research to lower the uncertainty of the decision. [32] The analysis of, expectations for, and representation of uncertainty in health economics has dramatically changed in the last 15 years.

Table 1. Dutch guidelines for pharmaco-economics as set of tools and subcriteria (items), adapted from www.cvz.nl [29, w102]

1. Perspective	The analysis should done and reported from the societal perspective, including costs, savings and health effects irrespective of who benefits and who looses
2.1 Comparator	The new technology should be compared with the standard technology recommended by health care professionals or the technology usually provided to patients (as derived from registries)
2.2 Indications	The indication should be clearly specified and the population considered in the economic analysis should be same as the population for which the new technology is considered
2.3 Subgroups	All relevant subgroups should be specified and explicitly considered in the analysis; all Subgroups should be clearly defined
3.1 Cost-utility	If quality of life is important, a cost-utility analysis should be performed
3.2 Cost-effectiveness	If mortality dominates the health effects of the disease considered, a cost-effectiveness study can be performed, using life-years gained as the preferred clinical outcome
4 Analytical period	The analytical period should be such to allow valid inferences to be drawn on consequences of the old comparator and the new technology regarding costs, savings and health
5.1 Identification of costs	All relevant costs should be identified: direct medical, direct non-medical, indirect non-medical and indirect medical and individually included/excluded in sensitivity analysis
5.2 Measurement of costs	Resource use has to be measured validly and adequately
5.3 Valuing resources	Adequate unit cost prices should be used to value resource use
6.1 Efficacy vs. effectiveness	Relevant measures of effect (morbidity and mortality) should all be identified validly and with highest achievable certainty
6.2 Quality of life	Quality of life should be measured validly and reliably
6.3 Utilities	Appropriate methods should be used to measure utilities
6.4 QALYs	Calculations of QALYs should done correctly and be reported transparently

7.1 Modelling	Use of a model is allowed for the analysis costs and effects of treatments to be compared, if sufficiently motivated
7.2 Reporting the model	Transparent reporting of the model is required, inclusive structure, cycles, transition probabilities, estimates and assumptions
7.3 Model validity	The validity of the model should be adequately investigated, tested and reported
8.1 Reporting totals	Totals for costs and effects of both the index drug and the comparator should be provided
8.2 Reporting incrementals	Incremental costs and effects between index and comparator should be reported in detail
9 Discounting	All relevant future effects (at 1.5%) and costs (at 4%) should be adequately discounted to current values
10.1 Deterministic SA[*]	To analyse uncertainty, all relevant deterministic uni- and multivariate SAs should be conducted adequately and transparently
10.2 Probabilistic SA[*]	To analyse uncertainty, all relevant probabilistic SAs should be conducted adequately and Transparently
11.1 Expert panel	If adequately motivated, expert panel opinions can be used
11.2 Consensus	It should be transparent how consensus was arrived at in the expert panel

[*]SA = sensitivity analysis.

Uncertainty analysis in health economics is focussed on dealing with the particular problems of the statistics of ratios that inherently arise with constructing confidence intervals around estimated cost-effectiveness ratios. The evolution of techniques is evident in transfusion safety interventions. Fieller's theorem has used to directly estimate the confidence interval of the estimated cost-effectiveness ratio. [33, 34] Bootstrapping has also been used to estimate the confidence interval of the cost-effectiveness ratio derived from clinical trial data comparing leukocyte reduced erythrocytes to buffy-coat depleted packed red cells in cardiac valve surgery patients. [35] More efficient methods are now available to evaluate uncertainty in health economics performed alongside clinical trials. The net-benefit framework in combination with regression methods offers a more convenient approach to perform health economics alongside clinical trials. [36, 37] In addition, second order Monte Carlo simulation of probability distributions (probabilistic sensitivity analysis) included in the models can be used to estimate the uncertainty intervals. In this context, the intervals are known as credible intervals representing specific cost-effectiveness ratio estimates from the distribution of the results obtained during the Monte Carlo simulation. Second order Monte Carlo simulation is considered as the minimum acceptable level of sensitivity analysis that should be conducted for health economic analyses.

Decisions on allocation of scarce health care resources are first and foremost made on the cost-effectiveness of the intervention. [30, 31] If the interventions are mutually exclusive, the additional costs of an intervention divided by the health gains of an intervention as compared with the next least expensive intervention are reported as incremental cost-effectiveness ratios Interventions that are dominated (more costly and less effective) are rejected. Also, interventions can be rejected by extended dominance, i.e., by combinations of interventions that are more effective and less costly. From the remaining interventions, the intervention which has the highest ICER below the cost-effectiveness threshold can be regarded as the optimal intervention. Generally, mean costs and effects of interventions are presented on the cost-effectiveness plane. Connecting all the cost-effective (non-dominated) interventions yields the cost-effectiveness acceptability frontier (CEAF). [38]

The cost-effectiveness acceptability curve (CEAC) was designed to inform decision makers on the uncertainty surrounding the decision to accept a new technology over the current standard relative to the cost-effectiveness threshold or willingness to pay. [39] The use of the CEAC to display uncertainty in health economic evaluations has been challenged. [40] Main objection against the use of the CEACs is the possibility of misinterpretation of CEACs by decision makers and analysts caused by the inability to distinguish dramatically different joint distributions of incremental costs and effects with CEACs. However, it is argued that the CEACs remain a valuable tool to inform decision makers on the probability that an intervention is cost-effective for a range of willingness to pay thresholds. [41] Decision makers should not use CEACs to inform them on optimal allocation of resources.

Nevertheless, CEACs in combination with arbitrary significance rules have been used to demonstrate decision makers' preferences. [42]

Generally, mean incremental costs and effects of interventions are presented on the cost-effectiveness plane. Connecting all the cost-effective (non-dominated) interventions yields the cost-effectiveness acceptability frontier, which is sometimes referred to as the efficiency frontier. [38] To simultaneously display the optimal decision along with the uncertainty surrounding this decision a cost-effectiveness acceptability frontier (CEAF) can be constructed from the CEAC and the ICERs of the evaluated interventions in the cost-effectiveness frontier. [43]

The CEAF is created from the CEAC of interventions that are optimal for a particular range of willingness to pay or cost-effectiveness thresholds. [32]

The optimal intervention has an ICER below the threshold willingness to pay, is part of the cost-effectiveness frontier and is as such not rejected by (extended) dominance.

Using CEACs or CEAFs to inform decision makers on the consequences of an incorrect decision and the need for further research to reduce decision uncertainty is inappropriate. In this case, the expected value of perfect information (EVPI) can be estimated to investigate whether it is worthwhile to invest in more research to reduce decision uncertainty. [30, 31]

Because an infinite sample gives perfect information that would eliminate all possibilities of making the wrong decision, the EVPI also equates to the expected costs of uncertainty. [30, 31]

The EVPI is determined by the probability of a wrong decision being made and on the consequences of that wrong decision. [30-32] Extensive discussions of the appropriate use of uncertainty in health economics can be found in journals dedicated to health economics, decision making and statistics in medical research. [32, 35, 39, 42-47]

Hardly any papers can be found in general medical journals using the EVPI approach.

Apparently, a fast growing knowledge gap is appearing between the state-of-the-art methodology of uncertainty evaluation in health economics and the level which readers and reviewers of general medical journals can grasp.

For health economics evaluations of blood safety and transfusion medicine minimum acceptable standards should include second order Monte Carlo simulation and presentation of results in a cost effectiveness acceptability frontier framework.

7.1. Best Practices in Health Economic Modelling

Perhaps no other word in the policy analyst's lexicon inspires greater confusion among lay observers the term *model*. [48] Models are critical and necessary tools for conducting health economic analyses. Often, health economic models are regarded as 'black boxes' with lack of transparency being a common criticism. Recently, common approaches and standards of practice been developed. Efforts to create standards stem from the reality that models are difficult to replicate, and so reporting on the model structure, function and data inputs are extremely critical for face validity within health economic assessments. A substantial new effort to promulgate appropriate techniques for health economic modelling has recently concluded. The results are series of best practices guidelines. These best practices guidelines are broadly written but fully applicable to economic analyses of transfusion safety interventions. [201-207]

7.2. Threshold Considerations in Transfusion Safety

While a general metric of US$ 50,000/QALY, also known as the willingness to pay, has long been considered a *de facto* indicator of a cost-effective intervention. [49] WHO and the World Bank suggest that the threshold for acceptability to gain one QALY should be closer to three times the GNI, which is currently approximately €100,000/QALY for The Netherlands, yet a ratio or threshold of €100,000/QALY (~US$125,000/QALY) has little meaning in the transfusion safety context. A large number of blood safety interventions have been adopted with cost-effectiveness ratio results above and sometimes exceedingly far above any suggested threshold. The obvious and often stated lesson is that thresholds for acceptable costs per QALY gained that may be applicable in other health care settings simply do not apply in blood safety. [50] This observation is likely a reflection of a broader societal desire to prevent transfusion-transmitted infection and appears to be applicable regardless of type of health care system (single payer government-funded, market-driven, or somewhere in between). Even in developing country settings, acceptable cost-effectiveness ratios for blood safety exceed those of other health care interventions. The threshold willingness to pay for optimal safety in blood transfusion is expected to remain substantially higher than the threshold for medical therapies. [1, 2, 50] The underlying reason for this may be the perception of the risks concerning transfusion and associated consequences by the general public, elected representatives and health regulators. [51, 52]

Additional factors that contribute to the willingness to pay for interventions with cost-effectiveness ratios outside of norms in health care include uncertainty as to whether a blood collector or the government is responsible when transfusion recipients become infected with a pathogen that could have been prevented by expensive technology. [53] This uncertainty may further tip the balance more to a maximal safety policy. The model of regulation and implementation in western countries promotes the adoption of expensive technologies. For example, the Dutch government is responsible for the policy with regard to the safety of cellular blood products and the budget required by Sanquin Blood Supply Foundation (Sanquin) to provide the required safety level.

Subsequently, Sanquin is responsible for the operational performance of the safety measures in place. This regulatory and implementation structure contributes to very high willingness to pay for each QALY that is gained. However, this approach to transfusion safety at any costs is clearly understood to be unsustainable and a new paradigm is emerging. The recent consensus conference on risk-based decision making for blood safety suggests a new framework and decision-making process is needed, which addresses as much the science of blood safety as the ethics, social values, economics, public expectations, and historical context. [54] This approach, if it takes root, will mean that economic evaluations are necessary before adoption of new interventions and thresholds for acceptability will need to be more transparent in transfusion safety.

Risk assessment and governance in combination with health economics may be a more appropriate strategy of risk management for blood transfusion safety. [55, 56] This is even more so when the risk of transmission and health consequences of transfusion transmitted infections are known. For instance, in the case of HBV, HCV and HIV, risk assessment and governance in combination with health economics is more justified than using (simply) the precautionary principle.

Accepting a certain threshold for safety in transfusion medicine, whether it is a health economic or a transmission risk threshold implies that theoretically some transfusion recipients could become infected who would not be infected if all available technology was implemented. Imagine a theoretical threshold of one infected transfusion recipient every five years in The Netherlands. Compare this threshold to one infected transfusion recipient every ten years if all available technology is implemented. One unfortunate transfusion recipient every ten years would bear the burden of a policy decision which probably saved millions of Euros during these ten years. These savings could potentially gain more health in other sectors of the health care system which would benefit the Dutch society more than allocating these funds to blood transfusion safety. Therefore, taking decisions informed by risk assessment and governance in combination with health economics without offering a no-fault compensation is a challenging ethical question. No-fault compensation is on and off the agenda of the Dutch government since the 1990s. [1, 2, 53, 57]

8. Brief Review on Health Economic Studies in Blood Transfusion Technologies

We analyzed published literature on economic evaluations of blood transfusion technologies using the set of tools represented by the health economic guidelines; i.e., the set of guidelines that can be seen more or less as universal for health economic evaluations. [w101]

8.1. Health Economics of Blood Transfusion Safety – Diminishing Returns on Investment in the Developed World?

Blood transfusion is a safe medical intervention in very high Human Development Index (HDI) countries[1], improving blood transfusion safety with regard to pathogen transmission or

---

[1] See Chapter 15 – HDI Ranking.

prevention of non-infectious threats to transfusion safety requires substantial monetary investment with very little health gain. The last decade has seen the adoption of nucleic acid amplification testing technologies (NAT) for both cellular and plasma derived blood components[2].

Depending on the setting (NAT) for HIV, HBV, HCV in addition to HAV, West Nile virus, and Parvovirus B19 have been adopted using various pooled or individual donation testing strategies. Relative to serological screening for HBV, HCV and HIV, NAT displayed cost-effectiveness ratios at least over 500 times the GNI for The Netherlands and at least 50 times the GNI for the US. Individual donation multiplex NAT may dominate minipool NAT for HBV, HCV and HIV in The Netherlands owing to increased effectiveness, mainly caused by a shorter window period of the individual donation for each virus in the multiplex assay compared to the window period of the minipool format of the NAT assay. The relationship between the individual and minipool cost will determine which strategy dominates the other in high HDI countries. NAT added to serological tests for HBV, HCV and HIV yielded marginal health gains at considerable cost. The cost-effectiveness of adding NAT to serological screening has consistently been found to be very poor in several evaluations. [5, 7, 58-61]

Very little health gains are to be expected of reducing the risk of HBV, HCV or HIV transmission by pathogen inactivation of platelets. Health gains from pathogen inactivation are mainly to be expected from reducing the risk of bacterial contamination sepsis. [62-64]

Incremental to bacterial culturing currently in place, the cost-effectiveness ratio of pathogen inactivation (€554,000 per life-year gained) will certainly be over three times the GNI threshold for the Netherlands and the US. This will be even more so if the most recent estimates for sepsis risk reduction due to bacterial culturing are used in the evaluation. With respect to non-infectious threats in transfusion, leukocyte reduction in cardiac valve surgery patients with or without coronary artery bypass grafting was shown to be cost-saving from the societal perspective. [36]

The probability that leukocyte reduction was cost-saving was 69%. Most health gains and cost reductions were found in patients receiving more than 3 units of red blood cell concentrates (RBC). On leukocyte reduction of blood, former Dutch Health minister Borst–Eilers tried to take an informed decision based on an advice by the Health Council and on additional health technology assessments. [1, 65] Despite this effort, the Dutch House of Representatives voted unanimously for a resolution to implement universal leukocyte reduction primarily for the prevention of variant Creutzfeldt-Jakob transmission and also for the reduction of the immunological side effects. [66] Universal leukocyte reduction was introduced in The Netherlands in 2001. [67]

Studies have supported the use of leukocyte reduction in cardiac valve surgery patients and especially those who require four or more units of RBCs. The health gains and associated costs of universal leukocyte reduction are yet still debated. [68]

In general, marginal health gains are achieved by methods intended to enhance the safety of blood components in very high HDI countries[3].

Three factors determine the low value for money of methods for enhancing blood transfusion safety:

---

[2] See Chapter 11 – Management of Blood Safety – Prevention and Precaution.
[3] See Chapter 15 – HDI ranking.

1) the risk of pathogen transmission is very small;
2) the costs of new methods to improve safety are high; and
3) the incubation time is long relative to the survival of transfusion recipients. [69]

The average age of the transfusion recipient in very high HDI countries is approximately 65 years. This would give a remaining life-expectancy of each person in the general population between 10 and 15 years. Due to underlying diseases, blood transfusion recipients are assumed to have an increased risk of mortality resulting in a further reduced remaining life-expectancy. Therefore, preventing the transmission of HBV and HCV, both with an incubation time of approximately 20 years, would give little health gains in the transfused population in high HDI countries.

The precautionary principle is often applied to decisions in blood transfusion safety[4]. The precautionary principle is of particular value when the blood supply system is faced with an emerging threat and knowledge is uncertain. [70] However, using the precautionary principle for decision making is still heavily debated. [71]

Moreover, as many as 19 different definitions have appeared in literature. According to the European Union definition, the application of the precautionary principle must be proportional, non-discriminatory, comparable, cost-effective, and subject to revision. [72] Sometimes the precautionary principle is wrongly regarded equivalent to a 'zero risk' policy. However, the proportionality included in many definitions of the precautionary principle precludes this. [70, 72]

Nevertheless, the precautionary principle is regularly associated with a high willingness to pay for blood transfusion safety. [73] Quality defects of pharmaceutical and medicinal products are never tolerated, whatever the costs to prevent. Moreover, societies are even less likely to accept adverse effects of medication. Rofecoxib and Cerivastatin are examples amongst other drugs that were recently withdrawn from markets due to side-effects. Aprotinin, which was withdrawn from the market but re-introduced for specific indications, provides another example.

The perception of the safety of blood components in combination with the increasing cost of blood transfusion due to safety measures make alternatives to blood transfusion highly valued medical interventions. [74] Adverse effects of alternatives to blood transfusion could easily offset any achieved health gains. This is clearly demonstrated by the demise of aprotinin due to end-organ damage. Therefore, transfusion triggers should first and foremost be used to determine the medical necessity for a transfusion. [75-77] Provided that the interventions are used in a systematic approach, often referred to as patient blood management measures to reduce exposure to allogeneic blood transfusions may be cost-saving for hospitals[5]. If reduced hospital stay can be further substantiated, alternatives to blood transfusion may become cost-effective from the societal perspective. The use of alternatives to blood transfusion in combination with progressively implementing more clear transfusion triggers have caused a declining trend in the number of issued RBCs in The Netherlands. [75, 78]

However, a declining economy of scale may cause increasing unit costs of RBCs in the future. Amongst other reasons, e.g., Sanquin Blood Supply Foundation anticipates to the

---

[4] See chapter 11 – Management of Blood Safety – Prevention and Precaution.
[5] See chapter 9 – Patient Safety and Quality Management at the Clinical Interface.

declining trend of blood transfusion utilisation by concentrating facilities. [1] One question with respect to the high willingness to pay for alternatives to blood transfusion remains whether it is ethical to ask donors to donate blood while methods exists to reduce the utilisation of blood transfusions despite the sometimes high costs involved. Although blood donation caries very few risks, it is not free of risks. [78, 79]

In very high HDI countries societies are willing to pay more for blood transfusion safety than for interventions in other areas of the health care system. Increased costs of blood transfusion in combination with costs and consequences of (perceived) adverse effects of blood transfusion may further increase the use of alternatives to blood transfusion. New threats to the blood supply are constantly lurking. The last decades the blood supply was challenged by various pathogens and diseases, such as West Nile virus, Chagas, Chikungunya and variant-Creutzfeldt-Jakobs disease. The source of the cellular blood components is of utmost importance for the resulting blood transfusion safety especially for emerging pathogens. The voluntary non-remunerated and regular donor pool is the corner stone of blood transfusion safety. Although a health economic evaluation of voluntary non-remunerated donors is hard to perform, the value of voluntary non-remunerated donors should not be questioned. [80, 81]

8.2. Cost-Effectiveness of Interventions Ensuring Blood Transfusion Safety in Africa, an Example of the Use of Health Economics in Quality Management

The risk of HIV, HBV and HCV transmission by blood transfusion in sub Saharan Africa is (very) high compared to high HDI countries. Since budgets for interventions to improve blood transfusion safety are limited, insight in the effects and costs of the interventions is important for the sub Saharan setting.

In this example we show a cost-effectiveness evaluation of interventions improving blood transfusion safety in Angola, Benin, Botswana, Côte d'Ivoire, Ethiopia, Kenya, Mozambique, Namibia, Rwanda, Uganda and Zambia.

The interventions included: donor management; quality of testing; quality of result administration and introducing additional tests. The results of this example were presented at the AABB Annual Meeting and ISBT International Congress in 2006. [82, 83]

The health gains and costs of improving blood transfusion safety were explored in three scenarios:

- In the NONE scenario (no screening, no donor management) the risk of transmission is the prevalence in the general population.
- The CURRENT scenario reflects the status of the blood transfusion services according to the Global Database on Blood Safety (GDBS; WHO, 2004). False negatives due to technical and administrative errors are estimated at 5.2% (one-fifth of the residual risk estimated for Kenya). [84]
- In the BEST scenario antibody/HBsAg screening is 100%, there are no technical and administrative errors and donor management outcomes are comparable to the developed world (prevalence in donors 1/333 of prevalence in the general population

for HIV and 1/167 for HCV and HBV, extra 5 US$ per donation). In this scenario a higher standard of quality management is modelled specifically.

In addition to the BEST scenario, additional antigen tests were evaluated. The residual risks of HIV, HBV and HCV transmission were derived from the GDBS and window periods for the test (table 1). Residual risk of infection was estimated by

$$Re\,sidual\,Risk\;=\;\frac{PREVALENCE * Window\,period}{Latency} \tag{1}$$

Health gains were expressed as disability averted. Survival was transformed into DALYs using remaining gender specific life expectancies (Life Tables, WHOSIS, 2001) and standard (Markov) models for HIV, HBV and HCV. For HIV, one secondary infection to partners of the recipient and 0.5 of the donor was included. DALYs were expressed as: $\Delta D = D_{Exp}-D_0$, where D_{Exp} is the expanded blood safety system and D_0 the comparative blood safety system. Health gains were discounted at 3%, age weighting is included. Net costs are expressed in 2006 US$. Cost of tests can be found in Table 2. Net costs expressed as: $\Delta C = C_{Exp}-C_0$, where C_{Exp} is the total costs of expanded blood safety system and C_0 the total costs of the comparative blood safety system. Once the difference in disability (ΔD) and the difference in net costs (ΔC) had been estimated, the incremental cost-effectiveness ratio (ICER) = $\Delta C / \Delta D$ in US$/DALY was estimated.

The total number of residual infections in the included countries for the evaluated scenarios is displayed in Table 3. The number of residual infections for HIV also includes secondary infections. As can be observed from this table, a drastic reduction of the number of residual infections is achieved by the both the Current and Best scenario. Additional testing, This health economic evaluation showed that CURRENT scenario is cost-saving compared to the NONE scenario preventing disability (gaining health) and saving money, see Table 4. Improving the blood transfusion services from the CURRENT to the BEST scenario by improving mainly quality management shows a cost-effectiveness ratio of 56.24 US$ per DALY averted.

In addition to the BEST scenario, HIV p24 and HCV-antigen testing shows an incremental cost-effectiveness ratio (ICER) of 63,947 US$ and ID-NAT Multiplex of 164,655 US$ per DALY averted.

Table 2. Window periods and test costs

Test	Window period (days)			Total Costs (US$)
	HIV	HBV	HCV	
Ab	22	59	50.9	9
Ag/Ab	16	NA	12.5	11
ID-NAT/Ab	7	38	7	25

Ab = antibody; Ag/Ab = combi-test antigen and antibody; ID-NAT/Ab = individual donation nucleic acid amplification and antibody.

Figure 1 is an example of a sensitivity analysis. In this particular example several parameters were varied in the health economic evaluation of including antigen testing

(Ag/Ab) or individual NAT in addition to the Best scenario incremental to the Best scenario. The variation of the parameters is specified in Figure 1. It was shown that the outcomes were sensitive to test costs and the inclusion of secondary infections.

Table 3. Total number of residual infections in the included countries for the evaluated scenarios

Virus	None	Current	Best (-DM[*])	Best (+DM[*])	Ag/Ab	ID-NAT
HIV	97,095	2,795	528	3.51	2.55	1.12
HBV	29,397	1,724	216	1.30	1.30	0.25
HCV	4,982	1,622	31.6	0.19	0.039	0.026

[*]DM = Donor Management HIV prevalence in donors 1/333 of the prevalence in the general population, for HCV and HBV 1/167.

Table 4. Total costs and disability adjusted life-years averted for the investigated scenarios

Scenario	ΔC (million US$)	ΔD (DALY)	ICER (US$/DALY)
Base case			
Current vs None	-82.25	1,950,939	Cost-saving
Best vs Current (- DM[*])	1.059	53,534	19.77
Best vs Current (+ DM[*])	3.624	64,434	56.24
Ag/Ab vs Ab @ Best (+ DM)	1.214	18.97	63,947
ID-NAT vs Ab @ Best (+ DM)	9.713	58.98	164,655
Sensitivity analyses			
Best (+DM) vs Best (-DM)	2.565	10,900	235
Ag/Ab vs Ab @ Best (- DM)	3.779	10,919	346
ID-NAT vs Ab @ Best (- DM)	12.278	10,959	1,120

[*]DM = Donor Management HIV prevalence in donors 1/333 of the prevalence in the general population, for HCV and HBV 1/167.

This brief health economic evaluation shows that the Current level of blood transfusion safety provided in the included countries is cost-saving. Investing in improving quality and donor management would be a sensible strategy according to this example.

Improving quality and donor management sharply reduced the residual risks of viral transmissions. In 2006, the weighted Gross National Income (GNI) of the selected countries was US$ 398.64. At 56.24 US$ per DALY averted, the ICER is much lower than the GNI threshold for cost-effectiveness.

Therefore, it may be concluded that according to World Bank and WHO definitions, improving quality and donor management is a cost-effective strategy in this example.

Introducing additional more sensitive tests alongside antibody testing on top of an improved donor management and quality system is associated with high costs and limited reduction of transmission risks with an unfavourable health economic profile, displaying ICERs over 3x GNI per capita.

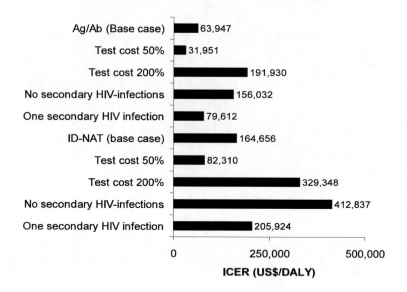

Figure 1. Sensitivity analysis for including antigen testing in addition to the Best scenario (including improved donor management).

8.3. Health Economics of Blood Transfusion Safety in Developing and Transitional Countries – Where to Put the Money?

Blood donation screening for HIV-antibody is a cost-effective method to prevent HIV infection in low, medium and high HDI countries. [85] Similar to (very) high HDI countries, more sensitive tests added to HIV-antibody, HCV-antibody and HBsAg screening are generally not cost-effective for low to medium HDI countries. More than three times the GNI or GDP per capita is needed to save one DALY for NAT for instance. However, compared to very high HDI countries, the ratio of GNI or GDP to the cost-effectiveness ratio is considerably lower. This difference is explained by the average young age of the transfusion recipient and higher risks of viral transmission. This very high HDI approach of using NAT in blood bank screening is not shown to be cost-effective to enhance HIV screening in a cross-section of African countries, see example in section 8.2. Antigen screening used in combination with antibody screening for HIV and HCV may be a cost-effective option for some countries.

Blood supply systems in very high HDI countries provide a very high level of product safety with regard to transfusion transmitted infection. Exporting these systems to developing countries would appear to be an attractive solution to improve blood transfusion safety in low, medium or high HDI countries. [86] However, the costs of maintaining the level of safety are very high. The costs of transfusing two units of RBC in The Netherlands exceed the GNI per capita in the majority of the low HDI countries. Blood supply systems in economy restricted countries are gradually moving from hospital based blood banks heavily depending on family and replacement donors to a more centralised system relying on voluntary non-remunerated donors. In general, the unit costs of blood components from consolidated blood supply systems are higher than from hospital based blood banks. [87] Most consolidated blood supply systems in African countries receive external funding (e.g., EU. PEPFAR, WB). [87] The dependence on external funding hampers the sustainability of the consolidated blood supply systems[6]. An alternative hospital based screening strategy is using pre-donation rapid test screening in combination with minipool NAT on HBV, HCV and HIV. [88] Pre-donation rapid tests for HBV, HCV and HIV in combination with post-donation NAT cost less and prevent more loss of health than post-donation serological screening.

The contribution of human error to the risk of pathogen transmission is reported very low in very high HDI countries. [89] In low HDI countries. However, scarce data indicate that human error can cause up to 20% of the HIV transmission risk. [83, 89] An overview of interventions improving transfusion safety in a selection of African countries revealed that interventions reducing human error in screening and processing of blood donations were cost-effective. (see example in section 8.2) Also, a considerable part of the prevented disease burden and associated health care cost found with pre-donation screening described was attributed to the reduction of human error. [88] Because of the lack of data, we designed a prospective study to investigate the contribution of human error to pathogen transmission in low HDI countries. [91] The study yielded useful and interesting observations, although the original goals of the research plan were not reached. We found that infectious disease marker screening was not performed within the required time after blood donation. Furthermore, collection and storage conditions of samples were not according to specifications. Also, volume variations, poor labelling and haemolysis of the blood samples were noticed. All these factors caused the failure to achieve the goals of the research plan. Nevertheless, the problems encountered do also indicate that human error augmented by absence of a working quality system will contribute to pathogen transmission in low HDI countries. [91] These conditions which lead to conditions conducive to bacterial growth also point to our current very limited understanding of the contribution of bacterial transmission by transfusion on post-transfusion DALYs in low and medium HDI countries.

Enhancing blood transfusion safety in low HDI countries by introducing more sensitive hi-tech tests is not cost-effective. Nevertheless, transfusion recipients in low HDI countries, whom are mainly children and young women (pregnancies), face a substantially higher probability of HBV, HCV and HIV and other infections compared to transfusion recipients in very high HDI countries. Directions for cost-effective improvements in transfusion safety in low HDI countries can be discerned. For some regions it may be worthwhile to investigate if pre-donation screening in combination with in-house NAT is also cost-effective in their situation. Preliminary data indicates that investments in donor management to motivate low risk voluntary non-remunerated donors to donate blood are cost-effective. Also, investments in laboratory performance and quality systems to achieve a reduction of human error may prevent considerable disease burden in transfusion recipients. Still, the insufficient supply of safe blood is regarded as the greatest threat to blood transfusion safety in low HDI countries. [92]

---

[6] See Chapter 14 – Quality Management in Transfusion Medicine in Resource Restricted Countries.

9. Future Perspectives

The cost-effectiveness of preventing HBV, HCV and HIV and other known pathogens with screening is well studied in very high HDI countries. However, health economic evaluation is still needed in case of emerging pathogens to provide decision makers insight in the costs and consequences of adopting new screening strategies. [57, 65, 93-95] Health economics of donor related interventions, such as temporary exclusion or motivating specific low risk donor groups to donate, are scarce and more research is warranted in this important area of blood transfusion safety. [50, 95] Health economic evaluations can also be used when new technologies become available to inactive pathogens in red blood cell concentrates or whole blood. [96] Artificial oxygen carriers are currently being developed, some of which are investigated in phase III clinical trials. [97] The application of artificial oxygen carriers in clinical practice should be preceded by full health economic evaluations which weigh the benefits, adverse effects and costs of these oxygen carriers against those of blood transfusion. Currently, transfusing the wrong ABO blood type causes the greatest disease burden in most high HDI countries including The Netherlands. [98-102] Health economic evaluations of available measures to prevent these mis-transfusions, such as barcode assisted transfusion, could motivate decision makers to develop legislation and make budget available to introduce these safety barriers in clinical practice. [101, 102] In low and medium HDI countries transfusion of the wrong blood type may be of even greater concern. The quality of blood grouping performed in the laboratory of the blood bank is as essential for the safety of the blood transfusion as screening donations for pathogens. The costs and consequences of replacing error prone manual blood grouping by more sophisticated techniques in low HDI countries may be worthwhile to explore. [91]

For low to medium HDI countries, further research in the health economics of improving blood transfusion safety by screening strategies for HBV, HCV and HIV is needed to inform decision makers. Special attention should be focused in these evaluations to the sustainability and technical feasibility of the proposed screening strategies. The sustainability and affordability should also be considered from the perspective of the payer, which is often the family of the patient in low HDI countries. Health economics of donor related interventions, such as using donor management to motivate regular voluntary non-remunerated donors, is of particular importance in low and medium HDI countries, see section 8.2.

As science progresses and new evidence comes available, economic models require updating. The time to publication of the results of a health economic evaluation is considerable. Often, estimates used in the health economic evaluation can become quickly outdated which subsequently outdates the results of the health economic evaluation. Sometimes, updates of health economic evaluations appear as brief reports which lack sufficient detail for proper interpretation. These problems can be overcome by disseminating health economic evaluations on internet as well as in peer-review journal. In fact, all peer-reviewed journals should stimulate authors to publish their models adjoining technical appendices online to promote the transparency of health economic models. Adherence to best practices in health economic modelling will improve the transparency of both models and the reporting of models. The use of health economic methods in HTAs will increase in importance because of the presence of competing interventions in blood safety and transfusion. The recognition of the need to change the decision-making paradigm in transfusion safety coupled with need to make decisions with scarce resources will bring HTAs that include health economics to greater prominence.

References

[1]   Dutch Ministry of Health, Welfare and Sport. *Ministrieel Plan Bloedvoorziening 2001*. 2000, Sdu Uitgevers, Den Haag, NL

[2]   Dutch Ministry of Health, Welfare and Sport. *Ministrieel Plan Bloedvoorziening 2007*. 2006, Sdu Uitgevers, Den Haag, NL

[3]   AuBuchon, J. P., Birkmeyer, J. D. Safety and cost-effectiveness of solvent-detergent-treated plasma. In search of a zero-risk blood supply. *JAMA: The Journal of the American Medical Association* 1994; 272: 1210-1214.

[4]   Klein, H. G. Will blood transfusion ever be safe enough? *JAMA: The Journal of the American Medical Association* 2000; 284:238-240.

[5]   Van Hulst, M., de Wolf, J. T. M., Staginnus, U., Ruitenberg, E. J., Postma, M. J. Pharmaco-economics of blood transfusion safety: review of the available evidence. *Vox Sang*. 2002;83:146-155.

[6]   Van Hulst, M., Smit Sibinga, C. Th, Postma, M. J. Health economics of blood transfusion safety--focus on sub-Saharan Africa. *Biologicals* 2010; 38:53-58.

[7]   Custer, B. Economic analyses of blood safety and transfusion medicine interventions: a systematic review. *Transfus. Med. Rev*. 2004;18:127-143.

[8]   Postma, M. J. Public Health Aspects of Vaccines in The Netherlands: methodological issues and applications. *J. Public Health* 2008;16:267-273

[9]   Vegter, S., Rozenbaum, M. H., Postema, R., Tolley, K., Postma, M. J. Review of Regulatory Recommendations for Orphan Drug Submissions in the Netherlands and Scotland: focus on the underlying pharmacoeconomic evaluations. *Clinical Therapeutics* 2010;9:1651-1661

[10] Blankart, C. R., Stargardt, T., Schreyögg, J. Availability of and Access to orphan Drugs. *Pharmacoeconomics* 2011;29:63-82

[11] Custer, B., Busch, M. P., Marfin, A. A., Petersen, L. R. The cost-effectiveness of screening the US blood supply for West Nile virus. *Ann. Intern. Med*. 2005;143:486-492.

[12] Busch, M., Walderhaug, M., Custer, B., Allain, J. P., Reddy, R., McDonough, B. Risk assessment and cost-effectiveness/utility analysis. *Biologicals* 2009;37:78-87.

[13] Van Hulst, M., Slappendel, R. and Postma, M. J. The Pharmacoeconomics of alternatives to allogeneic blood transfusion. *Transfusion Alternatives in Transfusion Medicine* 2004;6:29-36.

[14] Hjelmgren, J., Berggren, F., Andersson, F. Health economic guidelines--similarities, differences and some implications. *Value Health* 2001;4: 225-250.

[15] Siegel, J. E., Torrance, G. W., Russell, L. B., Luce, B. R., Weinstein, M. C., Gold, M. R. Guidelines for pharmacoeconomic studies. Recommendations from the panel on cost effectiveness in health and medicine. Panel on cost Effectiveness in Health and Medicine. *Pharmacoeconomics*. 1997;11:159-168.

[16] Weinstein, M. C., Siegel, J. E., Garber, A. M., et al. Productivity costs, time costs and health-related quality of life: a response to the Erasmus Group. *Health Econ.* 1997;6:505-510.

[17] Russell, L. B., Gold, M. R., Siegel, J. E., Daniels, N., Weinstein, M. C. The role of cost-effectiveness analysis in health and medicine. Panel on Cost-Effectiveness in Health and Medicine. *JAMA: The Journal of the American Medical Association* 1996;276: 1172-1177.

[18] Weinstein, M. C., Siegel, J. E., Gold, M. R., Kamlet, M. S., Russell, L. B. Recommendations of the Panel on Cost-effectiveness in Health and Medicine. *JAMA: The Journal of the American Medical Association* 1996;276:1253-1258.

[19] Brouwer, W. B., Koopmanschap, M. A., Rutten, F. F. Productivity costs in cost-effectiveness analysis: numerator or denominator: a further discussion. *Health Econ.* 1997;6:511-514.

[20] Brouwer, W. B., Koopmanschap, M. A., Rutten, F. F. Productivity costs measurement through quality of life? A response to the recommendation of the Washington Panel." *Health Econ.* 1997;6:253-259.

[21] Owens, D. K. Interpretation of cost-effectiveness analyses. *J. Gen. Intern. Med.* 1998;13: 716-717.

[22] WHO. *Investing in Health Research and Development: Report of the Ad Hoc Committee on Health Research Relating to Future Intervention Options.* 1996, WHO, Geneva, CH

[23] World Bank. *World Development Report 1993.* New York NY, US: Oxford University Press, 1993.

[24] Jefferson, T., Demicheli, W. H. O., Mugford. *Elementary Economic Evaluation in Health Care.* London, UK, BMJ Publishing Group, 1996.

[25] Barton, G. R., Briggs, A. H., Fenwick, E. A. L. Optimal Cost-Effectiveness Decisions: the Role of the Cost-effectiveness Acceptability Curve (CEAC), the Cost-effectiveness Fronties (CEAF), and the Expected value of Perfect Information (EVPI). *Value in Health* 2008;11:886-897

[26] Boersma, C., Broere, A., Postma, M. J. Quantification of the Potential Impact of Cost-effectiveness Thresholds on Dutch Drug Expenditures Using Retrospective Analysis. *Value in Health* 2010;13:853-856

[27] Knies, S., Ament, A. J. H. A., Evers, S. M. A. A., Severens, J. L. The transferability of economic evaluations. *Value in Health* 2009;12:730-738

[28] Welte, R., Feenstra, F., Jager, H., Leidl, R. A decision chart for assessing and improving the transferability of economic evaluation results between countries. *Pharmacoeconomics* 2004;22:857-876

[29] Hoomans, T., van der Roer, N., Severens, J. L., Delwel, G. O. Cost-effectiveness of new drugs impacts reimbursement decision making but room for improvement. *Ned Tijdschr Geneeskd.* 2010;154:A958

[30] Claxton, K. The irrelevance of inference: a decision-making approach to the stochastic evaluation of health care technologies. *J. Health Econ.* 1999;18:341-364.

[31] Claxton, K. Bayesian approaches to the value of information: implications for the regulation of new pharmaceuticals. *Health Econ.* 1999;8:269-274.

[32] Barton, G. R., Briggs, A. H., Fenwick, E. A. Optimal Cost-Effectiveness Decisions: The Role of the Cost-Effectiveness Acceptability Curve (CEAC), the Cost-

Effectiveness Acceptability Frontier (CEAF), and the Expected Value of Perfection Information (EVPI). *Value Health* 2008; 11:886-897. (Epub. 2008 May 16).

[33] Fieller, E. C. Some problems in interval estimation. *J. R Stat. Soc. Ser. B.* 1954;16:175-183.

[34] Briggs, A. H., O'Brien, B. J., Blackhouse, G. THINKING OUTSIDE THE BOX: Recent Advances in the Analysis and Presentation of Uncertainty in Cost-Effectiveness Studies. *Annu. Rev. Public Health* 2002; 23:377-401.

[35] Van Hulst, M., Bilgin, Y. M., van de Watering, L. M., et al. Cost-effectiveness of leucocyte-depleted erythrocyte transfusion in cardiac valve surgery. *Transfus. Med.* 2005;15:209-217

[36] Hoch, J. S., Briggs, A. H., Willan, A. R. Something old, something new, something borrowed, something blue: a framework for the marriage of health econometrics and cost-effectiveness analysis. *Health Econ.* 2002; 11:415-430.

[37] Ramsey, S., Willke, R., Briggs, A., et al. Good research practices for cost-effectiveness analysis alongside clinical trials: the ISPOR RCT-CEA Task Force report. *Value. Health* 2005; 8:521-633.

[38] Gold, M. R., Siegel, J. E., Russel, L. B., Weinstein, M. C. *Cost-Effectiveness in Health and Medicine.* 1996. New York, NY, US: Oxford University Press

[39] Van Hout, B. A., Al, M. J., Gordon, G. S., Rutten, F. F. Costs, effects and C/E-ratios alongside a clinical trial. *Health Econ.* 1994;3:309-319.

[40] Groot Koerkamp, B., Hunink, M. G., Stijnen, T., Hammitt, J. K., Kuntz, K. M., Weinstein, M. C. Limitations of acceptability curves for presenting uncertainty in cost-effectiveness analysis. *Med. Decis. Making* 2007;27:101-111.

[41] Fenwick, E., Briggs, A. Cost-effectiveness acceptability curves in the dock: case not proven? *Med. Decis. Making* 2007;27:93-95.

[42] Briggs, A. H., Goeree, R., Blackhouse, G., O'Brien, B. J. Probabilistic analysis of cost-effectiveness models: choosing between treatment strategies for gastroesophageal reflux disease. *Med. Decis. Making* 2002; 22:290-308.

[43] Fenwick, E., O'Brien, B. J., Briggs, A. Cost-effectiveness acceptability curves--facts, fallacies and frequently asked questions. *Health Econ.* 2004;13:405-415.

[44] O'Hagan, A., McCabe, C., Akehurst, R., et al. Incorporation of uncertainty in health economic modelling studies. *Pharmacoeconomics.* 2005;23:529-536.

[45] Glynn, S. A., Briggs, A. H., Polsky, D. Quantifying stochastic uncertainty and presenting results of cost-effectiveness analyses. *Expert Rev. Pharmacoeconomics Outcomes Res.* 2001;1:89-100.

[46] Briggs, A. H., Wonderling, D. E., Mooney, C. Z. Pulling cost-effectiveness analysis up by its bootstraps: a non- parametric approach to confidence interval estimation. *Health Econ.* 1997;6:327-340.

[47] Koerkamp, B. G., Hunink, M. G., Stijnen, T., Weinstein, M. C. Identifying key parameters in cost-effectiveness analysis using value of information: a comparison of methods. *Health Econ.* 2006;15:383-392.

[48] Roberts, M., Russell, L. B., Paltiel, A. D., Chambers, M., McEwan, P., Krahn, M., On Behalf of the ISPOR-SMDM Modeling Good Research Practices Task Force. Conceptualizing a Model: A Report of the ISPOR-SMDM Modeling Good Research Practices Task Force-2. *Med. Decis. Making.* 2012;32:678-689.

[49] Dutch Council for Public Health and Health Care. *Fair and Sustainable Care.* 2007. Sdu, The Hague, NL

[50] Custer, B. S. Good evidence begets good policy: or so it should be. *Transfusion* 2012; 52:463-465.

[51] Finucane, M. L., Slovic, P., Mertz, C. K. Public perception of the risk of blood transfusion. *Transfusion* 2000;40:1017-1022.

[52] Lee, D. Perception of Blood Transfusion Risk. *Transf. Med. Reviews* 2006; 20:141-148.

[53] Derckx, V. L. Een bloedserieus dilemma: optimale versus maximale veiligheid van de bloedvoorziening. *Tijdschrift voor Gezondheidsrecht* 2001;25:502-516.

[54] Leach Bennett, J., Blajchman, M. A., Delage, G., Fearon, M., Devine, D. Proceedings of a consensus conference: Risk-Based Decision Making for Blood Safety. *Transfus. Med. Rev.* 2011;25:267-292.

[55] Van Asselt, M. B. A. *Risk Governance: Over Omgaan Met Onzekerheid En Mogelijke Toekomsten.* 2007 Maastricht, NL.

[56] De Hollander, A. E. M., Hanemaaijer, A. H. *Coping Rationally With Risks.* 2003, RIVM, Bilthoven, NL

[57] Dutch Health Council. *Leukodepletion of Blood Products.* 2000. Health Council, The Hague, NL

[58] Kleinman, S. H., Busch, M. P. Assessing the impact of HBV NAT on window period reduction and residual risk. *J. Clin. Virol.* 2006;36 Suppl. 1:S23-S29.

[59] Custer, B., Chinn, A., Hirschler, N. V., Busch, M. P., Murphy, E. L. The consequences of temporary deferral on future whole blood donation. *Transfusion* 2007;47:1514-1523.

[60] Jackson, B. R., Busch, M. P., Stramer, S. L., AuBuchon, J. P. The cost-effectiveness of NAT for HIV, HCV, and HBV in whole-blood donations. *Transfusion* 2003;43:721-729.

[61] Marshall, D. A., Kleinman, S. H., Wong, J. B., et al. Cost-effectiveness of nucleic acid test screening of volunteer blood donations for hepatitis B, hepatitis C and human immunodeficiency virus in the United States. *Vox Sang.* 2004;86:28-40.

[62] Postma, M. J., van Hulst, M., De Wolf, J. T. M., Botteman, M., Staginnus, U. Cost-effectiveness of pathogen inactivation for platelet transfusions in the Netherlands. *Transfus. Med.* 2005;15:379-387.

[63] Janssen, M. P., van der Poel, C. L., Buskens, E., Bonneux, L., Bonsel, G. J., van Hout, B. A. Costs and benefits of bacterial culturing and pathogen reduction in the Netherlands. *Transfusion.* 2006;46:956-965.

[64] Custer, B., Agapova, M., Martinez, R. H. The cost-effectiveness of pathogen reduction technology as assessed using a multiple risk reduction model. *Transfusion.* 2010;50:2461-2473.

[65] Dutch Health Council. *Pathogen Reduction in Blood Products.* 2003. Health Council, The Hague, NL

[66] Hermann and Buijs. Motie om de verwijdering van witte bloedcellen uit transfusiebloed in te voeren. 27401 36. 2000. Accessible by: *http//:zoek. officielebekendmakingen.nl/h-tk-20002001-3717-3717-1.html*

[67] Vaststelling van de begroting van de uitgaven en de ontvangsten van het Ministerie van Volksgezondheid, Welzijn en Sport (XVI) voor het jaar 2001; Brief minister met standpunt inzake advies 'Variant van de ziekte van Creutzfeldt-Jakob en

bloedtransfusie' (Gezondheidsraad). 27400 XVI 83. 2001. Accessible by: *http//:zoek.officielebekendmakingen.nl/ kst-27400-XVI-83.html*

[68] Vamvakas, E. C., Blajchman, M. A. Transfusion-related immunomodulation (TRIM): an update. *Blood Rev.* 2007;21:327-348.

[69] Cobain, T. J., Vamvakas, E. C., Wells, A., Titlestad, K. A survey of the demographics of blood use. *Transfus. Med.* 2007;17:1-15.

[70] Grandjean, P. Implications of the precautionary principle for primary prevention and research. *Annu. Rev. Public Health* 2004;25:199-223.

[71] Peterson, M. The precautionary principle should not be used as a basis for decision-making. Talking Point on the precautionary principle. *EMBO reports* 2007;8:305-308.

[72] Grandjean, P. Seven deadly sins of environmental epidemiology and the virtues of precaution. *Epidemiology* 2008;19:158-162.

[73] Shander, A., Hofmann, A., Gombotz, H., Theusinger, O. M., Spahn, D. R. Estimating the cost of blood: past, present, and future directions. *Best. Pract. Res. Clin. Anaesthesiol.* 2007;21:271-289.

[74] Fergusson, D., van Walraven, C., Coyle, D., Laupacis, A. Technologies to minimize blood transfusion in cardiac and orthopedic surgery. Results of a practice variation survey in nine countries. International Study of Peri-operative Transfusion (ISPOT) Investigators. *Int. J. Technol. Assess Health Care* 1999;15:717-728.

[75] Eindhoven, G. B., Diercks, R. L., Richardson, F. J., et al. Adjusted transfusion triggers improve transfusion practice in orthopaedic surgery. *Transfus. Med.* 2005;15:13-18.

[76] Hebert, P. C., Wells, G., Blajchman, M. A., et al. A multicenter, randomized, controlled clinical trial of transfusion requirements in critical care. Transfusion Requirements in Critical Care Investigators, Canadian Critical Care Trials Group. *N Engl. J. Med.* 1999; 340:409-417.

[77] Anonymous. *Clinical Guideline Blood Transfusion.* 2011,The Dutch Institute for Healthcare Improvement (CBO). Utrecht, NL

[78] Sanquin Blood Supply Foundation. *Sanquin Annual Report 2006.* 2007, Sanquin Blood Supply Foundation Amsterdam, NL

[79] Sorensen, B. S., Johnsen, S. P., Jorgensen, J. Complications related to blood donation: a population-based study. *Vox Sang.* 2008;94:132-137.

[80] *The Clinical Use of Blood. Handbook* 2002, WHO Geneva, CH.

[81] Friele, D., Dute, J. C. J., Coppen, R., Volkers, A. C. *Tweede Evaluatie Wet Inzake Bloedvoorziening.* 2008, ZonMW, Den Haag, NL.

[82] Van Hulst, M., Dhingra-Kumar, N., Smit Sibinga, C. Th, Postma, M. J. Cost-effectiveness of interventions ensuring blood transfusion safety in Africa *Transfusion.* 2006;46 Supplement:169A-169A.

[83] Van Hulst, M., Dhingra-Kumar, N., Smit Sibinga, C. Th, Postma, M. J. Cost-effectiveness of interventions ensuring blood transfusion safety in Africa. *Vox Sang.* 2006; 91 Supplement 3:300-301.

[84] Moore, A., Herrera, G., Nyamongo, J., et al. Estimated risk of HIV transmission by blood transfusion in Kenya. *Lancet.* 2001;358:657-660.

[85] Foster, S., Buve, A. Benefits of HIV screening of blood transfusions in Zambia. *Lancet* 1995;346:225-227.

[86] Ouattara, H., Siransy-Bogui, L., Fretz, C., et al. Residual risk of HIV, HVB and HCV transmission by blood transfusion between 2002 and 2004 at the Abidjan National Blood Transfusion Center. *Transfus. Clin. Biol.* 2006;13:242-245.

[87] Bates, I., Manyasi, G., Medina, L. A. Reducing replacement donors in Sub-Saharan Africa: challenges and affordability. *Transfus. Med.* 2007; 17:434-442.

[88] Van Hulst, M., Owutsu-Ofori, S., Sarkodie, F., et al. Cost-effectiveness of pre-donation screening blood donors with rapid tests and subsequent nucleic acid amplification testing of blood donations in a resource-poor setting. *Vox Sang.* 2006;95 Supplement 1:261.

[89] Busch, M. P., Watanabe, K. K., Smith, J. W., Hermansen, S. W., Thomson, R. A. False-negative testing errors in routine viral marker screening of blood donors. For the Retrovirus Epidemiology Donor Study. *Transfusion* 2000;40:585-589.

[90] Van Hoogstraten, M. J., Consten, E. C., Henny, C. P., Heij, H. A., van Lanschot, J. J. Are there simple measures to reduce the risk of HIV infection through blood transfusion in a Zambian district hospital? *Trop. Med. Int. Health* 2000;5:668-673.

[91] Van der Schaaf, I. P., van Hulst, M., van der Tuuk Adriani, W. P. A., Postma, M. J., Smit Sibinga, C. Th. Safety of the blood supply: an attempt to predict the value of the current infection marker screening in an African country. In: vqan Hulst, M., editor *Health Economics of Blood Transfusion Safety.* Academic Thesis University of Groningen, 2008. Buijten en Schipperheijn Amsterdam, NL

[92] WHO. *Global Database on Blood Safety; Report 2001-2002.* 2004 World Health Organization, Geneva, CH.

[93] Dutch Health Council. *Should Blood Donors Be Tested for Variant Creutzfeldt-Jakob Disease?* 2006, Health Council, The Hague, NL.

[94] Custer, B., Johnson, E. S., Sullivan, S. D., et al. Quantifying losses to the donated blood supply due to donor deferral and miscollection. *Transfusion* 2004;44:1417-1426.

[95] Custer, B., Tomasulo, P. A., Murphy, E. L., et al. Triggers for switching from minipool testing by nucleic acid technology to individual-donation nucleic acid testing for West Nile virus: analysis of 2003 data to inform 2004 decision making. *Transfusion* 2004;44:1547-1554.

[96] Alter, H. J. Pathogen reduction: a precautionary principle paradigm. *Transfus. Med. Rev.* 2008;22:97-102.

[97] Kocian, R., Spahn, D. R. Haemoglobin, oxygen carriers and perioperative organ perfusion. *Best Pract. Res. Clin. Anaesthesiol.* 2008; 22:63-80.

[98] *Patient dies after wrong blood transfusion* (In Dutch). 2008, NRC Handelsblad, Rotterdam, NL.

[99] Williamson, L. M., Lowe, S., Love, E. M., et al. Serious hazards of transfusion (SHOT) initiative: analysis of the first two annual reports. *BMJ* 1999;319:16-19.

[100] TRIP Foundation. *Transfusion Reactions In Patients, Annual Report 2006.* 2007 TRIP Foundation, Den Haag, NL.

[101] AuBuchon, J. P., Littenberg, B. A cost-effectiveness analysis of the use of a mechanical barrier system to reduce the risk of mistransfusion. *Transfusion* 1996;36: 222-226.

[102] Davies, A., Staves, J., Kay, J., Casbard, A., Murphy, M. F. End-to-end electronic control of Eddy the hospital transfusion process to increase the safety of blood transfusion: strengths and weaknesses. *Transfusion* 2006;46:352-364.

Websites

[101] www.ispor.org
[102] www.cvz.nl: HPV-vaccine, rotavirus vaccine, ivabradine, oseltamivir, baraclude and rasagiline may serve as just some examples
[103] www.gr.nl
[104] www.EUnetHTA.eu

ISPOR-SMDM Best Practice Guidelines

[201] Hollingworth, W., Caro, J. J., Tsevat, J., McDonald, K. M., Wong, J. B.; ISPOR–SMDM Modeling Good Research Practices Task Force. Model Transparency and Validation: A Report of the ISPOR-SMDM Modeling Good Research Practices Task Force-7. *Value Health.* 2012;15:843-850. doi: 10.1016/j.jval.2012.04.012.

[202] Briggs, A. H., Weinstein, M. C., Fenwick, E. A., Karnon, J., Sculpher, M. J., Paltiel, A. D. ISPOR-SMDM Modeling Good Research Practices Task Force. Model Parameter Estimation and Uncertainty: A Report of the ISPOR-SMDM Modeling Good Research Practices Task Force-6. *Value Health.* 2012;15:835-842.

[203] Pitman, R., Fisman, D., Zaric, G. S., Postma, M., Kretzschmar, M., Edmunds, J., Brisson, M. ISPOR-SMDM Modeling Good Research Practices Task Force. Dynamic Transmission Modeling: A Report of the ISPOR-SMDM Modeling Good Research Practices Task Force-5. *Value Health.* 2012;15:828-834.

[204] Karnon, J., Stahl, J., Brennan, A., Caro, J. J., Mar, J., Möller, J. ISPOR-SMDM Modeling Good Research Practices Task Force. Modeling using Discrete Event Simulation: A Report of the ISPOR-SMDM Modeling Good Research Practices Task Force-4. *Value Health.* 2012;15:821-827.

[205] Siebert, U., Alagoz, O., Bayoumi, A. M., Jahn, B., Owens, D. K., Cohen, D. J., Kuntz, K. M. ISPOR-SMDM Modeling Good Research Practices Task Force. State-Transition Modeling: A Report of the ISPOR-SMDM Modeling Good Research Practices Task Force-3. *Value Health.* 2012; 15:812-820.

[206] Roberts, M., Russell, L. B., Paltiel, D., Chambers, M., McEwan, P., Krahn, M. ISPOR-SMDM Modeling Good Research Practices Task Force. Conceptualizing a Model: A Report of the ISPOR-SMDM Modeling Good Research Practices Task Force-2. *Value Health.* 2012; 15:804-811.

[207] Caro, J. J., Briggs, A. H., Siebert, U., Kuntz, K. M. ISPOR-SMDM Modeling Good Research Practices Task Force. Modeling Good Research Practices-Overview: A Report of the ISPOR-SMDM Modeling Good Research Practices Task Force-1. *Value Health.* 2012;15:796-803.

In: Quality Management in Transfusion Medicine   ISBN: 978-1-62618-665-1
Editor: Cees Th. Smit Sibinga   © 2013 Nova Science Publishers, Inc.

Chapter XIII

Knowledge Management and Blood Transfusion

René J. Jorna[1,] and Niels R. Faber[2,†]*

[1]Professor of Knowledge Management and Cognition
Fryske Akademy, Leeuwarden, The Netherlands. Faculty
of Economics, Business/Behavioural and Social Sciences;
University of Groningen Groningen, The Netherlands
[2]Saxion University of Applied Sciences,
Deventer, The Netherlands

Abstract

Knowledge Management (KM) mainly is about organizstional issues. It concerns secondary processes or tasks in an organisation, not in the first place primary processes or tasks. When we look at blood transfusion medicine, much knowledge in terms of content is not useful. Chemical, physiological or medical analyses focus on the content of blood and blood products. The advantage of knowledge content and knowledge management is primarily based on managerial issues and possibilities. In combination with databases, management information systems and knowledge systems improvement of these secondary processes can easily be realized. In this contribution we start with the various usages of data, information and knowledge, which we discuss for two developed and three under-developed countries. In using criteria of the role of the government, the payment to donors, the use and existence of ICT and the application of organisational forms, we compare the countries with one another and make some general remarks about the use and advantage of knowledge management.

---

* René J. Jorna, PhD: Professor of Knowledge Management and Cognition, Fryske Akademy, P.O. Box 54, 8900 AB Leeuwarden, NL. Tel: +31-58-2343026. Faculty of Economics, Business/Behavioural and Social Sciences; University of Groningen, P.O. Box 800, 9700 AV Groningen, NL. Tel:+31-50-3633625/7020; E-mail: r.j.j.m.jorna@rug.nl.
† Niels R. Faber, PhD: Saxion University of Applied Sciences, P.O. Box 501, 7400 AM Deventer, The Netherlands. Tel: +31-6-1089.5520; E-mail: n.r.faber@gmail.com.

Keywords: Knowledge technology, primary and secondary processes, organisational forms, databases (or DBMS), conservation and storage of blood

1. Introduction

In all countries over the world with a reasonably developed or even underdeveloped medical system, blood transfusion is relevant. Blood transfusion connects donors with recipients. In giving blood and in receiving blood, besides medical and chemical issues, organisational and managerial structures are more strongly discussed. One of the increasing organisational debates is about how to deal with knowledge and information, whether in behavior or digitally of individuals and of collectives.

In its basic structure a donor gives blood that can be used by a patient or recipient. Although simple, as soon as the donor and the recipient are not in the same place at the same time, all kinds of areas of complication arise. We mention six of them: the organisation(s), medical and chemical issues, storage(s), knowledge and informational issues, developed and underdeveloped countries and systems, and transportation and conservation of blood. We explain and illustrate the six complications, below. However, we first start with the processes and elements of the blood transfusion system (Figure 1).

The processes in blood transfusion, taking apart the really rare situation that donor and recipient are at the same place and the same time and even more rare have the same type of blood group, includes chemical and medical analyses, transportation, storage, certification, preparation and pre-operation treatment. In medical as well as in organisational fields knowledge is becoming increasingly essential. The blood of donors consists of blood itself and of the substance realized by the process of plasma- phaeresis.

Both methods have their pros and cons in terms of speed, transportation and storage. One should know that no more than 150 years ago blood type analyses and many chemical procedures were not available and not even discovered or detected. In explaining the history of blood types from Vesalius (15th century) to Landsteiner (19th century), we refer to a different chapter.

Looking at the blood donor and the blood recipient in both cases, it is a human individual and not an organisation that is the focus. Blood donors are usually not organized and neither are blood recipients. The whole process for the blood donor is structured in a private hospital or community setting, sometimes guided by the Red Cross or the Red Crescent. For recipients it is normally structured in a hospital. There is one other important organisation in this process and that is the Blood Bank, in the Netherlands Sanquin Blood Supply Foundation and in Belgium the Belgian Red Cross Society.

In these organisations blood and other preparations or components are analyzed and stored. Since the beginning of the 50s techniques became available to store blood for a longer period of time. Depending on the country, being a blood donor does usually not lead to a fee and neither does a blood recipient have to pay. The basic idea is that donation and reception of blood is free (Figure 1).

Medical and chemical analyses are normally done after the donation of blood is realized. Also before blood donation, a donor has to fill in a questionnaire and some small medical tests are submitted.

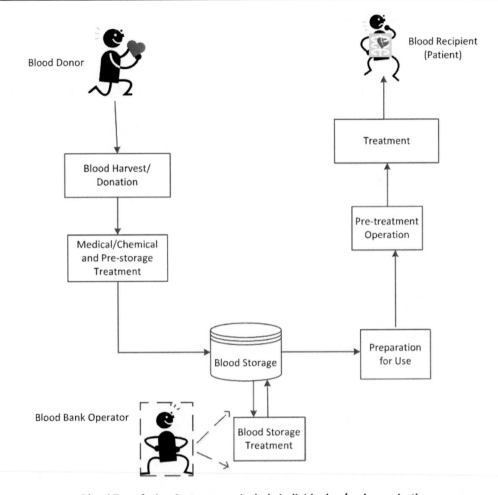

Blood Transfusion System: may include individual or/and organization

Figure 1. The vein-to-vein flow of blood transfusion.

A similar process, but in a different context, takes place in hospitals when recipients get blood. In principle, tests and analyses are open and transparent, in any case to the donor and to the patient.

The physical distance between donor and recipient was very important in the past. This has changed the last 25 years. When blood is well preserved and kept in cold places, transport is not an issue anymore. Chemical and physiological processes have improved in such a way that given standard conditions blood or its components can be sent all over the world.

Besides transportation and conservation, for various reasons storage of blood is still very important. Because it cannot be predicted how much of all blood groups and Rhesus factors have to present, blood establishments have to store conservative amounts of blood. The simplest situation is storing and preparing blood group O. This group can be used within limits for all other blood groups. On the other hand this is not ideal in terms of the Rhesus factor.

Concerning knowledge and information, in practice, the various types of knowledge are used in combinations. They depend on the domains and content of knowledge, on the tasks to be executed and on other people one with whom one cooperates. It neither is the case that someone's type of knowledge exclusively is sensory or coded or theoretical. They are always present together, but with different emphasis. Sometimes the mixture of coded and sensory is dominant, in other situations it is the combination of coded and theoretical. [1-4] We explain this in section 2 in detail.

The big issue in the donor and recipient processes is the differences in developed and underdeveloped countries and medical systems. Developed countries have working legal en financial systems. To a certain extent this is different in underdeveloped countries. It is not that in these countries crime and extreme corruption are the common procedures, but the medical field and the organisational structures are less developed, there. We will give examples of two developed and three underdeveloped countries to illustrate our points in section 3. In section 4 we discuss ICT, information, and Knowledge Management (KM) for Transfusion Medicine (TM). In section 5 we focus on the future and some recommendations for TM.

2. Knowledge Management and Its Relation with Blood Transfusion

When addressing the topic of knowledge management, one important barrier needs to be overcome. Namely, taking a stance amidst the various interpretations that exist in the knowledge management realm. The reason behind the existence of various interpretations is a historical one. McElroy [5] indicates that the knowledge management discipline grew from two distinct roots, during differing periods in time. The first and earliest root of knowledge management emerged from the field of information and communication technology. This root does not distinguish between knowledge and information. In fact, the information technological perspective views knowledge and information to be similar, and information technology suitable to process it. An important presupposition of this perspective is the notion that all knowledge already exists; the only task for knowledge management is to ensure that knowledge is available at the right person, at the right time, and in the right quality. [6] The second root of knowledge management emerged in the 1990s from the field of organisational learning. This field emphasises the learning ability of organisations and people and recognizes the role humans play within. In the organisational learning perspective, humans are the carriers of knowledge at the individual, group, and organisational level. The organisational learning root of knowledge management links to the notion that it is humans who are managed. Humans are carriers of knowledge at the individual level. The group and organisation levels provide communication and co-ordination mechanisms along which individuals create and exchange knowledge and attune their activities. How functions of knowledge creation and exchange take place, and how activities are synchronized is described in various models of knowledge management and will be discussed in the remainder of this chapter (section 3).

In the next sub-section (2.1), we address knowledge management cycles, in which we explain how the two main processes of knowledge creation and knowledge exchange are formed. Next (2.2), we discuss various models of knowledge management, describing the main functional components of knowledge management. Finally, knowledge management strategies and metrics for knowledge management processes are addressed.

2.1. Knowledge Management Cycles

As the term indicates, the field of knowledge management concerns the management of knowledge. Although this seems trivial, a closer look reveals that understanding what knowledge management is, is not clear at all. In order to pinpoint what knowledge management is all about, we first need to understand what the term knowledge in this particular context means, and consequently that what is managed. The triplet data, information, and knowledge commonly is used to explain what knowledge is and how it can be distinguished from other, relating concepts. [6, 7] The concept of data pertains to observable signs or symbols. These signs and symbols directly relate to signals. When structured, data becomes information. Information enables answering of questions of 'what', 'who', 'when, 'where', and 'how'. In this sense, information resides at a higher level of aggregation and complexity than data. The third and final level of the triplet concerns knowledge. To information, knowledge adds meaning and interpretation. The knowledge level [see 8] enables to answer questions of 'why' things are as they are. In summary, in the context of knowledge management, the object that is managed is knowledge, or interpretations and meanings.

From the above description of knowledge as interpretation and attribution of meaning, the question arises, what thing is it that give interpretation or attributes meaning. Interpretation and the attribution of meaning are cognitive activities [9], implying the need of some cognitive architecture to execute these. From this stance, the processing of knowledge in terms of creation, sharing, storage, etc. is considered a human ability exclusively [see also 10]. Where the object that is managed in knowledge management concerns knowledge in terms of interpretations and meaning, individuals are the managed subjects. The objective of knowledge management in this regard is to ensure that individuals are able to perform the tasks for which they are responsible, in an organised and co-ordinated way.

A knowledge management cycle describes the main processes or functions of knowledge management in relation to the managed object knowledge. Various cycles have been recorded. Dalkir [7] provides an overview including cycles from Nickols [11], Wiig [12], McElroy [5], Bukowitz and Williams [13] and Meyer and Zack [14]. Although knowledge management cycles differ from each other in appearance, at least three main processes are present in all. These main processes of knowledge management are

(i) knowledge capture and creation,
(ii) knowledge sharing and dissemination, and
(iii) knowledge acquisition and application. [7 p. 43]

The process of knowledge capture and creation relates to the process of obtaining new knowledge. Both processes centre on an organisation that aims to obtain new knowledge. Knowledge capture concerns the obtaining of new knowledge from outside into the organisation. In contrast, knowledge creation concerns the generation of new knowledge from within the organisation.

Knowledge sharing and dissemination is the process of distributing the newly obtained knowledge within an organisation. Dalkir [7] indicates that the process of knowledge sharing and dissemination forms the first step in contextualizing knowledge. Newly obtained knowledge is adapted to the context in which it will be used. First, individuals within the organizstion who are in need of the new knowledge are selected. Second, the new knowledge is transformed such that it connects to the knowledge these individuals already possess.

The final process of acquisition and application also is the final step in contextualization of newly obtained knowledge. Knowledge acquisition relates to processes of learning new knowledge by individuals. During the learning process, individuals attempt to relate this new knowledge to the knowledge already residing in their minds. In knowledge application, knowledge that is acquired is put into practice. These processes comprise what Dalkir [7] labels the integrated knowledge management cycle. The cycle is integrated in the sense that all knowledge management functions identified in literature are capture in the three processes.

Contributing to the objective of ensuring that an organisation is able to function and hence the individuals within are able to execute their tasks, an implementation of knowledge management needs to incorporate all three main processes of creation, sharing, and application.

As indicated in the previous section, implementing knowledge management is not an easy undertaking. Various models of knowledge management have been conceptualized. In order to choose which model to apply. Insight into available models is a prerequisite. A selection of models is presented in the next section.

2.2. Models of Knowledge Management

Essentially, knowledge management models describe the way knowledge management can or should be arranged within an organisational context, in order to effectively manage knowledge within. Dalkir [7] provides a comprehensive overview of six different knowledge management models. Important dimensions underlying each of these models are

(i)   an epistemological dimension and
(ii) an ontological dimension.

The epistemological dimension concerns the conceptualisation of knowledge that is central in the knowledge model. Conceptualisations relate to the identified knowledge typology, and the lifecycle of knowledge. Knowledge and informational issues concern what people individually and in groups do and what kinds of information systems they use to be supported. Knowledge concerns content and types of knowledge. Content of knowledge is about domain and field and this content is expressed in a form or type. To formulate this explicitly, content and type of knowledge bring us directly to the expression of knowledge, which in many situations is language. Content of knowledge refers to domains, e.g., the construction of houses, physics, the working of computers or health care. In the case of blood medical and chemical content and theory have to be used and if necessary further developed. Most tests are more or less standard, but in the 80s in the last century a disease later labeled as HIV asked for new tests and much medical new research including new theory. One should understand that concerning content knowledge of the primary processes (all aspects of blood) is as important as the secondary processes of and in the organisation).

Knowledge according to type is the denomination of how this knowledge content is presented. The various aspects of knowledge make it almost impossible to define types of knowledge unambiguously. Based on the work of Boisot [3], we developed three (semiotically inspired) types of knowledge:

a) Sensory or tacit,
b) (en)Coded, and
c) Theoretical (or tacit) knowledge. [8]

The first type concerns sensory (or tacit) knowledge or just behavior. It starts from a perception of difference. The situation is well known: when you eat a fruit you never ate before, your reaction to the new taste will be something like: "*Well, it reminds me of ...*" and you name a fruit you know. Essential is to recognize the situation in terms of a situation you already know. It should be clear that the bigger the sensory 'problem' is, the more difficult to find an analogy. We believe that sensitiveness in sensory knowledge is often underestimated but of the utmost importance. We hypothesize that creative people also are the ones with a big talent for expressing sensory knowledge. The sensory - or as some would call it the tacit - perspective underlies what Michael Polanyi has coined 'personal knowledge'. [2, p11] He described the process involved in this knowledge type as being "aware of that from which we are attending to another thing, in the appearance of that thing". Sensory knowledge is bodily knowledge: "*when we make a thing function as the proximal term of tacit knowing, we incorporate it in our body - or extend our body to include it - so that we come to dwell in it*". Boisot identifies this knowledge as the domain of the 'ineffable'. [3, p62] It cannot be coded, it is about concrete experiences, and it can be shared only with those who are physically co-present. Quantification of sensory knowledge is possible through looking at details. The more detailed a sensory experience is, the richer it is. Knowledge of details is relative to domains. A professional will be able to perceive more when looking at a certain activity than an amateur will. Sensory knowledge can therefore mostly be measured through the analysis of behavior.

The second type, (en)coded knowledge, materializes when signs become codes. Certain aspects of remembered situations (visual, acoustic and tactile forms) evoke these situations. For example, concrete cows are replaced (represented) by the sound 'cow' and the category of 'cow' emerges. With the sign, codes emerge - a code being nothing else than a convention establishing a relation of substitution. The sign enables communication and makes communication easier and more efficient. The diffusion of knowledge becomes easier where signs (codes) are available. [3] Externalization requires coding. In terms of Boisot [3]: diffusion of the sign now takes place along the lines of a social community. Co-workers or partners do not have to be co-present. It is therefore extremely unlikely that coded knowledge is dominant in the early phases of innovation. Codes can be quantified by taking into account the number of elements and the combination rules a code consists of. Musical notation systems are more strongly coded (allow less ambiguity) than natural languages. Therefore, in the use of images and metaphors, coded knowledge comes closest to the non-coded sensory knowledge. More details on the weakness or strength of signs (codes) can be found in Goodman [15], who uses five syntactic and semantic requirements to distinguish weaker from stronger sets of signs [see 10 and 16].

A third kind of knowledge type emerges when a third aspect is added to the aspects of sensory difference and codification (substitution), that of structure or pattern. It arises when coded signs relate to the events represented, not based on a convention, but based on patterned or structural qualities. We then have theoretical knowledge. Scientific, ideological and religious knowledge are of this type. Can one be creative in this phase? Certainly one can learn. However, no longer is knowledge acquired through searching for perceptual analogies or categorizing. Knowledge is now the result of (scientific) inquiry - empirical as well as theoretical. This means that innovation, here, is much more difficult, because an enormous accumulation of past knowledge has to be re-interpreted. An attempt to quantify theoretical knowledge is to describe this type in terms of 'why' or 'because' chains. The longer the chain, the more abstract theoretical knowledge. Therefore, we believe that knowledge creation and therefore innovation at the start is more sensory than theoretical. One should note that not only scientific knowledge is theoretical. Ideologies or religions also provide complex 'why' chains and therefore are theoretical too.

Besides the three types mentioned, another common knowledge typology is that of tacit and explicit knowledge. [2] Tacit knowledge concerns that knowledge that is expressed through behaviour. This type of knowledge cannot easily be explained in words, but only shared by showing and observing. Explicit knowledge in contrast is easily explained in words and can be expressed verbally, written down on paper or be digitized. In practice the various types of knowledge are used in combinations. They depend on the domains and content, on the tasks to be executed and on other people one works together with. It neither is the case that one's knowledge only is sensory or coded or theoretical. They are always present together, but with different emphases. Sometimes the mixture of coded and sensory is dominant, in other situations it is the combination of coded and theoretical.

Other knowledge typologies exist, distinguishing types based on e.g., their level of detail, their level of diffusion within a group, or based on that what it expresses (e.g., procedural versus factual knowledge). Concerning the lifecycle of knowledge in particular the way knowledge is created and stored forms the centre of the knowledge model. For instance, the model by von Krogh and Roos [see 7, p50] takes a connectionist approach regarding the knowledge lifecycle. This approach upholds the notion that knowledge is created in interactions between individuals. The connectionist perspective contrasts to the cognitive perspective, which explains knowledge creation through the manipulations of mental representations within the human mind.

In contrast with the epistemological dimension, the ontological dimension distinguishes between at least two levels of aggregation, namely the level of the individual and the level of the collective. Concerning the level of the collective, a refinement into group and organisation is justified. The distinction lies in the level of formalisation of interactions between members. A group concerns any bunch of individuals who interact and communicate. When interactions and communications of a group take place in a co-ordinated fashion, the group becomes an organisation.

Both dimensions of epistemology and ontology are addressed in the models discussed by Dalkir [7]. Briefly we address three of the recently presented models, namely the models by van Krogh et al. [17], von Krogh and Roos [18], Nonaka and Takeuchi's SECI model [19], and Boisot's I-Space model. [3] The von Krogh and Roos model takes a connectionist approach towards knowledge. [18] It does not adopt a specific knowledge typology. Subsequently, in their model knowledge creation starts with the individual, requiring mechanisms to be in place that stimulate individuals into knowledge creation. Also, group level mechanisms are required in order to realise knowledge sharing throughout the organisation. In the model by Nonaka and Takeuchi [19], a similar approach is presented.

However, their model adopts the tacit/explicit typology of knowledge. They explain knowledge creation also to start from the individual in a tacit form. Through a series of operations tacit knowledge is shared between individuals (socialization), made explicit (externalization), combined with already existing, explicit knowledge (combination), and connected to individuals' tacit knowledge (internalization) [for more details see 19]. Boisot's I-Space model of knowledge management also adopts the ontological distinction between individual and group/organisational levels. In the I-Space the ontological dimension is labeled un-diffused (individual level) and diffused (group/organisational level). Epistemologically, the I-Space model distinguishes between the level of detail of knowledge, and the extent to which knowledge is (en)codified. The latter resembles the distinction between tacit and explicit knowledge, in which tacit equals uncodified and explicit equals (en)codified knowledge. Similar to Nonaka and Takeuchi, does Boisot recognise a process of development of knowledge through the various types and ontological levels. Again knowledge is created at the individual level, a process that is recognized as scanning. This knowledge is concrete and highly uncodified. At the individual level, knowledge simultaneously becomes more (en)codified through codification, and more abstract through abstraction (i.e., decontextualized and applicable to more situations). When a certain level of abstraction and codification is reached, the process of diffusion ensures that knowledge is shared with individuals within the group or organisation. These individuals subsequently absorb the new knowledge, which transforms the (en)codified into uncodified knowledge again. The final process involves the conversion of abstract into concrete knowledge (impacting). This final step ensures that multiple individuals within the group or organisation are able to apply the new knowledge in their practice.

A more recent insight in the field of knowledge management is that knowledge management should be seen as a process of supporting or enabling knowledge processing. This position contrasts to a perspective of knowledge management that influences knowledge directly. The newer perspective on knowledge management is shared by among others McElroy [5] and von Krogh and Roos [18], and von Krogh, Ichijo, and Nonaka [19]. McElroy [5] explicitly uses the term knowledge processing, as the system that is controlled by knowledge management activities. Knowledge processing involves the main processes of knowledge capture and creation, knowledge sharing and dissemination, and knowledge acquisition and application. Von Krogh, et al. [17] utilise the term knowledge enabling as replacement of the term knowledge management, to express the notion that knowledge management is more about enabling and supporting than about traditional forms of management. Regardless of the epistemological perspective that is adopted in a knowledge management model, this recent insight is of relevance. Changing knowledge directly or neurologically remains impossible thus far.

A knowledge management perspective on blood transfusion medicine shows interesting differences relating to knowledge content and type in the distinct process steps (see Figure 1). For instance, knowledge about blood type and rhesus factors is of importance during all stages of the process. However, this importance has different connotations to the actors involved. For instance, the blood donor only needs to report his/her blood type (if known). The nurse who receives the blood needs to make sure that the blood sample is correctly registered. During storage, knowledge about the blood type is important to make sure blood in stock is stored in complete separation from other types, and cross-contamination risks are removed. The actor transporting the blood between the various parts of the blood transfusion system is only concerned with maintaining proper conditions for transport. This person or organisation generally is unaware of the particularities of blood in transit. In the last stage of the blood transfusion process, in which the recipient is administered as donor blood, knowledge about the specific blood type of patient and the type of donor blood is crucial. Not only in order to make sure the proper type of blood is administered. Also, the nurse administering the donor blood needs to be able to recognise events during the administering of the blood in case mistakes have been made. The sketched situation in which different actors within the process of blood transfusion all possess different knowledge regarding the main topic, i.e. blood is not unique. A similar fragmentation of knowledge has been reported by Faber, Peters, and Jorna [20] in the paper industry, and by Peters [21] regarding a common thing asweather. The latter context illustrates our point nicely. To the layman weather consists of temperature (cold or warm) and precipitation (dry or wet). To sailors, wind and clouds carrying rain play an important factor in their perspective on the weather. Finally, the meteorologist probably has the most elaborate view on the weather, including atmospheric pressure, wind movements at different heights, etc. The notion that one domain has different meanings and hence involves different knowledge about it, is identified as knowledge crossover. [19]

Relating to the type of knowledge, also differences exist in the various stages of the blood transfusion process. Both the nurse responsible for collecting the blood and responsible to administering the blood heavily rely on sensory or tacit knowledge. Their task to collect blood from the blood donor or provide it to the blood recipient involves connecting a person to respectively the collection bag or the donor bag demands a well-trained skill. Such skill typically relies on sensory knowledge; it relies on motor abilities that are well trained, combined with deliberate behaviour. In order to perform their tasks properly, involved nurses need to be able to insert a needle into the donor or recipient's vein with a steady hand and without hesitation. Otherwise, complications during the collection or provisioning of blood may occur. Although sensory knowledge is their dominant knowledge type, nurses require some theoretical knowledge concerning the human body, for they need to be able to adequately respond to unanticipated events during treatment. In contrast to the sensory knowledge needed by nurses, the storage facility operator of the blood relies strongly on coded knowledge. The task of the storage facility operator is dictated by the mechanistic nature of the machines comprising the storage facility. In this sense, the task of the storage facility operator is much more formalized i.e., coded than the nurses' tasks described before. Using the information that accompanies a blood sample received from the donor, the storage facility operator is able to store this in the proper way. Next to coded knowledge, the storage facility operator needs a good deal of theoretical knowledge about behaviour of blood. For instance, the operator needs to know how long blood can be kept in store, or what happens in case of failures in the storage facility. Sensory knowledge is practically absent with storage facility operators. Similar to the fragmentation of knowledge throughout the process of the blood transfusion system, the spread of knowledge types over the actors performing different tasks varies between them.

Depending on the task, the actors rely more on sensory knowledge (i.e., those tasks that involve human-human interactions) or on coded and theoretical knowledge (i.e., those tasks in which machines have a leading part). Hence, depending on the nature of the task, and the way the task is organized, a specific knowledge type becomes dominant. Also in the blood transfusion system this dominance is observable and needs to be taken into consideration when developing, maintaining, or changing the system.

3. Characteristics in Organising Blood Transfusion: Cases in 5 Different Countries

In this section we generally describe a number of characteristics in 5 countries: 2 from developed and 3 from underdeveloped countries. The characteristics are

a) government or private;
b) working with a fee or for free; (fee means that the donor is paid, receives money)
c) the way blood is stored and transported;
d) the requirements and ways to do medical and chemical analyses;
e) Databases (DB), Management Information Systems (MIS)and Knowledge Systems (KS);
f) organisational forms and coordination mechanisms.

We begin with the 3 underdeveloped countries.

Case 1

A NIS (New Independent State) country in Central Asia (Kazakhstan), belonging to the high HDI group (HDI Human Development Index: 0.745), became independent in 1991 as a Republic. The social structure is based on the former Soviet Union society arrangement – education, health care, etc. Despite the high HDI ranking there is still a considerable poverty among the population. In 2006 the country experienced an HIV/AIDS outbreak through infected blood that was transfused. The health care structure was fragmented and far from up to date as was the blood supply - almost 100% family/replacement and paid donors, poor facilities and old fashioned equipment and testing methodologies and technologies, underdeveloped human capacity and largely the whole blood transfusion taking place in hospitals. Prevalence for virus markers of blood transmissible diseases (hepatitis B and C, and HIV/AIDS) were found considerable.

The World Bank initiated a comparative national assessment in four of the Central Asian Republics and reported on this in May 2008. The report stresses that the factors that increase the risk of communicable disease outbreaks and epidemics in Central Asia include

- high poverty levels in some countries;
- relatively poor access to basic water and sanitation services;
- underfunded and inefficient public health services;
- deteriorated health care infrastructure and medical equipment;
- weak public health laboratory networks;
- limited human resources in health systems;
- poor quality health services, including the unsafe use of blood and its products and unsafe injections in medical settings;

- local health systems that fail to use epidemiological information for decision-making and provide little feedback to those who collect data and issue reports using such data (significant manipulation of communicable disease data occurs in these countries:
  o   some disease cases are never reported, and even outbreaks of special pathogens have been controlled without reporting).

As a result the Ministries' early response was to adopt several measures with the support of international organisations, as follows:

- Legal and regulatory measures have been issued and adopted in some countries;
- Blood centers that did not use questionnaires to identify behavioral risk factors among potential donors are now starting to use them;
- New laboratory equipment has been installed in two republican blood centers;
- Blood centers that used re-usable vials have started using disposable bags; they are also using more reliable test-kits;
- Training workshops have been organized on blood safety for laboratory quality;
- Control, blood safety for epidemiologists, and blood banking and use for medical personnel. Also, full courses have been conducted in these countries for epidemiologists and blood service specialists;
- Additionally, national guidelines on the use of blood are being revised.

These measures reflect a gross underestimation of the existing enormous knowledge gap and therefore the need to focus on human capacity building and knowledge management in line with current 21st century state of the art of transfusion medicine. If we look at the characteristics we see the following (Table 1):

Table 1. Characteristics and Valuation (Kazakhstan:)

Characteristics	Valuation
Government or private	Organised by the state, not by private institutions
Fee of free	Mostly a fee is given to donors
Storage and transport of blood	Mostly done in hospitals
Medical and chemical analyses	Poor; mix of manual and mechanical
DB, MIS and Knowledge Systems	All these technologies are very poorly developed;
Organisational form and coordination mechanisms:	Organisational form is hierarchical and very bureaucratic; coordination mechanism is rules and authority.

Case 2

An Anglophone East African Republic (Uganda), belonging to the low HDI group of countries (HDI 0.446) became independent in 1962. In 1957, a centralized transfusion service - the Uganda Blood Transfusion Service (UBTS) was started at Nakasero. This supplied blood to the entire country for the following 20 years.

The period from 1977 to 1987 saw political unrest disrupting national infrastructures and aggravating the human resource crisis in the health sector. This resulted into reversion to the original unregulated hospital based transfusion service nationwide from before 1980.

Like any other low human development index (L-HDI) country, Uganda is still challenged by a low availability of voluntary non-remunerated blood donors (VNRBD); insufficient transport and storage facilities; low capacities in testing of donated blood and quality assurance in testing laboratories. Through a step-by-step approach these problems are being reversed using locally and internationally sourced technical and financial support.

In May 1987, the Republic of Uganda with the assistance of the Global Programme on AIDS (GPA) of the World Health Organisation (WHO) held a financial donor conference in Kampala. As a result, the Uganda AIDS Control Programme (ACP) was formed. The European Commission (EC) through its AIDS Task Force (ATF) made a pledge of 1.5 million Euros to rehabilitate the central blood bank at Nakasero and the collection, processing and distribution of 10,000 units of whole blood to be supplied to hospitals within 100 kilometers from Nakasero Blood Bank Center.

In the period 1989-2004, further funding from EC together with adequate technical advice and support enabled the UBTS to improve it's infrastructure by opening four regional blood banks in Mbarara, Fort-Portal, Gulu, Mbale and two satellites in Arua and Kitovu. This was accompanied by development and adoption of a National Blood Transfusion Policy, and the organisation and coordination of a national safe blood transfusion service based on voluntary non-remunerated blood donors. This period saw reduction of HIV and Hepatitis B sero-prevalence among donors.

A quality assurance program was instituted in the UBTS establishment, and opportunities for human resource development in-service skills oriented training were initiated.

The EC fund was phased out in 2004 amidst increasing demands for safe blood for an increasing population.

From 2004 - 2010, UBTS has enjoyed technical (TA provision) and financial support from the US PEPFAR project, focused on strengthening of the UBTS. This has been followed by renovation of existing and the establishment of new facilities, increased blood collection from 110,000 units in 2004 to 165, 500 units in 2009.

Blood testing for hepatitis C was started in 2005 in addition to HIV, Hepatitis B and Syphilis testing.

Hospital transfusion committees to oversee clinical use of blood are being created, and a major emphasis is put on quality systems essentials and human capacity building in the regional blood banks. It was only during this last episode that human capacity building was initiated in order to bridge the existing knowledge gap at senior and middle management level as well as with the work force.

Donor funding has been used to strengthen technical skills and facilities without paying adequate attention to the need for knowledge development and management. However, when appropriately and holistically utilized and supported by adequate provision of guidance and technical advice such funding can improve blood transfusion programs in the low HDI countries through creation of a competent (knowledge and skills) and sustainable human capacity. If we look at the characteristics we see the following (Table 2):

Table 2. Characteristics and Valuation (Uganda)

Characteristics	Valuation
Government or private	Government (financial support EC and US)
Fee of free	Mostly free
Storage and transport of blood	Still difficult and not always guaranteed
Medical and chemical analyses	Basically present and increasing
DB, MIS and Knowledge Systems	Very few of these systems are developed
Organisational form and coordination mechanisms:	Organisational form is hierarchical and very bureaucratic; coordination mechanism is rules and authority.

Case 3

A Southeast Asian country (Cambodia), belonging to the medium HDI group of countries (HDI 0.534) gained independence as a democratic and constitutional monarchy in 1953. The country suffered from 1975 to 1993 from a communist totalitarian regime (Khmer Rouge) and went through a brutal and devastating genocide. In 1993 the monarchy was rehabilitated and a multi-party democracy instituted.

There is a National Blood Policy since 2003, with attached priority strategies related to blood safety. However, there is no Strategic Plan for implementation.

There is also a National Blood Transfusion Centre (NBTC), which is hospital based, 5 National Hospitals, several NGOs and private clinics in the capital Phnom Penh.

There are also 21 hospitals based Provincial Blood Transfusion Centers of which only 4 are collected through mobile drives.

Donors are almost exclusively family/related (with hidden payment). There is no donor registry available and therefore no traceability of donors.

Almost all the blood collected is used as whole blood (> 89%). A few hospitals do have a Transfusion Committee, but little is known about the activities of these Committees. In 1999 a Guideline for Clinical use of Blood was developed to which in 2006 with Terms of Reference for the Referral Hospital Transfusion Committee (HTC) have been added. Given the identified need, little to nothing so far has been done with this Guide.

In 2007 GFATM-WHO launched an initiative to develop clinical guidelines for appropriate use of blood. An international expert consultant was asked:

1   In coordination with the National Blood Transfusion Center and the Hospital Transfusion Committee (s) to revise guidelines for clinical use of blood;
2   To provide technical advice to NBTC and the HTC on appropriate clinical use of blood;
3   To identify references and develop documents such as guidelines and procedures for medical doctors, laboratory technicians, nurses, as applicable, on the following aspects of the Blood Transfusion Services:
  3.1.   Blood and blood component therapy: general guidelines on indication and dosages;
  3.2.   Blood and blood component therapy: storage and administration;
  3.3.   Information about other blood products and alternatives for transfusion;

3.4. Request for blood and blood components: standard blood request form;

3.5. Request for blood and blood components: Minimum blood ordering schedule;

3.6. Administration of blood: SOPs in hospitals;

3.7. Monitoring blood use, including adverse events related to transfusion and report;

4   Discuss output to various stakeholders through participation in a consensus workshop on the clinical use of blood.

However, given the picture of the fragmented blood supply and transfusion system in Cambodia it would have been more appropriate to start developing a properly founded (legislation and regulations) and organized National Blood Transfusion system, vein to vein based on knowledge and skills.

Clinicians, prescribers of haemotherapy, need to have adequate knowledge on how to provide proper care to patients and own the knowledge. Only then will guidelines for their practice be followed and adhered to. The horse should not be behind but in front of the wagon.

A prominent missing part of the GFATM proposal is the aspect of human capacity building, the initiation of current knowledge and understanding the entire vein (donor) to vein (recipient) chain to guarantee good quality clinical practice using available blood components, rather than imposing guidelines while offering whole blood.

If we look at the characteristics we see the following (Table 3):

Table 3. Characteristics and Valuation (Cambodia)

Characteristics	Valuation
Government or private	Government with financial sponsors
Fee of free	Partly free, with hidden payment (family/friends)
Storage and transport of blood	Very little long time storages
Medical and chemical analyses	Only basically and following international rules
DB, MIS and Knowledge Systems	Mostly absent, except for some databases (DB)
Organisational form and coordination mechanisms:	Organisational form is primarily (professionally) bureaucratic; coordination mechanism is authority and rule following

Case 4

The Netherlands – a highly developed Western European country (HDI 0.910).

According to their own information, Sanquin Blood Supply Foundation started in 1998 as a merger of Dutch transfusion blood banks and the Central Laboratory of the Blood Transfusion Service of the Dutch Red Cross.(see http://www.sanquin.nl/en/about/about-sanquin/)

On the basis of the Law of Blood Supply, Sanquin is named the only organisation in the Netherlands to take care for the need of blood and blood products. The name Sanquin is a reference to the literal meaning of the word in French (sanguine) and Latin (sanguis). The 'g' is replaced by the 'q'. The correct pronunciation of Sanquin is 'Sankwien'. The logo of Sanquin is a pelican with a drop of blood on the breast. The image refers to the legend of the curly pelican (Pelecanus Crispus or Dalmatian Pelican). Since the Middle Ages the pelican is symbol for altruism and mercy. According to the legend this pelican picks in her breast to feed her hungry offspring with her own blood. The pelican stands for Sanquin, also a symbol for the unselfish blood donations of the Dutch donors. Below you see the board structure of the organisation (Figure 2). Sanquin is a non-profit organisation.

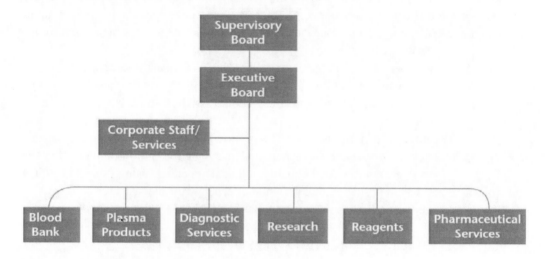

Figure 2. Board Structure of Sanquin Blood Supply Foundation.

Without the more than 400.000 donors in the Netherlands, Sanquin Blood Bank could not do her life-saving work that is the reason that Sanquin takes her tasks serious: provided that the merciful money donations are as safe and efficiently as possible to help as many patients as possible. This strategic task requires a well-oiled, technically high standard and very professional organisation.

Sanquin has constructive contact with a great number of patient societies, nationally and internationally

National
- Society for Immune Disorders;
- Dutch Society of Haemophilia Patients;
- Society for Muscle Diseases Netherlands;
- Patient Society for Hereditairy Angio-edema and Quincke's edema;
- ITP (Idiotypic Trombocytopenic Purpura);
- Netherlands Patient Association;
- Society for rare blood diseases (Hematoslife);
- Society AA and PNH;
- Society StiKa (Disease of Kawasaki);
- Dutch Patient Consumer Federation.

International
- – Patient Association for Hereditary Diseases;
- – Angio-edema Society;
- – European Haemophilia Consortium;
- – World Federation of Haemophilia;
- – US HAE Association (HAEA);
- – Thalassaemia International Federation.

Sanquin has the following research lines: Molecular Cell Biology, Phagocyte laboratory, Laboratory for Blood Transfusion Technology, Plasma Proteins, Laboratory of Cellular Haemostasis, Haematopoiesis, Laboratory of Adaptive Immunity, Experimental Immunohaematology, Immunopathology, Laboratory of Autoimmune Diseases, Blood-borne Infections, Transfusion Technology Assessment, Transfusion Monitoring, Transfusion Medicine, Donor Studies.

If we look at the characteristics of the Dutch blood transfusion system, we see the following (Table 4):

Table 4. Characteristics and Valuation (Netherlands)

Characteristics	Valuation
Government or private	Non-for-profit foundation
Fee of free	Free, reward system through Red Cross Society
Storage and transport of blood	Very well organized
Medical and chemical analyses	High quality, automated and centralized
DB, MIS and Knowledge Systems	Many databases, but not with the newest DB-technology; MIS only for management and KS mainly absent
Organisational form and coordination mechanisms:	The organisational form is primarily (professionally) bureaucratic and the coordination mechanism is authority and rule following.

Case 5

England and Wales – a highly developed Western European country (HDI 0.863).

The NBS is part of NHS Blood and Transplant, which is a National Health Service Special Health Authority. (see http://www.blood.co.uk/) The authority also includes the Bio Products Laboratory, which supplies blood products to hospitals and UK Transplant, which operates the national organ donor register. The service was formed in 1946 as the Blood Transfusion Service and is still often referred to as this.

The name change came about in 1991 to reflect the move away from a regionally based service to a nationally organized one. The service operates out of fifteen centers, and collects around 2.1 million donations per year and supplies 8,000 units of blood every day. Service directors proposed a reconfiguration and centralization strategy in 2006, based on the closure of most local processing and testing labs, and subsequent operation out of just three large 'supercenters' to serve the same geographical area. Staff is opposed to this strategy, and it is now in 2011 under review. The future organisation of NBS blood processing and testing is still to be agreed. About NHS Blood and Transplant: NHSBT is a Special Health Authority in

England and Wales, with responsibilities across the United Kingdom for organ donation and transplantation. The core purpose is to 'save and improve lives' through the provision of a safe and reliable supply of blood components, solid organs, stem cells, tissues and related services to the NHS, and to the other UK health services where directed. The supply of these critical products and services depends entirely on the loyalty of our donors.

NHSBT engages with millions of people throughout the country and connects directly with more people on a daily basis than any other single part of the NHS. In addition to supplying the lifesaving products that are needed by NHS patients they are proud that the activities support the incredible altruism and generosity of the donors and bring communities together across the country.

In these respects NHSBT is unique. They operate supply chains that are similar in nature to those found in the private sector but with characteristics that cannot be found anywhere else apart from similar services in other countries across the world.

As a result, comparing and benchmarking the effectiveness with other national services is a fundamental part of the strategic process.

The ambition is simple – to be demonstrably the best service of this type in the world. NHSBT is a relatively complex organisation with a number of distinct strategic operating units that include, along with the supporting corporate strategy:

- Blood Components;
- Organ Donation and Transplantation;
- Tissues;
- Diagnostic Services;
- Stem Cells, and
- Specialist Therapeutic Services.

The strategic plan of the NHSBT for 2012-17 focused on:

- Continuing to modernize the blood donation service so that enough donors are attracted to meet the needs of NHS patients and improving the interfaces with NHS hospitals so that their needs can be seen and provide services that are as accessible and effective as possible;
- As part of this we plan to integrate the management of hospital blood bank stocks and use this to facilitate better planning of the end-to-end blood supply chain from donor through to patient ;
- Delivering the 50% growth in deceased organ donation by 2013 that was targeted by the Organ Donation Task Force (ODTF) whilst bringing stakeholders together to identify the strategy and aspirations for organ donation and transplant in the UK beyond 2013;
- Building on the unique skills and capabilities in tissues, stem cells, diagnostic services and aphaeresis based therapies to support the provision of life changing treatments to NHS patients. The new plan requires a longer-term view, introduce more effective planning processes and provide more modern interfaces with both the donors and the hospitals that are served. As such, it is very different from the previous plan, which included a strong focus on consolidation and the removal of

excess capacity in the blood supply chain. To learn more go to: www.nhsbt.nhs.uk/strategic plan.

Since a few years the Battenburg markings are used on NBS vehicles. NBS vehicles are allowed the use of blue lights and sirens (known commonly "blues and twos") for the use of emergency blood transports (see Figure 3).

In some cases this will also require the use of a police escort for the transporting vehicle in order to safely and quickly navigate major road junctions. Escort is normally provided by several motorbike units.

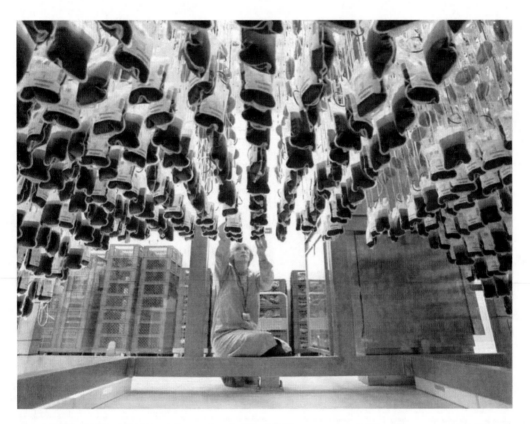

Figure 3. The NHS NBT blood processing facility in Filton operates 24/7 and processes 600,000 units of blood a day.

Concerning blood the NHS reduced the price of red cells to NHS hospitals from £140/unit in 2008-09 to £125/unit in 2011-12 through a continued focus on cost improvement and efficiency program. A successful winter stock build will result in no blood group falling below a three-day stock level for three consecutive days. 87% of platelets via component donation (target 80%) were collected against a continued upward trend in demand. The manufacturing productivity has risen by 69% and testing productivity by 65% since 2008-09, with productivity in both areas above target and in the top quartile of countries in the European Blood, If we look at the characteristics we see the following (Table 5):

Table 5. Characteristics and Valuation (England and Wales)

Characteristics	Valuation
Government or private	Government (NHSBT)
Fee of free	Free, reward system
Storage and transport of blood	Very well organized
Medical and chemical analyses	High quality, newest technologies, automated and centralized
DB, MIS and Knowledge Systems	Many databases, also advanced, standard MIS and very little KS
Organisational form and coordination mechanisms:	The organisational form is primarily (professionally) bureaucratic and the coordination mechanism is mainly authority and rule following.

Table 6 provides a comparative overview of the 5 countries.

Table 6. overview of 5 countries and 6 criteria

Countries → Criteria ↓	Kazakhstan	Uganda	Cambodia	Netherlands	UK (England and Wales)
HDI	0.745	0.446	0.534	0.910	0.863
Government or private	Government	Government (sponsors)	Government (sponsors)	Non-profit and private	Government
Fee or free	Fee (family)	Free	Fee and free (family)	Free	Free
Blood storage and transport	Low quality	Low quality	Low quality	High quality	High quality
Medical and chemical analyses	Medium	Low	Low	High	High
Databases Management Information Systems (MIS), Knowledge Systems (KS)	Only DB, little MIS and no KS	Only DB, little MIS and no KS	Only DB, little MIS and no KS	Large DB, much MIS and very little KS	Large DB, much MIS and very little KS
Organisational forms and coordination mechanisms	Professional bureaucracy and rules and authority	Professional bureaucracy and rules	Professional bureaucracy and rules	Professional bureaucracy and rules and authority	Professional bureaucracy and rules and authority

4. ICT, Information, and KM for Transfusion Medicine

As presented in section 2, a knowledge management perspective on any process in which humans perform various tasks, reveals knowledge as a necessity to ensure adequate execution of these tasks and consequently the process as a whole.

In order for each task performer to acquire required knowledge, s/he needs to obtain task related information. Through a mechanism of interpretation and by connecting it to existing knowledge, the task performer is able to extent his/her knowledge about the task at hand. The interrelatedness between information and knowledge has been described more formally in the Information Processing System hypothesis. [11] This hypothesis models humans as information processing systems, equipped with receptors and effectors to interact with their environment. Receptors enable the reception of information; effectors shape the ability to act (e.g., the ability to grasp, move, or speak).

The internal system of memory and cognitive processor enables the human to store knowledge and execute operations on this store. We will not discuss the Information Processing System more detailed, here. What is important from this hypothesis is the relation it describes between information, which resides in the world outside of humans, and knowledge, residing in humans' memory.

The Information Processing System hypothesis makes way to reason about how knowledge of people can be influenced, and how people's knowledge can be connected to enable meaningful interactions.

An important tool in knowledge management still is the use of information and communication technology (ICT). ICT for knowledge management comes in various shapes and sizes.

The available portfolio consists of e.g., decision support systems, databases, management information systems, or electronic communication systems. Each of these systems supports one or more of the stages of the knowledge management cycle. For instance, decision support systems are particularly suited to support knowledge acquisition and use. These systems incorporate particular information that is used in decision-making. Using this information, decision support systems provide support for individuals relating to specific problems concerning their task at hand.

In contrast, electronic communication systems are more versatile in their application.

In knowledge capture and creation, communication systems enable information exchange between individuals involved in the creation process.

During knowledge sharing and dissemination, communication systems are able to replicate information from one to many individuals. And in knowledge acquisition and use, communication systems enable individuals to consult others to help them in applying specific knowledge in their tasks.

Regarding the blood transfusion system's process as depicted in figure 1, various opportunities for ICT support can be distinguished. Whereas a more fine-grained way to provide ICT support surely is thinkable, we only provide a rough overview of the type of ICT support that suits the various process steps. From an ICT support perspective, we identify three distinct functions.

First, the front-office function, which concerns the nurses that retrieve blood from donors and provide blood to patients. Information wise, these tasks are recognised as administrative tasks. The donor and patient data are registered into some information system (e.g., a rudimentary database or simple information system).

In addition to name and address, the donor and patient's history is recorded. The latter is mandatory, in order to guarantee that the blood that is obtained from donors and provided to patients meets predetermined quality criteria. For instance, the blood donor should not carry a disease that renders the blood unusable such as hepatitis.

The second type of ICT support system concerns a back-end system that enables the matching of blood to a patient. Based on blood characteristics of both the patient and that in stock, a proper batch of blood for the patient is selected. To ensure a proper match is obtained, a knowledge system might be used.

Based on decision rules, a matching mechanism can be implemented. In addition to a content-wise matching mechanism, the ICT support for matching can be extended with a logistical module. Such a module enables the selection of the blood in stock that is closest to the patient who requires the blood.

The final type of ICT support we identify here concerns support for additional analyses and tests on the blood in storage. This task is not an immediate task in the blood transfusion system as described in Figure 1. It concerns an additional task that is performed within the storage facility. The additional analyses and tests help to obtain a greater understanding of specific properties of blood, and in this way help to enlarge the body of knowledge relating to blood.

5. The Future and Some Recommendations for Knowledge Management in Transfusion Medicine

For Transfusion Medicine (TM) we argue that training and education are very important in the under-developed as well as in the developed countries. This concerns secondary as well as primary processes and tasks. The primary processes concern blood and the chemical and physiological content that nurses and doctors have or need, secondary processes concern storage, transport, information, knowledge structures and communication in and between partners in blood donations and blood recipients. This is a very often forgotten part of transfusion medicine (also see chapter 14). Given this emphasis on training and education, we furthermore see at least three developments concerning

a) management and organisation,
b) supra-national structures and
c) various kinds of ICT-use.

Sub a) Management and organisation: structures are very much country and culture dependent. One management structure for every country is impossible. The same applies with respect to culture. Even within countries one sometimes sees various ways of doing things and of structuring, take for examples, England, Wales, Scotland and Ireland in relation to the UK. The same is the case with the various countries that resulted from the former Soviet Union or with the many provinces in India. The cultures are different and very often also the languages are different. Given the fact that cultures, languages and organisations are so different, the only useful process concerns a bottom-up strategy. Languages in various countries will remain different and so will cultures, but management structures in various countries may become similar, especially in countries that exchange blood and blood products. This may be possible between the Netherlands and Germany, Italy and Spain or France and Switzerland and so. A similar pattern may emerge between various countries in Asia of in Africa. This bottom-up approach can be completed by a top-down approach, a supra-national structure, in principle in line with already existing organisations, such as the

UN, the EC or the Commonwealth. This bottom-up approach can be combined with a kind of top-down approach as we see in the next issue.

Sub b) Supra-national structures. A supra-national blood organisation does not exist, yet. Close by for organs comes the Eurotransplant International Foundation, commonly known simply as Eurotransplant. It is an international non-profit organisation responsible for encouraging and coordinating organ transplants in its member countries. The headquarters of Eurotransplant are located in Leiden, the Netherlands. The organisation was created by Jon J. van Rood in 1967, and legally founded on May 12, 1969. Member states of Eurotransplant include the Benelux countries, Germany, Austria, Slovenia, Croatia. All transplant clinics, tissue-typing laboratories and hospitals where organ donations take place are included in the exchange. Eurotransplant helps coordinate work in these institutions, with the goal of efficiently allocating and distributing donated organs. The group also promotes research into transplantation and seeks to raise public awareness of the benefits of donation. As mediator between donor and recipient, Eurotransplant plays a key role in the allocation and distribution of donor organs for transplantation.

The mission statement and goals of Eurotransplant express its main target: to ensure an optimal use of available donor organs. The allocation system is based upon medical and ethical criteria. Through conducting and facilitating scientific research, Eurotransplant aims at a constant improvement of transplant outcomes. Eurotransplant aspires to achieve an optimal use of available donor organs in its member states Austria, Belgium, Croatia, Germany, Luxembourg, the Netherlands and Slovenia. The mission statement of Eurotransplant is that it is a non-profit service organisation for donation and transplantation through the collaborating transplant programs within the organisation. Eurotransplant provides services to transplant centers and their associated tissue typing laboratories and donor hospitals in its member states (see also www.eurotransplant.org/cms/). The organisational goals are:

1   To achieve an optimal use of available donor organs and tissues;
2   To secure a transparent and objective allocation system, based upon medical and ethical criteria;
3   To assess the importance of factors which have the greatest influence on waiting list mortality and transplant results;
4   To support donor procurement to increase the supply of donor organs and tissues;
5   To further improve the results of transplantation through scientific research and to publish and present these results;
6   To promote, support and coordinate organ donation and transplantation in the broadest sense of the term.

Comparable institutions as Eurotransplant are Scandiatransplant in Iceland, Norway, Finland, Denmark, and Sweden and Balttransplant in Estonia, Latvia and Lithuania.

A supra-national organizstion can use the ISO certificate. For example the ISO 9000 family addresses various aspects of quality management and contains some of ISO's best-known standards. The standards provide guidance and tools for companies and organisations that want to ensure that their products and services consistently meet customer's requirements, and that quality is consistently improved. There are many standards in the ISO 9000 family, including:

- ISO 9001:2008 - sets out the requirements of a quality management system;
- ISO 9000:2005 - covers the basic concepts and language;
- ISO 9004:2009 - focuses on how to make a quality management system more efficient and effective;
- ISO 19011 - sets out guidance on internal and external audits of quality management systems.

Similar criteria can also be used for blood banks and blood transport between countries.

Sub c) Kinds of ICT-use, DB, MIS and KS. We start with a database. *A database* (DB) is an organised collection of data, today typically in digital form. The data are typically organised to model relevant aspects of reality (for example, the availability of rooms in hotels), in a way that supports processes requiring this information (for example, finding a hotel with vacancies). The term database is correctly applied to the data and their supporting data structures, and not to the database management system (DBMS). The database data collection with DBMS is called a database system. The term database system implies that the data is managed to some level of quality (measured in terms of accuracy, availability, usability, and resilience) and this in turn often implies the use of a general-purpose database management system (DBMS). A general-purpose DBMS is typically a complex software system that meets many usage requirements to properly maintain its databases, which are often large and complex. The utilization of databases is now so widespread that virtually every technology and product relies on databases and DBMSs for its development and commercialisation. Even they may have DBMS software embedded. Also, organisations and companies, from small to large, depend heavily on databases for their operations.

Well known DBMSs include Oracle, IBM DB2, Microsoft SQL Server, Microsoft Access, PostgreSQL, MySQL, and SQLite. A database is not generally portable across different DBMS, but different DBMSs can inter-operate to some degree by using standards like SQL and ODBC together to support a single application built over more than one database. A DBMS also needs to provide effective run-time execution to properly support (e.g., in terms of performance, availability, and security) as many database end-users as needed. A way to classify databases involves the type of their contents, for example: bibliographic, document-text, statistical, or multimedia objects. Another way is by their application area, for example: accounting, music compositions, movies, banking, manufacturing, or insurance. The term database may be narrowed to specify particular aspects of organised collection of data and may refer to the logical database, to the physical database as data content in computer data storage or to many other database sub-definitions.

Most countries in the world use databases or RDBMS's and many suppliers as we discussed in the above can deliver such systems. They are already very sophisticated, as in the Netherlands and in the UK or very simple such as in Cambodia or Uganda. The important factor in many cases is the price or the available applications. The future trends will be more data, more structures and more (complicated) queries.

A *Management Information System* (MIS) is an organised approach to the study of the information needs of the organisation's management at every level in making operational, tactical, and strategic decisions. Its objective is to design and implement procedures, processes, and routines that provide suitably detailed reports in an accurate, consistent, and timely manner. In a management information system, modern, computerized systems continuously gather relevant data, both from inside and outside an organisation. This data is then processed, integrated, and stored in a centralized database (or data warehouse) where it is constantly updated and made available to all who have the authority to access it, in a form that suits their purpose.

From a management perspective, a MIS is not using contents of the primary tasks and processes, for example blood and blood products. As the title MIS already says these systems focus on the secondary or organisational tasks and processes. Depending on management requests MISs are useful or not useful enough. Most under-developed countries do not use MISs.

A *Knowledge System* (KS) or knowledge based system is an artificial intelligent tool working in a narrow domain to provide intelligent decisions with justification. Knowledge is acquired and represented using various knowledge representation techniques such as in rules, frames and scripts.

The basic advantages offered by such system are documentation of knowledge, intelligent decision support, self-learning, reasoning and explanation. Knowledge-based systems are systems based on the methods and techniques of Artificial Intelligence.

Their core components are: a knowledge base, an acquisition mechanism and an inference mechanism. Knowledge Base Systems (KBS) go beyond the decision support philosophy to indicate the expert system technology into the decision-making framework. Expert Systems (ES) have been the tools and techniques perfected by artificial intelligence (AI) researchers to deduce decision influences based on the codification of knowledge. The codification of knowledge uses the principles of knowledge representation (part of the large theoretical ideas of knowledge engineering). Typically such codification uses rules like IF-THEN rules to represent logical implications. While for some authors [9] expert systems, case-based reasoning systems and neural networks are all particular types of knowledge-based systems, there are others who consider that neural networks are different, and exclude it from this category.

Because KS or KBS are knowledge content dependent, these systems are not developed or available at this moment, not even in the developed countries. Here, much gain can be realized in the next 10-20 years.

Combining blood transfusion with various aspects of knowledge management makes two things clear. In the first place, KM is not about the content of blood or medical and chemical issues. It is about various kinds of secondary or organisational processes and tasks. To be honest it should be so, unless we are talking about expert systems and knowledge technology, bur KM does not deal with these systems to begin with. In the second place many organisational issues can precisely use the new developments in ICT and KM. The use of KM in an organisation can and must use digital innovations, whether they relate to databases and RDBMS's or to find matching possibilities between donors and recipients. From a general perspective here is a world to win.

References

[1] Jorna, R. J. (2007). Knowledge Dynamics: A Framework to Handle Types Knowledge. In: J. F. Schreinemakers and T. M. van Engers (Eds.) *Advances in Knowledge*

Management, Vol. 3: 15 Years of Knowledge Management. Würzburg, Germany, Ergon Verlag. pp. 25-48.

[2]   Polanyi, M. (1966). *Personal knowledge: towards a post-critical philosophy*. Routledge and Paul Kegan, London UK.

[3]   Boisot, M. (1995). *Information space: a framework of learning in organisations, institutions and culture.*, Routledge, London UK.

[4]   Jorna, R. J., Faber, N. R. (2011). Innovation and Knowledge Management for Sustainability: Theoretical Perspectives. In: F. Nobre (Ed.), *Technological, Managerial and Organizational Core Competencies: Dynamic Innovation and Sustainable Advantage*. Hershey, Pennsylvania, US: IGI Global.

[5]   McElroy, M. W. (2003). *The new knowledge management: complexity, learning, and sustainable innovation*. Butterworth-Heineman. London UK

[6]   Schreiber, A., Akkermans, H., Anjewierden, A., et al. (2000). *Knowledge engineering and management: the CommonKADS methodology*. The MIT Press. Cambridge. MA, US

[7]   Dalkir, K. (2005). *Knowledge management in theory and practice*. Butterworth-Heineman. London UK

[8]   Newell, A., Simon, H. A. (1972). *Human problem solving*. Englewood Cliffs, NJ, Prentice-Hall.

[9]   Wilson, R. A., Kiel, F. C. (1999). *The MIT Encyclopaedia of cognitive science*. Cambridge, Mass: The MIT Press. Cambridge, MA, US

[10]   Jorna, R. J. (2006). *Sustainable innovation: the organisational, human, and knowledge dimension*. Sheffield UK: Greenleaf Publishing.

[11]   Nickols, F. (1996). Cooperative development of a classification of knowledge management functions. In: P. Murray, *Knowledge Praxis*. 1997. Accessible through URL: http://www.media-access.com/ classification.html

[12]   Wiig, K. (1993). *Knowledge management foundations*. Arlington, TX, US, Schema Press.

[13]   Bukowitz, W., Williams, R. (2000). *The knowledge management fieldbook*. London UK, Prentice Hall.

[14]   Meyer, N., Zack, M. The design and implementation of information products. *Sloan Management Review*, 1996;37:43-59.

[15]   Goodman, N. (1981/1968). *Languages of art*. Brighton: The Harvester Press.

[16]   Jorna, R. J. (1990). *Knowledge representation and symbols in the mind: an analysis of the notion of representation and symbol in cognitive psychology*. Stauffenberg Verlag, Germany.

[17]   Von Krogh, G., Ichijo, K., Nonaka, I. (2000). *Enabling knowledge creation: how to unlock the mystery of tacit knowledge and release the power of innovation*. Oxford UK, Oxford University Press.

[18]   Von Krogh, G., Roos, J. A perspective on knowledge, competence and strategy. *Personnel review* 1994;26:31.

[19]   Nonaka, I., Takeuchi, H. (1995). *The knowledge-creating company: how Japanese companies create the dynamics of innovation*. New York NY, US, Oxford University Press.

[20] Faber, N. R., Peters, K., Jorna, R. J. (2006). Technology for knowledge crossover: a tool for a sustainable paper industry. *International Conference on Organisational Semiotics 2006 – ACM SIG Proceedings*. New York, NY, US

[21] Peters, K. (2006). Integrating separate knowledge domains with a decision support system: applying chemical knowledge in the paper industry. *Master thesis, University of Groningen, NL.*

In: Quality Management in Transfusion Medicine   ISBN: 978-1-62618-665-1
Editor: Cees Th. Smit Sibinga   © 2013 Nova Science Publishers, Inc.

Chapter XIV

Quality Management in Transfusion Medicine in Resource Restricted Countries

Jean C. Emmanuel,[1,*] *Isaac Kajja*[2,†]
and Lawrence Marum[3,‡]

[1]BTS Consultants, Borrowdale, Harare, Zimbabwe
[2]Makerere University, Department of Orthopaedics, Kampala, Uganda
[3]Centers for Disease Control and Prevention – Zambia, Lusaka, Zambia

Abstract

In order to provide a safe, accessible, adequate and affordable supply of blood and blood products, every country must have a coordinated National Blood Service. This Service may be provided by one organisation or made up of multiple organisations, which are nationally coordinated. The globally accepted model for the provision of labile blood components is based on voluntary non-remunerated blood donation and the service provider is ethically and morally obligated to ensure that the products and services are available on a not for profit basis, particularly in respect to the blood donated. A clear distinction should be made between labile blood components/products and pharmaceutically derived medicinal plasma products, stabile blood products.

Provision of adequate and safe blood products remains a goal, yet to be achieved in many resource-restricted countries, despite continued international technical and financial support. The establishment of nationally coordinated Blood Services supported by the country's Health Authorities, with appropriate legal frameworks, is critical to an equitable supply of safe blood products to the private and public sector health facilities in all countries. Additionally, the development and implementation of appropriate Quality

* Jean C. Emmanuel, MD MCPCP(Z): BTS Consultants. PO Box BW 1681, Borrowdale, Harare, Zimbabwe. Tel: +263 4 883537 and mobile +263 774687297; E-mail: emmanuelj@ btsconsultants.org.
† Isaac Kajja, MD, PhD: Makerere University, Department of Orthopaedics. P.O. Box 7072 Kampala, Uganda. Tel: +256-772443473. E-mail: kajja133@gmail.com.
‡ Lawrence Marum, MD, FAAP, MPH: Centers for Disease Control and Prevention – Zambia. PO Box 31617, Lusaka, 10101 Zambia. Tel: +260-977-770-958. E-mail: LMarum@ cdc.gov.

Management Standards is essential to the safe and effective operation of these Services. Progress in achieving total quality systems in many resource restricted countries have been due to a lack of government support, lack of political stability; adequate facilities; insufficient budget; no effective leadership and management; cultural attitudes and misconceptions; and challenging environment and infrastructural issues.

Keywords: Coordinated sustainable National Blood Services, Quality and safety of blood, Quality Management in blood services, Developing a culture of quality, Adopt lessons from successful services

1. Introduction

Blood transfusion is an important part of health care; in resource restricted countries. Lack of access to safe transfusion limits progress in meeting the United Nations Development Programme (UNDP) 8 Millennium Development Goals (MDGs), which were endorsed and adopted in 2000, by 198 member states, to eradicate poverty and multiple deprivations, especially goal 4 reducing child mortality, goal 5 to improve maternal health and goal 6 to combat HIV/AIDS, malaria and other diseases. [1]

In 2000, Blood Transfusion Safety was accorded high priority by the World Health Organisation (WHO), making it one of its 7 Priority Areas of Work. WHO has, since 1975, tabled relevant resolutions, endorsed by all Member States, supporting the implementation of blood safety activities. [2] Developed countries have implemented mechanisms and strategies to ensure blood safety, responding rapidly to the threat to the safety of the blood supply, although some countries were penalised for not reacting sufficiently rapidly. This lead to the much publicized and sensationalised ⎡Blood Scandals⎦ which involved many countries in the 1990s. [3]

The potential of blood to transmit infectious agents is well documented. HIV has proved the single most important transfusion transmissible infection in focusing international and national health authorities on the importance of ensuring a safe supply of blood and plasma products for all potentially infectious agents, which can be transmitted through these products.

The spread of HIV among populations was accelerated through blood transfusions in the Americas and Europe in the early 1980s, in Africa throughout the 1980s and 1990s and China in the 1990s. This global epidemic has strained resources and health systems in an unprecedented way.

In Africa, which continues to have a disproportional prevalence of HIV globally, the slow introduction of HIV screening, inconsistent supplies of test kits, inadequate quality controls and less than 100% testing of donated blood was a major early contributor to this rapid spread, in particular in Sub-Saharan Africa. [4-6]

WHO, through the Global Programme on AIDS (GPA), established in 1987, developed wide-ranging strategies in all areas of HIV/AIDS Prevention and Control, including blood safety. GPA played an important global role in developing short and medium term plans to strengthen blood safety systems in resource restricted countries through capacity building, provision of reagents, equipment and facilitating bilateral and multi-bilateral funding agreements with international organisations, foundations and financing through donor countries.

Progress has been made in developing appropriate standards for blood donor screening, blood testing strategies and capacity building.

In most resource restricted countries categorised by the United Nations Development Programme (UNDP) as Medium and Low Human Development Index countries (MHDI and LHDI)[1], the majority of blood collected and transfused is still provided through individual hospital blood banks, which are within a hospital laboratory system, both in the public sector and private sector hospitals. This leads to a lack of coordinated service provision and logistical difficulties and ultimately uniform quality management.

These blood banks are part of a hospital structure and are organisationally and financially accountable to hospital administration and take their place alongside all other support departments as part of the hospital structure..

These blood banks, like other hospital departments, cannot be subject to selective legislative and dedicated fiscal budgets and additionally cannot adequately provide for the needs of patients in private sector hospitals.

The blood bank's prime responsibility is to ensure that the requirements of the hospital are met, with hospital laboratory staff providing all technical, nursing and logistical support necessary within the framework of the hospital laboratory's budget, facilities and infrastructure. In spite of extensive efforts to provide capacity building for technical and nursing staff, trained personnel are often moved to other areas of work within the respective government and hospital departments. In addition, the needs of the private sector and other public sector hospitals cannot be met through these organisational structures.

Recognising the importance of quality, WHO, in 2000, developed the Quality Management Programme (QMP), which was used as the platform for declaring Blood Safety as one of the seven priority areas of work. WHO developed an interactive training tool 'Quality Management Training for Blood Transfusion Services – Facilitator's Toolkit'. [7] Support to blood services in medium and low human development index countries was a key attendant strategy. However, even services in high human development index countries (advanced or developed countries) were encouraged and reminded of the need to re-examine the processes and procedures for quality, to improve and maintain all aspects of quality management and also to extend their support and expertise to MHDL and LHDI countries in the goal of ensuring global blood safety.

At the present time there is a lack of an independent database to assess accurately the true state of Blood Services or Establishments, and the safety and adequacy of hospital blood supplies, especially in MHDI and LHDI Countries. Credible and accurate global, regional and national epidemiological data is available through collection of information from national and international experts and authorities. However, lamentably, data for blood safety, especially in low resource countries, is collected, in the main, through questionnaires directed to Government Ministries of Health. The data provided are limited by incompleteness or inaccuracy in the absence of strong national data collection and coordination of systems and may be influenced by political and cultural taboos or aspirational factors rather than a true reflection of blood safety. Global blood data must be collected in the same credible manner as

---

[1] See Chapter 15 – Annex 4: HDI ranking.

that collected for infectious diseases in order to address the true need and assess achievements therein.

The WHO Quality Management Programme (QMP) is a global programme that is designed to assist and support countries, particularly MHDI and LHDI countries, to improve the safety and adequacy of blood transfusion by: a) building capacity in quality management in all aspects of blood transfusion through an integrated approach of training and assessment; and b) supporting the establishment of sustainable national quality systems in blood establishments and transfusion services. As WHO is not able, within its mandate, to carry out independent audit and accreditation of national blood supply and in-hospital blood services (vein-to-vein), this gap has been addressed by other internationally recognized organisations and societies working in close collaboration with WHO. These include AABB (formerly the American Association of Blood Banks), the International Red Cross/Red Crescent Society and member societies, and the International Society for Blood Transfusion (ISBT) and regional societies such as the Africa Society for Blood Transfusion (AfSBT). Bilateral and multilateral funding from the European Union (EU) and the US President's Emergency Plan For AIDS Relief (PEPFAR) has expanded capacity for auditing and accreditation of blood services in resource restricted countries. However, increased investment of financial and human resources by national governments within a sustainable fiscal budgetary policy, is necessary to sustain these improvements, as has been shown in a number of notable country examples.

2. Quality Management

A safe and adequate blood supply cannot be assured without quality, which involves every member of staff. An integrated culture of quality has to be created and all staff must be fully aware and implement quality practices at all levels at all times. A fundamental objective of every service is to appoint a dedicated, trained and experienced team responsible for developing a realistic plan of action for establishing an effective and sustainable quality system.

Quality Management, in all its facets, is a key component and goal of every effective programme. In order to ensure quality and safety at all levels of service provision, on a sustainable basis, a National Blood Service requires the following:

1 A well organized and managed structure within an approved and registered legal framework,
2 Adequate infrastructure and facilities,
3 Approved fiscal budgets for public responsibility patients and cost recovery on a 'fee for service' basis for private patients on medical health insurance;
4 Skilled, competent and motivated leadership, qualified financial and medical direction, and dedicated staff with social benefits and career structures.

However, without the commitment and support of National Health Authorities in ensuring that there are independent and effective regulatory bodies, with the authority to inspect or audit, approve, accredit and license these Services, the quality programme will not be effective. Existing Health Care Regulatory bodies may need specific capacity building in order to fulfil this specific function and this should be carried out together with the dedicated Quality staff in the service. External Quality Assurance (EQA) plans, proficiency testing and international and regional accreditation, such as the AfSBT, AABB and International Organization for Standardization (ISO) certification offer, are objective measures that regulatory authorities may use to assess quality of blood services.

There are a small number of National Blood Services in resource restricted countries, which have these requirements in place and have established Quality Management Departments, dedicated to implementing Quality Standards in the respective areas of work, in the National Blood Service and in promoting quality standards in the hospital blood banks in the private and public sector hospitals, which are customers of their products. This strategy has been developed through capacity building partnerships for technical, nursing, clinical and administrative staff. In addition national policies and guidelines are promoted to ensure compliance at each level of the transfusion chain including clinical guidelines and practices. [8] As stated, the highest levels of the most serious transfusion transmitted infections (HIV; Hepatitis B and C and malaria) occur in in Sub-Saharan Africa, where most of the LHDI Countries are situated. Paradoxically, it is in this area, in which at least 5 model blood services are found and which national structures have been developed with quality management departments. These blood services have achieved various stages of achievement towards international and regional accreditation in quality management. The example countries, confirmed as LHDI in the latest UNDP HDI Ranking for 2011 for Low Human Development, are the National Blood Services in: Zimbabwe ISO Certified]; Malawi [AfSBT Accreditation in process]; Uganda; Zambia; and Kenya. In the same region the Blood Service in Namibia, ranked as Medium HDI Country, has achieved Level 3 AfSBT Accreditation (June 2012), following inspections from experts from AABB and AfSBT.

However, the majority of resource-restricted countries continue to rely on hospital based laboratory blood banking systems. These systems are unable to meet quality standards on a sustainable basis, due to a lack of structure and finance related to functional requirements as these are part of hospital laboratory departments, which have a primary responsibility to meeting the hospitals needs and subject to hospital budgets and priorities.

In order to improve Quality Management Systems (QMS), even in resource limited countries, lessons should be learned from the limited successful model Blood Services in these countries, which, with assistance from international and regional organisations and societies, have developed strategies and activities to establish and maintain sustainable Quality Management through well organized and managed Services. Quality has been described as a journey and resource restricted countries need to take the first steps on this journey and develop sustainable strategies to reach their goals.

2.1. Investment in Development of Quality Systems

Studying successful, appropriate and comprehensive model Blood Services, in the journey to Quality, is a first step in identifying respective country requirements, which should be developed following well-defined guidelines and recommendations towards establishing a national quality management system.

From 1988 through to the present time, the European Commission (EC) has provided support to many countries to improve blood safety with a focus on developing a national Centre, which would coordinate blood services and provide Quality Management in screening, processing, storing and distributing blood for transfusion. While this was focused on blood donation and the laboratory components of the system, these projects laid the foundation for quality systems. [9] Establishment of blood centres, in some countries followed, gradually replacing hospital blood banks moving from hospital-based blood banks to a consolidated and centralised system. In 1998, in Kenya and Tanzania, following the tragic bombings of a foreign embassy, funding for blood safety programmes was accelerated, but was not sufficient to meet national needs on a sustainable basis. More recently, substantial funding has been provided by the United States of America, through the President's Emergency Plan For AIDS Relief (PEPFAR) and also through the Global Trust Fund for AIDS, Tuberculosis and Malaria for developments at country level. Funding agreements with 14 countries were established through PEPFAR in 2005, with 80% of funding going to a national service and 20% to a technical assistance partner. This funding was predicated on the understanding that recipient countries commit to establish effective organisational and management structures, which are sustainable beyond the funding agreements and have dedicated and adequate fiscal budgets and that there is measured progress to achieve targets for the provision of an adequate supply of safe blood. As this effort has matured and expanded to other countries, an emphasis on host country ownership and investment has helped to encourage the establishment of sustainable and integrated Blood Services. [10, 11]

The process of development from a fragmented situation of uncoordinated hospital blood banks to a nationally coordinated, quality managed Blood Service may take several paths. Assessments of various aspects of blood safety in the existing system are first steps in order to determine the weaknesses and vulnerabilities of a national programme. Objectives for such assessments may include the following questions:

- Is the supply of blood adequate to meet local and national needs?
- Is the laboratory screening of blood for TTIs and blood grouping adequate?
- Are blood donors motivated and selected in a consistent and effective manner?
- Is the processing and storage of blood adequate to ensure quality and safety?
- Is distribution of blood adequate to meet needs at all private and public health facilities?
- Are standards applied for prescribing and monitoring transfusion?
- Are there reporting systems for adverse events and review of outcomes?
- Is there archiving of blood samples and accessibility of data for quality assurance?

3. Supply of Blood and Blood Products

In low-income countries (LHDI) there is still a reliance on hospital blood banks and family replacement (hidden paid system) and paid donors in more than one-third of the blood supply. [12] Quantifying the collection and use of blood for transfusion at hospital, regional or national level is a useful starting point to determine the adequacy and distribution of existing blood resources. Donations per 1,000 population and transfusions per hospital bed per year can be measured for a hospital catchment area, for a district or region, or at a national level. [13]

Comparing blood orders (prescriptions) and transfusions within a facility is also useful, but must be qualified by assessing whether blood was actually required to assess unmet demand. Estimating a country's need for blood and blood components requires an understanding of the disease burden for conditions requiring transfusion, the coverage of health services and capacity of the health system to utilize these products for transfusion. Quality management in resource-limited settings requires a dynamic response to changing conditions of need and demand, coverage and capacity.

3.1. Blood Donor Selection and Services

Ensuring safety of the blood supply requires both appropriate selection of low risk and loyal donors and effective, quality controlled laboratory screening. The effectiveness of both aspects of this screening process was seen in Kenya, where PCR testing to detect window period' infections did not detect additional HIV infections compared to antigen-antibody testing. [14, 15].

Quality management of blood collection involves a robust donor screening process and donor services to encourage an adequate pool of low-risk, regular, lifelong blood donors.

3.2. Laboratory and Manufacturing Practices

Good Manufacturing Practices (GMP) will guide a Blood Service toward comprehensive quality management, which includes blood collection, infectious disease testing, production of components and storage and distribution (cold chain).

The International Organization for Standardization (ISO), certification, could also be considered by blood establishments in resource-limited settings, if budgets are available. AABB has developed simplified models to assess deficiencies and facilitate a developmental process of improvement. [16]

3.3. Clinical Transfusion Practice

Improving quality of prescribing and bedside transfusion practice is especially critical in resource-limited settings. Appropriateness of prescription improves efficiency when blood supply is limited and reducing inappropriate prescription lowers risk to patients. Timeliness is critical since patients often come late to a facility where transfusion is possible. Malaria and complications of pregnancy represent 75% of the need for blood in many settings in Africa and Southeast Asia; integrating transfusion guidelines and good clinical practices for these conditions may reduce the need for transfusion and improve outcomes. Blood components, where available, should be used appropriately. Practical standards and record keeping for monitoring transfusions are especially important when human resources are limited. Hospital Transfusion Committees at hospitals should be established and meet regularly.

3.4. Monitoring and Evaluation

Data collection and reporting are critical in the development of the systems for monitoring and evaluation that are necessary for quality management and improvement. This includes review of blood collection, screening, processing, distribution and clinical use. In addition, the archiving of blood unit specimens allows for quality control activities and better understanding of adverse outcomes. These data contribute information for a quality improvement process to identify gaps, weaknesses and vulnerabilities in a Nationally supported Blood Service. Hospital Transfusion Committees, which involve all partners in the transfusion process, are essential in achieving the goal of an effective and well-monitored transfusion process. Reporting and monitoring any adverse events, in a non-punitive environment, will improve the safety and efficacy of transfusions and are part of the quality management system.

4. Accreditation Levels for Blood Services

Quality management is an accepted priority at all levels of development in every country. In order to assist and support countries to achieve these goals, funding agencies, International and Regional Societies and Associations representing Blood Services have worked together to develop capacities to meet agreed goals and standards. In particular AABB and the African Society for Blood Transfusion (AfSBT) have worked together to develop a 3 Step Accreditation Scheme, which incorporates internationally recognised and established processes and procedures for evaluation of the development of blood services through 3 levels, with level 3 being full accreditation. The 3 levels of accreditation will allow for quality standards to be audited even in those countries with low levels of financial resources and at the same time act as an incentive to aim at establishing an appropriate and sustainable blood service, which will provide quality blood components.

Together with a team of standards-writing experts from AABB, AfSBT has developed the Quality Standards document, a guidance document to aid understanding of individual standards, and compliance charts addressing specific requirements for steps 1 through 3.

AfSBT will issue a certificate of compliance to blood services which meet the Standards as required for steps 1, 2 and/or 3. The programme has been endorsed by AABB, ISBT and WHO, which fully support this programme and are participants in the AfSBT Accreditation Committee.

This Step-Wise Accreditation programme is now ready for pilot testing. [17]

5. Culture of Change and Quality Improvement

At a glance, total quality management (TQM) of transfusion services appears difficult to achieve and beyond the budgetary reach of many resource restricted countries. It should be noted that quality is a journey not a destination, even limited resources may be utilised effectively to achieve the beginning of a quality system. However, there are intrinsic factors that hinder development and implementation of quality services within these settings.

Table 1. Step-Wise Accreditation Programme. Courtesy of Africa Society for Blood Transfusion (AfSBT)

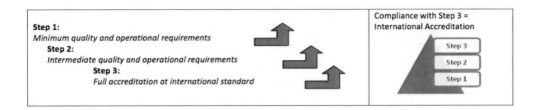

These include presence of leadership; knowledge gap of the importance of quality at all levels from the highest to the lowest level; cultural inclinations and prejudices; lack of infrastructure, dedicated department with staff ; adequate finance and the ability to implement necessary change to achieve and maintain quality in all areas of work by all staff from the cleaners through to leadership level; and most important is to have in place a conducive work environment, which includes career and social benefits in order to retain skilled and experienced staff, which are the most valuable resource.

5.1. Effect of Leadership

In many developing countries, lack of leadership and limited management capacity have negatively impacted on total quality management (TQM) in a number of ways. The WHO Aide-mémoire for Ministries of Health on Developing a National Blood System identifies leadership and governance as critical elements and provides practical advice for a National Blood Service [18]:

- The WHO Global Data Base has identified that national blood policies are not yet developed in many of these countries and where they are formed, are not properly implemented. In such settings there is no basis for standardization of quality systems in the vein-to-vein chain; [19]
- Legislation governing blood services is inadequate or absent in resource restricted countries;
- Limited budgetary allocations to publicly financed transfusion services contribute to shortages of blood and insufficient quality management programmes; [20]
- In some of these countries the professional staff involved in blood transfusion has limited skill, training or experience in leadership and management. The lack of a dedicated professional and competent staff in a blood service leads to inconsistencies in quality;
- Poor administration and management of human and financial resources.

Leadership is also required in the establishment and nurturing blood donor services as a component of quality management plans. Failure to mobilize the required numbers of voluntary non-remunerated blood donors who form a safe and consistent supply of the badly needed blood for the disease burden in these countries leads to inconsistency and shortages. [18, 19]

Leadership and management in the laboratory of blood establishments ensure that Good Manufacturing and Laboratory Practices are continuously met. The prevention of transfusion transmissible infections, contamination or degradation of blood during screening, processing, storage and distribution of blood components is impossible without oversight of critical control points and assurance of in-process controls.

In the hospital setting, lack of oversight and accountability results in poor planning for quality assurance, failure to set hospital transfusion standards, lack of quality training, monitoring and mentoring strategies, including haemovigilance through Hospital Transfusion Committees.

Practices along the entire transfusion chain are not locally generated and evidence- based. Leadership is lacking in order to collate and examine these practices. This leads to adoption of 'borrowed' approaches of which quality assurance is not sustainable, and which cannot be critically tested in the attendant setting to ensure quality improvement.

5.2. Effect of Culture

Quality assurance (QA) is influenced by cultural beliefs and practices of political and religious leaders, professional staff and each section of the community resulting in an impact on each step of the transfusion chain and influences donor motivation and blood donation. Political decision makers may not appreciate the importance of transfusion as a critical component of health care. Without the leadership of a nationally coordinated blood service and strong advocacy from stakeholders to influence decision makers, it is unlikely that quality standards will be met. The concept of quality assurance and management in blood transfusion is not formally and philosophically incorporated into the structure and functioning of health care systems of many developing countries. When it is not consistently being implemented and supported through a culture of quality, it will lead to a poor policy of quality of care, which will be reflected in every facet of the organizational values and policies of a countries health care.

In many cultures the head of family or village, and even the school head, rather than the individual, decides on who should, or should not, donate blood. This limits the availability and access to the safety and consistency of blood donation. Reliance on a particular population group as a blood source, such as secondary school students, also threatens the blood supply, during school vacation and examination times, as suitable alternative blood donors are not easily identified, mobilized, or accessible. [11] Creating a culture of altruistic, non-remunerated and anonymous donation of blood requires the support of community leaders (traditional, cultural, religious and/or political). The lack of trained and experienced blood donor programme staff, in most of the developing countries transfusion services affects the level of quality and effectiveness of motivating and retaining safe and regular blood donors. The blood donor department requires more that 50% of the budget requirements of the blood service and its efficacy is improved through economies of scale, which is directly related to numbers and centralisation of collections. Quality can best be implemented through effective organisation and good leadership management practices. [20]

Blood services depend on the implementation of national procurement guidelines and effective provision of an unbroken supply of reagents, devices and services essential for the collection, processing, testing, storage and distribution of blood and blood components. In many situations, there are procurement and provision delays for funding of equipment and reagents, which are essential for an adequate, unbroken supply of products for the blood service/establishment and for clinical patients. As a result of bureaucracy these delays can be caused by inefficiency in tendering and ordering procedures, which will be further compromised if there are no contingency funds available to act as a bridging financial safety net. The outcome is that quality and staff morale are affected and patient care is compromised.

Developing countries, which have adopted a centralized model of leadership and management with effective financial direction, have demonstrated the importance of financial management. Hospital blood banks dependent on hospital administration, often lack the ability to overcome unforeseen delays in the supply chain and financial delays, which results in an inability to ensure access and availability of blood to the hospital, let alone to demands from other hospitals. Hospitals in larger urban areas are normally structured to act as referral hospitals for the rural hospitals and consequently are allocated a larger proportion of the available national budget finance and resources. Consequently rural hospitals are often left to manage with insufficient resources and lack the political power and advocacy of the central hospital administration. This affects the ordering culture exhibited by the hospital clinical staff, which results in supply driven orders, over ordering and high levels of hospital ward blood expiry rates. [21]

The paternalistic cultural practice exhibited by clinicians in many developing country hospitals – "*the doctor knows it all*" – does not provide the patient (customer) with an opportunity to seek an explanation, discuss or understand the reasons for the procedures.

The result is that informed consent to accept or refuse a transfusion is a matter seldom afforded the individual patient in an elective setting. This challenges the conventional requirement for quality of care, in addressing customer issues.

5.3. Environment

Environmental aspects impact on quality management due to the lack of infrastructure and facilities, which are taken for granted in advanced and developed countries, are rarely provided for in resourced limit environments. Regular supplies of quality electricity, without back-up generators, and an adequate water supply, which are basic essentials for effective laboratory services, are often irregular and sometimes absent for long periods of time. Humidity and tropical rain, without proper air conditioning and sound structural facilities, hamper the provision of quality products; absence of reliable commercial suppliers, or their in-country agents, and the need to seek services from distant supply source; negotiating with national authorities for much needed and scarce foreign currency; dealing with customs and excise bureaucratic requirements to access goods; all lead to shortages and delays in delivery of reagents, spares, maintenance of equipment and provision of devices (blood bags).

Inadequate and incompetent staff complement results in staff being overworked with little or no time for capacity building and reorientation, with the development of dispirited staff and low morale.

Heavy tropical rains and bad road conditions interfere with accessibility to and from donor sites and delivery of blood to remote district hospitals. Donated blood may be stored and transported without an appropriate cold chain and affect the quality of the components to be produced. Inconsistent power supply and lack of adequate backup systems may further compromise the cold chain.

The education (teaching and training) curricula are not well defined or provided in a comprehensive manner with the result that staff competency is lacking or severely compromised. Lack of opportunities for continued professional development for individuals at all levels of staff lead to dissatisfaction and a high turnover rate of staff, which seek alternative and better remuneration in allied and diverse technical fields of work or are enticed to work in the private sector.

Many hospital blood banks are housed in small rooms, which are inadequate and not fit for purpose. The facilities are dilapidated and in need of maintenance and are inadequate to house the equipment or working space needed to ensure that a quality system can be implemented.

Even if external funding is provided for the provision of reagents, essential equipment and devices, the facilities and infrastructure are inadequate.

In many instances funding agencies require that national authorities provide the infrastructure and manpower as these are often outside the terms of the financing agreements.

The current attitudes and perceptions of many of the staff working in resource limited countries are in need of education, capacity building and technical support in order to develop a quality culture which is set at achieving the goal of total quality management. (Figure 1 and 2)

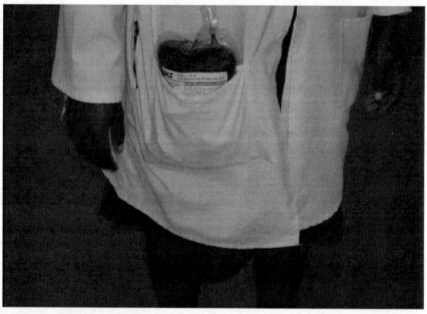

Figure 1. A clinical student carrying a unit of blood from a hospital blood bank to the patient in the pocket of in his white protective coat.

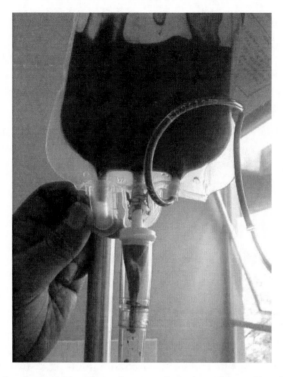

Figure 2. A unit of blood at the bedside, where the nurse has pierced the spike of the administration set through the tube of the inlet port.

Conclusion

In order for Blood Services, or Establishments, to meet the national requirements for access to safe, adequate and affordable blood components for the private and public sector, the services must be clearly identified entities, with an approved legislative frame work, which must be adequately financed, effectively managed and organised by qualified and experienced financial managers, with medical direction, trained technical, nursing and required support staff.

Infrastructure, facilities and budget can then be transparently and accurately quantified and justified, which will be the tools used to table annual fiscal and other budgets approved through the Ministries of Health and the respective Financial Directorates.

The Step Wise Accreditation Scheme, developed by AfSBT, will assist country assessments and objectively document progress and shortcomings impartially and unequivocally, to ensure that Quality Systems are sustainable and effective. Strategies, which only promote blood donation, will be of little use if facilities and systems are not in place and the clinical interface and bedside practice are not addressed.

Collection of data to establish an accurate and credible database, by independent evaluation, will be an important tool in the step-wise accreditation strategy and will serve as an advocacy document to encourage policy makers and national health authorities to support and implement WHA Resolutions and WHO recommendations to ensure blood safety and quality systems, as endorsed by successive Ministers of Health from all Member States, in the numerous World Health Assembly Resolutions, since 1975.

Although there is a trend for some health services to be devolved into public-private sector partnerships, the evidence from successful Blood Services and Establishments demonstrates that an organization established as a separate national entity, with a well-developed business plan (even though not-for-profit), autonomy from individual hospital administration and budgets and registration by appropriate legal and regulatory frameworks, are critical for achieving effective and sustainable quality blood transfusion services that meet all national needs

References

[1]   http://www.un.org/millennium/declaration/ares552e.pdf

[2]   Resolutions relating to blood safety adopted by WHO governing bodies. http://www. who.int/bloodsafety/BTS_Resolutions Adopted.pdf-WHO/WHA Resolutions on Blood and Blood Product Safety; WHA 28.72 (1975)

[3]   Blood Feuds, Feldman E. and Bayer R., editors – Oxford Press, UK 1999, ISBN 0-19-512929-6];

[4]   Jager, H., Jersild, C., Emmanuel, J. C. Safe Blood Transfusions in Africa; - *AIDS* 1991;5 (suppl. 1):S163–S168

[5]   Reducing HIV Transmission Through Blood; - Emmanuel, J. C., Britten, A. F. H. *AIDS Prevention Handbook*, 1992;

[6]   Moore, A., Herrera, G., Nyamongo, J., et al. Estimated risk of HIV transmission by blood transfusion in Kenya. *Lancet* 2001;358:657-660;

[7]   Quality Management Programme Facilitator's Tool Kit 2004, WHO/ EHT/04.13 Geneva, CH;

[8]   The Clinical Use of Blood. *Handbook – WHO/BTS/99.3 Geneva*, CH 2001– ISBN 92 4 154539 9;

[9]   Safe Blood in Developing Countries – The Lessons from Uganda, Winsbury R editor. *Development Studies and Research*, EC Brussels, BE 1995- ISBN 92-827-5281-X;

[10]   Pitman, J., Marum, L., Basavaraju, S., McIntyre, A. Progress toward strengthening blood transfusion services – 14 countries, 2003-2007. *MMWR* 2008;57:1273-1277

[11]   Holmberg, J., Basavaraju, S., Reed, C., Drammeh, B., Qualls, M. Progress toward strengthening national blood transfusion services – 14 countries, 2008-2010. *MMWR*, 2011;60:1578-1582;

[12]   WHO Blood safety and availability, Fact sheet 279, June 2012. Accessible from http:// www.who.int/mediacentre/factsheets/fs279/en/ index.html;

[13]   Blood safety and availability: facts and figures from the 2007 Blood Safety Survey. Geneva, Switzerland: World Health Organization; 2009. Downloadable from http://www.who.int/mediacentre/factsheets/fs279/ en/index.html;

[14]   Basavaraju, S. V., Mwangi, J., Nyamongo, J., et al. Reduced risk of transfusion-transmitted HIV in Kenya through centrally coordinated blood centres, stringent donor selection and effective p24 antigen-HIV antibody screening. *Vox Sang* 2010; 99: 212—219; Okonji, J., Basavaraju, S., Mwangi, J., et al. Comparison of HIV-1 detection in

plasma specimens and dried blood spots using the Roche COBAS Ampliscreen HIV-1 test in Kisumu, Kenya. *J. Virol. Methods* 2012; 179 21-25.

[15]   AABB Quality Manuals for Blood Safety; Accessible from http://www.aabb.org/pages/ Products.aspx?category=BOOK

[16]   Africa Society for Blood Transfusion (AfSBT) Step-wise Accreditation Document; accessible from - http://www.afsbt.org/index.php?option=com_contentandview= articleandid=37andItemid=73

[17]   http://www.who.int/bloodsafety/publications/am_Developing_a_national_blood_ system.pdf

[18]   WHO Global Database on Blood Safety. Report 2004-2005; WHO/EHT/08.07 downloadable from http://www.who.int/bloodsafety/global_database/GDBSReport 2004-2005.pdf

[19]   Global Blood Safety and Availability. Facts and figures from 2007 survey, WHO Geneva CH accessible from http://www.who.int/bloodsafety/global_database/GDBS_ Summary_Report_2008.pdf

[20]   Basavaraju, S., Pitman, J., Henry, N., Harry, C., Hasbrouck, L., Marum, L. The need for computerized tracking systems for resource-limited settings: the example of Georgetown, Guyana. *Transfus. Med.* 2009;19: 149-151.

In: Quality Management in Transfusion Medicine
Editor: Cees Th. Smit Sibinga

ISBN: 978-1-62618-665-1
© 2013 Nova Science Publishers, Inc.

Chapter XV

Annexes

Cees Th. Smit Sibinga

Annex 1 – Flow Charts

1   Blood procurement (Blood Establishment)

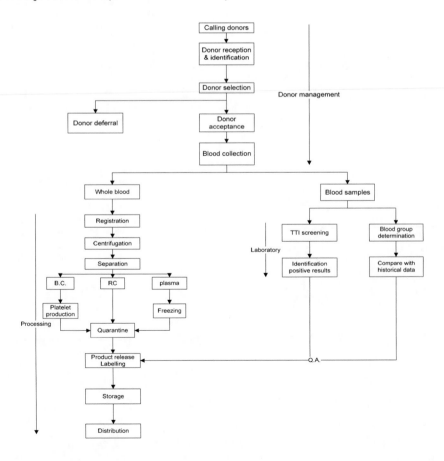

2   Donor management (collection)

Donor Management

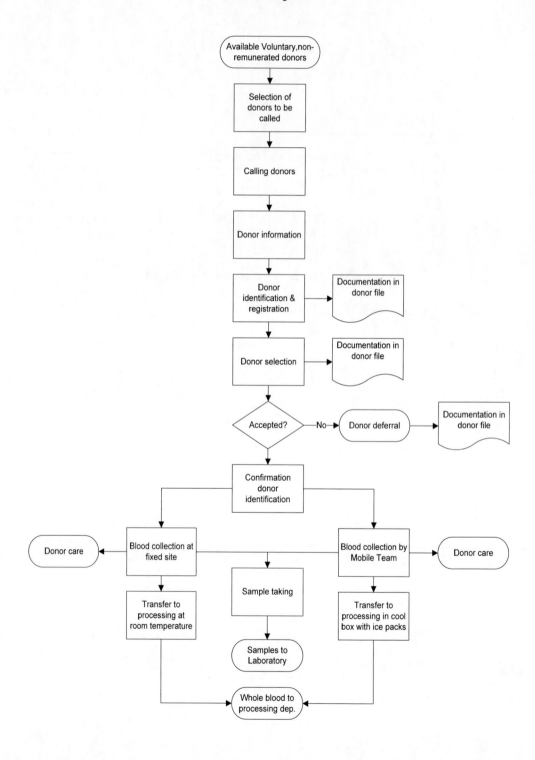

3 Blood processing (component production, storage and distribution)

Blood processing

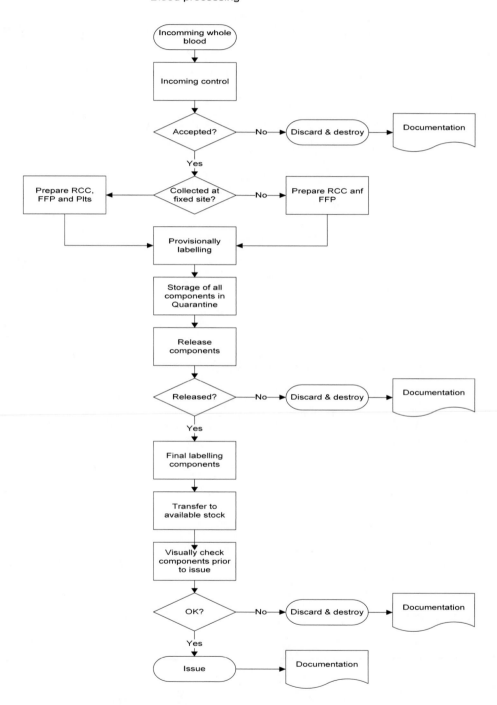

4   Routine (mandatory) quality control/testing

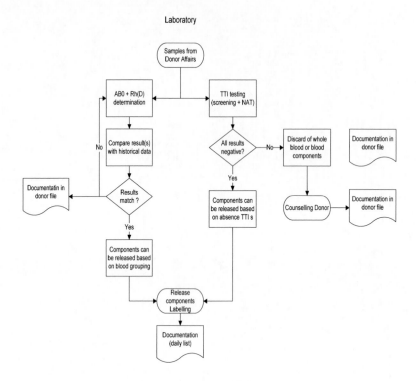

5   In-process quality control/component specifications

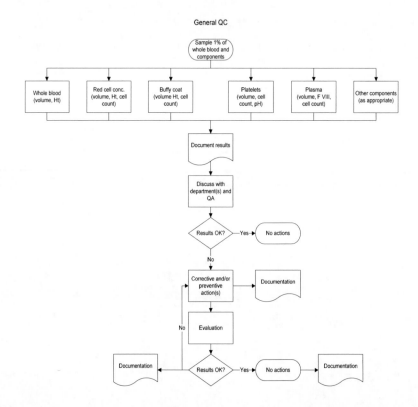

6 Platelet quality control

Platelets QC

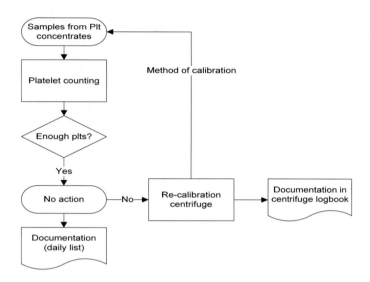

7 External Quality Assessment Scheme structure

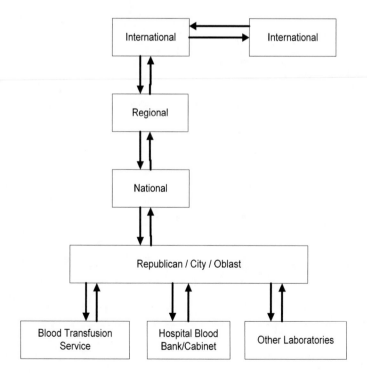

8 In-hospital transfusion process

In Hospital Transfusion Flow

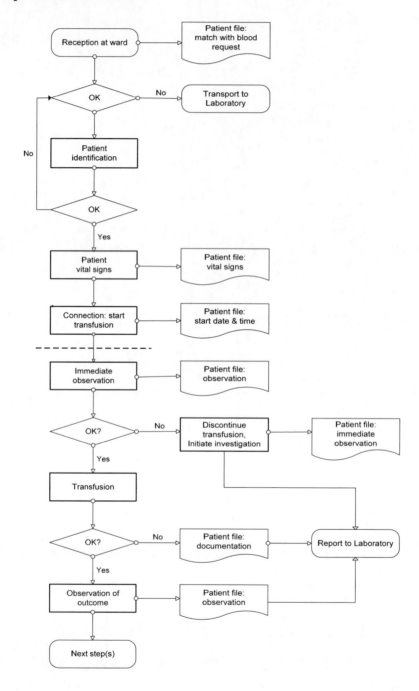

Annex 2 – Check Lists
(Quality System Essentials)

1. Checklist for QSE Supporting Documents

Documents that Support the Processes of the QSEs

PROCESSES: Facilities may use this list as a checklist to verify that they have these processes in place in their facility. Facilities may find a need to add more processes to this list based on facility-specific, local, and state requirements.
ORGANIZATION • Blood Establishment/Hospital Transfusion Service Organization Chart • Executive/Senior Management Authority and Responsibilities • Medical Director Authority and Responsibilities • Annual Quality Plan • Emergency Operations Plans • Management Review Process • Justification of Exceptions to Established Policy, Processes, or Procedures
RESOURCES • Job Description Development and Maintenance Process • Hiring Process • Education (Teaching and Training) Process • Competence Assessment Process • Performance Appraisal Process • End of Employment Process • Finance and accounting process
EQUIPMENT • Equipment Selection Process • Equipment Installation Process • Calibration Process and Schedule • Maintenance Process and Schedule • Alarm Response Process
SUPPLIER AND CUSTOMER ISSUES • Supplier Selection Process • Purchasing Process • Receiving, Inspection and Testing Process • Supplier Audit and Evaluation Process
PROCESS CONTROL • Change Control Process (Process Validation Process) • Test Method Implementation Process • Quality Control Programmes, Schedules, and Procedures • Proficiency Testing (Internal and External) Process • Work Operations Processes – Donor Handling and Blood Collection – • Donor Qualification Process • Blood Donor Informed Consent Process

- Whole Blood Collection Process
- Aphaeresis, Blood/Component Collection Process
- Confidential Unit Exclusion Process
- Care of Donors Process
Component Preparation/Blood Processing –
- Component Preparation Processes (red cells, platelets, plasma, cryoprecipitate, etc)
- Quarantine/Disposition of Units from Prior Collection Process
- Blood Component Quarantine Release and Final Labeling Process
- Blood Component Final Inspection Before Distribution Process
- Consignee Notification of Nonconforming Units Process
Quality Control (Laboratory Testing) –
- Donor Blood Testing Processes (serology, infectious diseases)
- Donor Notification of Abnormal Findings/Test Results Process
Handling, Storage and Distribution (Cold Chain) –
- Handling, Storage, and Distribution Processes
Clinical Handling and Use –
- Donor Unit Blood Type Confirmation Process
- Recipient Consent Process
- Blood Component Request Process
- Urgent Requirement for Blood and Components Process
- Pretransfusion Sample Collection Process
- Pretransfusion Compatibility Testing Processes (incl. component selection)
- Blood Component Final Inspection Before Issue Process
- Reissue of Blood and Components Process

(Continued)

- Blood Component Administration Process
- Adverse Reaction Investigation Process
- Rh Immune Globulin Process
- Dispensing and Use of Tissue Processes
- Therapeutic Phlebotomy Process
- Therapeutic Aphaeresis Process

DOCUMENTS AND RECORDS
- Document Master List
- Document Creation, Review, and Approval Process
- Annual Review Process
- Document Distribution and Archiving Process
- Record Filing Process
- Record Storage and Distribution Process
- Record Retention Schedule
- Record Copying Process
- Record Destruction Process
- Computer System Validation Process
- Computer Downtime Process
- Computer Back-up Process

DEVIATIONS, NONCONFORMANCES, AND COMPLICATIONS
- Evaluation of Nonconforming Blood, Components Process
- Blood Component Deviation Reporting to Competent Authority Process

| • Evaluation of Nonconforming Derivatives and Critical Materials Process |
| • Evaluation of Nonconforming Services Process |
| • Fatal Donor and Transfusion Recipient Reaction Process |
| • Suspected Transfusion Recipient Complications Reporting and Evaluation Process |
| • Look-Back Process |
| • Transfusion-Transmitted Disease Reporting and Investigation Process |
| **ASSESSMENTS** |
| • External Assessment Process |
| • Internal Assessment Process |
| • Quality Reporting Process (to executive management for review) |
| • Blood Utilization Review Process |
| **PROCESS IMPROVEMENT** |
| • Event (incident, error, accident, nonconformance) Management Process |
| • Complaint Management Process |
| • Corrective Action Process |
| • Preventive Action Process |
| • Quality Indicator Process |
| **FACILITIES AND SAFETY** |
| • Dressing Code Plan |
| • Entrance Restriction and Control Plan |
| • Infection Control Plan |
| • Chemical Hygiene Plan |
| • Radiation Safety Plan |
| • Disaster Plan (fire, weather, armed conflict, other) |
| • Hazardous Waste Disposal Plan |

2. Checklist for Ongoing Competence Testing

Ongoing Competence Assessment Process

What happens	Who's responsible	Applicable documents
Job requirements are established	BB/TS supervisor	Current job descriptions
Test results reviewed	BB/TS supervisor	Employee's worksheets
Other work reviewed	BB/TS supervisor	Other work records such as: worksheets, QC records PT results, calibration results
Assessment exercises developed and assigned	BB/TS supervisor	Direct observations Unknown specimens Quizzes, case studies, problem cases
Assessment exercises performed	Employee	Worksheets and answer sheets
Direct observation of work duties and maintenance	Employee performs Supervisor observes	Direct observation checklists
Determination if criteria for competence were met	BB/TS supervisor	Competence assessment documentation summary form
Training needs identified	BB/TS supervisor and employee	
Remedial measures developed and initiated	BB/TS supervisor	Remedial action plan
Remedial measures performed	Employee	Worksheets and answer sheets
Documentation filed	BB/TS supervisor	Employee file

Adapted from: A model quality system for the transfusion service.
Bethesda, MD: American Association of Blood Banks, 1997.

3. Competence Testing Flow Chart

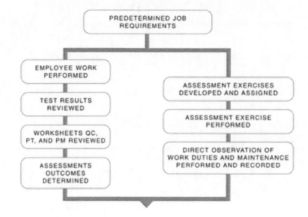

Ongoing Competence Assessment Process. (Continued).

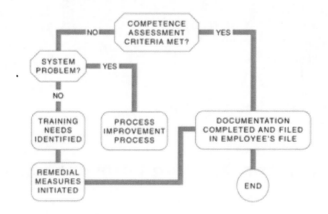

Adapted from: A model quality system for the transfusion service.
Bethesda, MD: American Association of Blood Banks, 1997.

Ongoing Competence Assessment Process.

Annex 3 – Quality Terminology

The use of terminology is commonplace in quality.

It is essential that all words and phrases used are clearly defined to ensure that there are no misunderstandings or any confusion about their use. However, it is acknowledged that definitions are often a source of intense debate, and consequently care has been taken to use accepted definitions from ISO 9000, but not all of the terms used within the materials are defined within the most recent ISO standard. In these cases the most commonly accepted international definitions have been used in the absence of any other formal definitions.

In situations where there is any doubt about the meaning of any of the terms used within the materials, reference should be made to this glossary and the definition given; this definition is the one that should be applied.

Quality Terminology

A –	
Acceptable quality level (AQL)	The maximum percentage or proportion of nonconformities in a lot or batch that can be considered satisfactory as a process average.
Acceptance sampling	Statistical quality control technique used in deciding to accept or reject a shipment of input or output.
Accreditation	Procedure by which an authoritative body gives formal recognition that a body or person is competent to carry out specific tasks
Accident	Undesirable, unexpected and unintended event
Accuracy	Agreement between the results obtained and the true value.
Accreditation	To recognize as conforming with a standard.
Active data gathering	A method for gathering data that involves approaching respondents to get information.
Actively solicited customer feedback	Proactive methods for obtaining customer feedback such as calling customers on the telephone or inviting customers to participate in focus groups.
Activity network diagram	Also knows as a PERT diagram, an activity network diagram is a tool used in controlling projects
Aesthetics	A dimension of quality that refers to subjective sensory characteristics such as taste, sound, look, and smell.
Affinity diagram	A tool that is used to help groups identify the common themes that are associated with a particular problem.
Alignment	Term that refers to optimal coordination among disparate departments and divisions within a firm.
Annuity relationship	This occurs when a business receives many repeat purchases from a customer. The income is received steadily over time from a single customer.
Appraisal costs	Expenses associated with the direct costs of measuring quality.
Assessment	Investigation and determination of the quality or value of a performance or situation
Assurance	A dimension of service quality that refers to the knowledge and courtesy of employees and their ability to inspire trust and confidence
Attribute	A binomial state of being.
Attributes data	Data that is counted in discrete units such as dollars, hours, items, and yes/no options. The alternative to attributes data is variables data, which is data that is measured on a continuous and infinite scale such as temperature or distance. Charts that use attribute data include bar charts, pie charts, Pareto charts and some control charts.
Attrition	The practice of not hiring new employees to replace older employees who either quit or retire.
Audit	Systematic, independent and documented examination to determine whether activities comply with planned and agreed quality system Systematic , independent and documented process for obtaining evidence and evaluating it objectively to determine the extent to which audit criteria are fulfilled - ISO 9000
Audit client	Person or organization requesting an audit - ISO 9000

Quality Terminology. (Continued)

A –	
Audit conclusions	Outcome of an audit decided by the audit team after consideration of all the audit findings - ISO 9000
Audit criteria	Set of policies, procedures or requirements against which collected audit evidence is compared - ISO 9000
Audit evidence	Records, verified statements of fact or other information relevant to the audit - ISO 9000
Audit findings	Identified compliances and non-compliances against the standards used for the audit Results of the evaluation of the collected audit evidence against audit criteria - ISO 9000
Audit plan	Description of the activities and arrangements for an audit – ISO 9000
Audit program	Set of audits to be carried out during a planned timeframe - ISO 9000
Audit scope	Extent or range of a given audit - ISO 9000
Audit team	The individual(s) performing the audit One or more auditors conducting an audit, one of whom is appointed as leader - ISO 9000
Auditee	Process, department, organization being audited Organization being audited - ISO 9000
Auditor	Person qualified and competent to conduct audits - ISO 9000
Availability	A product or service's ability to perform its intended function at a given time and under appropriate conditions. It can be expressed by the ratio operative time/total time where operative time is the time that it is functioning or ready to function.
Average chart (X-bar chart)	A control chart in which the average of the subgroup, represented by the X-bar, is to determine the stability or lack thereof in the process. Average charts are usually paired with range charts or sample standard deviation charts for complete analysis.
Award audits	Site visits relating to award programmes
B –	
Bar chart	A chart that compares different groups of data to each other through the use of bars that represent each group. Bar charts can be simple, in which each group of data consists of a single type of data, or grouped or stacked, in which the groups of data are broken down into internal categories.
Basic events	Term used in fault tree analysis. Basic events are initiating faults that do not require events below them to show how they occurred. The symbol used for a basic event is a circle.
Basic prototype	Nonworking mock-up of a product that can be reviewed by customers prior to acceptance.
Basic seven (B7) tools of quality	These are the fundamental methods for gathering and analyzing quality-related data. They are: fishbone diagrams, histograms, Pareto analysis, flowcharts, scatter plots, run charts, and control charts.
Bathtub-shaped hazard function	Reliability model that shows that products are more likely to fail either very early in their useful life or very late in their useful life.

B –	
Benchmark	An organization that is recognized for its exemplary operational performance in one or more areas and is willing to allow others to view its operations and tour its facilities.
Benchmarking	The process of finding a company that is superior in a particular area, studying what it does, and gathering ideas for improving your own operation in that area.
Best-of-the-best	Term used to refer to outstanding world benchmark firms
Best-in-class	Term used to refer to firms or organizations that are viewed as the best in an industry on some meaningful criterion.
Blood	Whole blood collected from a donor and processed either for transfusion or for further manufacturing
Blood component	A therapeutic constituent of blood (red cells, white cells, platelets, plasma) that can be prepared by various methods
Blood component release	A process which enables a blood component to be released from a quarantine status by the use of systems and procedures to ensure that the finished product meets the release specifications.
Blood cold chain	The maintained storage of blood and products at the appropriate storage temperature and conditions from the point of collection to the point of use – 'vein to vein'
Blood Establishment	Any structure or body that is responsible for any aspect of the collection and testing of human blood or blood components, whatever their intended purpose, and their processing, storage, and distribution when intended for transfusion. This does not include hospital blood banks.
Blood Service	Synonymous to Blood Establishment
Blood usage review (BUR)	An activity that includes the planned, systematic, ongoing measurement, assessment, and improvement of the ordering, distributing, handling, dispensing, administration, and monitoring of the use of blood and blood components in a health care facility.
Brainstorming	A tool used to encourage creative thinking and new ideas. A group formulates and records as many ideas as possible concerning a certain subject, regardless of the content of the ideas. No discussion, evaluation, or criticism of ideas is allowed until the brainstorming session is complete.
Breakthrough thinking	A management technique which emphasizes the development of new, radical approaches to traditional constraints, as opposed to incremental or minor changes in thought that build on the original approach.
Business process redesign or Reengineering	A management method which stresses the fundamental rethinking of processes, questioning all assumptions, in an effort to streamline organizations, and to focus on adding value in core processes.

Quality Terminology. (Continued)

C –	
Calibration	The set of operations which establish, under specified conditions, the relationship between values indicated by a measuring instrument or measuring system, or values represented by a material measure, and the corresponding known values of a reference standard. Comparison of a measurement standard or instrument of known accuracy with another standard or instrument of lesser accuracy in order to confirm, delete, correlate, report or eliminate by adjustment, any variation in the accuracy or the item being compared.
Capability	Ability to an organization, system or process to realize a product that fulfils the requirements for that product - ISO 9000
Care mapping	Medical procedure for a particular diagnosis in a diagrammatic form that includes key decision points used to coordinate care and instruct patient.
Categorizing	The act of placing strengths and weakness into categories in generic internal assessment.
Cause and Effect diagram (fishbone or Ishikawa diagram)	A tool used to analyze all factors (causes) that contribute to a given situation or occurrence (effect) by breaking down main causes into smaller and smaller sub-causes. It is also known as the Ishikawa or the fishbone diagram.
CEO	Chief executive officer
Certification audit	Audits relating to registration (e.g., ISO 9000 audits).
Chain of customers	A philosophy that espouses the idea that each worker's "customer" is the next worker in the chain of people that produce a finished product or service.
Change	In the context of quality management, this means to move from one state of operation to another state of operation.
Change management	The management of moving from one state of operation to another state of operation.
Characteristic	Distinguishing feature - ISO 9000
Check sheet	A customized form used to record data. Usually, it is used to record how often some activity occurs.
Check list	A list of important steps that must take place in a process or any other activity. A list of things to do.
Clean area	An area with defined environmental control of particulate and microbial contamination constructed and used in such a way as to reduce the introduction, generation and retention of contaminants within the area. Note: The different degrees of environmental control are defined in the EU Supplementary Guidelines for the Manufacture of sterile medicinal products.
Clean/contained area	An area constructed and operated in such a manner that will achieve the aims of both a clean area and a contained area at the same time.
Clinical practice guideline	A general term for statements of an accepted medical procedure/ intervention for a particular diagnosis.

C –	
Common causes	Inherent causes of variation in a process. They are typical of the process, not unexpected. That is not to say that they must be tolerated; on the contrary, once special causes of variation are largely removed, a focus on removing common causes of variation can pay big dividends.
Compensate	(1) To pay or remunerate for some work; (2) To make up for some lack of ability or acuity
Competence	Demonstrated personnel attributes and demonstrated ability to apply knowledge and skills
Competence assessment	The objective measurement of an individual's ability to perform a specific job or task. Synonymous with competence evaluation and competence testing.
Complaint-recovery process	Process associated with resolving complaints.
Complementary products	Products that use similar technologies and can coexist in a family of products.
Compliance	Meeting required standards
Component reliability	The propensity for a part to fail over a given time.
Computer-aided design (CAD)	A system for digitally developing product designs.
Computer-aided inspection (CAI)	A system for performing inspection through the use of technology. For example, some systems use infrared to detect defects.
Computer-aided testing (CAT)	Technology for taking tests or examinations.
Computer-based training	A form of training that uses specialized software, known as courseware, to address specific topics.
Concept design	The process of determining which technologies will be used in production and the product.
Concession	Authorization to use or release a product that does not conform to specified requirements - ISO 9000
Concurrent engineering	The simultaneous performance of product design and process design. Typically, concurrent engineering involves the formation of cross-functional teams. This allows engineers and managers of different disciplines to work together simultaneously in developing product and process designs.
Conformance or conformity	Fulfillment of a requirement or specification - ISO 9000
Consistency	Doing the same thing time after time, makes the outcome more predictable and allows for reduced variation in products and processes
Consultant audits	Inspections that are performed by consultants to determine how an organization should be changed for improvement.
Consumer's risk	The risk of receiving a shipment of poor quality product and believing that it is good quality.
Contact personnel	The people at the "front lines" who interact with the public in a service setting.
Contingency theory	A theory that presupposes that there is no theory or method for operating a business that can be applied in all instances.

Quality Terminology. (Continued)

C –	
Continual improvement	Recurring activity to increase the ability to fulfil requirements
Continuous improvement	On-going improvement of any and all aspects of an organization including products, services, communications, environment, functions, individual processes, etc.
Continuous quality improvement	The ongoing improvement process at the centre of all quality systems: plan, do, check and act; as encapsulated in the Deming Cycle
Contract	Formal agreement of intention to supply a product or service in accordance with agreed specifications. Binding agreement.
Contract review	Systematic activities carried out by the purchaser to ensure that contractual requirements for quality have been met and are adequately defined, free from ambiguity and can be realized by the supplier.
Contrition	Forgiveness for error or mistake.
Control chart	A chart that indicates upper and lower statistical control limits, and an average line, for samples or subgroups of a given process. If all points on the control chart are within the limits, variation may be ascribed to common causes and the process is deemed to be "in control." If points fall outside the limits, it is an indication that special causes of variation are occurring, and the process is said to be "out of control."
Control factors	Variables in a Taguchi experiment that are under the control of the operator. These can include things such as temperature or type of ingredient.
Control limit	A statistically-determined line on a control chart used to analyze variation within a process. If variation exceeds the control limits, then the process is being affected by special causes and is said to be "out of control." NB: A control limit is not the same as a specification limit.
Control process	A process involving gathering process data, analyzing process data, and using this information to make adjustments to the process.
Conversion process	Aligning the inputs of a process together to form a product or service.
Correction	Action taken to eliminate a detected nonconformity - ISO 9000
Corrective action	Action taken to eliminate the cause of a detected nonconformity or other undesirable situation - ISO 9000 Remedial action taken to rectify a non-compliance or other situation in which an error has occurred.
Cost of poor quality	The costs incurred by producing products or services of poor quality. These costs usually include the cost of inspection, rework, duplicate work, scrapping rejects, replacements and refunds, complaints, and loss of customers and reputation.
Count chart (c chart)	An attributes data control chart that evaluates process stability by charting the counts of occurrences of a given event in successive samples. (A chart used to monitor the number of defects in a production process).

C –	
Count-per-unit chart (u chart)	A control chart that evaluates process stability by charting the number of occurrences of a given event per unit sampled, in a series of samples.
Cp	Commonly used process capability index defined as [USL (upper spec limit) - LSL (lower spec limit)] / [6 x sigma], where sigma is the estimated process standard deviation.
Cpk	Commonly used process capability index defined as the lesser of USL - m / 3sigma or m - LSL / 3sigma, where sigma is the estimated process standard deviation.
Criteria	Elements against something can be measured.
Critical control points (CCP)	Key elements that need documentation
Criticality	A term that refers to how often a failure will occur, how easy it is to diagnose, and whether it can be fixed.
Cross-functional teams	Teams with members from differing departments and vocations.
Cross-training	Training an employee to do several different jobs.
Cumulated sum chart	Control chart that shows the cumulative sum of deviations from a set value in successive samples. Each plotted point indicates the algebraic sum of the last point and all deviations since. NB: PathMaker does not support cumulative sum charts.
Current Good Manufacturing Practice (cGMP)	Part of quality assurance that ensures that products are consistently manufactured to, and controlled by, the quality standard appropriate to their intended use; encompasses both manufacturing and quality control procedures.
Customer	Organization or person that receives a product - ISO 9000 Any recipient who uses and can be affected by a product or service one produces. A customer can be external (outside the organization) or internal to the organization.
Customer benefits package (CBP)	The package of tangibles and intangibles that make up a service.
Customer contact	A characteristic of services that notes that customers tend to be more involved in the production of services than they are in manufactured goods.
Customer coproduction	The participation of a customer in the delivery of a service product. For example, in many restaurants it is not uncommon for customers to fill their own drinks.
Customer dissatisfaction	Customer's opinion of the degree to which a transaction has failed to meet the customer's needs and expectations - ISO 9000
Customer-driven quality	Term that refers to a proactive approach to satisfying customer needs.
Customer expectations	(1) What customers expect from a service provider; (2) A part of the SERVQUAL questionnaire.
Customer future needs projection	Predicting the future needs of customers and designing products that satisfy those needs.

Quality Terminology. (Continued)

C –	
Customer perceptions	(1) How customers view products or services; (2) The second part of the SERVQUAL survey.
Customer rationalization	The process of reaching an agreement between marketing and operations as to which customers add the greatest advantage and profits over time.
Customer-related ratios	Ratios that include customer satisfaction, customer dissatisfaction, and comparisons of customer satisfaction relative to competitors.
Customer-relationship management	A view of the customer that asserts that the customer is a valued asset that should be managed.
Customer retention	The percentage of customers who return to a service provider or continue to purchase a manufactured product.
Customer satisfaction	Customer's opinion of the degree to which a transaction has met the customer's needs and expectations - ISO 9000
Customer service surveys	Instruments that consists of a series of items (or questions) that are designed to elicit customer perceptions
D –	
Decision matrix	A tool used to evaluate problems, solutions, or ideas. The possibilities are listed down the left-hand side of the matrix and relevant criteria are listed across the top. Each possibility is then rated on a numeric scale of importance or effectiveness (e.g. on a scale of 1 to 10) for each criterion, and each rating is recorded in the appropriate box. When all ratings are complete, the scores for each possibility are added to determine which has the highest overall rating and thus deserves the greatest attention.
Deduction	An approach to theory development based on modelling.
Defect	Failure of a product or procedure to meet part or all of its given specification Non-fulfilment of a requirement related to an intended or specified use - ISO 9000
Deficiency	See non-compliance EMEA
Deficiencies, critical	See non-compliance EMEA
Deficiencies, major	See non-compliance EMEA
Deficiencies, other significance	See non-compliance EMEA
Deming cycle	The Plan-Do-Check-Act cycle, a four-stage approach to problem-solving. It is also sometimes called the Shewhart cycle.
Dependability	Collective term used to describe the availability performance and its influencing factors: reliability performance, maintainability performance, and maintenance support performance - ISO 9000
Design and development	Set of processes that transforms requirements into specified characteristics and into the specification of the product realization process - ISO 9000
Design control	A set of steps focused on managing the design of a product

D –	
Design for disassembly	A method for developing products so that they can easily be taken apart.
Design for maintainability	A concept that states that products should be designed in a way that makes them easy for consumers to maintain.
Design for manufacture (DFM)	The principle of designing products so that they are cost effective and easy to make.
Design for remanufacture	A method for developing products so that the parts can be used in other products. Associated with green manufacturing.
Design for reuse	Designing products so they can be used in later generations of products.
Design of Experiments (DOE)	DOE is the science of designing sets of experiments which will generate enough useful data to make sound decisions without costing too much or taking too long.
Design review	The process of checking designs for accuracy.
Development plan	A plan that identifies the skills that will be required for a particular employee to move up in an organization.
Deviation permit	Authorization to depart from the originally specified requirements of a product prior to realization, for a limited quantity of product or period of time, and for a specific use - ISO 9000
Diagnostic journey or remedial journey	A problem-solving approach in which a problem is investigated by looking first at symptoms, and gradually working back towards root causes. Once root causes have been established, experimentation and tracking are used in the remedial journey - the finding of a cure for the roots of the problem.
Distance learning	Training that is conducted in one location and is observed in a distant location through telecommunications technology.
Distribution	The act of delivery of blood and blood components to other blood establishments, hospital blood banks and manufacturers of blood and plasma derived products. It does not include the issuing of blood or blood components
Document	All the written instructions, records and actions involved in providing a product or service Information and its support medium - ISO 9000
Document control	Formal control of the issue, use and review of authorized documents within the quality system
Documentation hierarchy	A scheme documenting the quality system, using the following levels: Level 1 (A) – Philosophy and Principles (*the what*) Level 2 (B) – Principles and Strategy (*the when, where and who; cross-functional quality processes*) Level 3 (C1) – Practice (*the how, i.e., procedures and work instructions at the task level*) Level 4 (C2) – Evidence (*the records and forms; outcome documents*)
Donation	Blood and blood components collected from an individual and intended for transfusion to another individual (allogeneic) or to the same (autologous).

Quality Terminology. (Continued)

D –	
Donor	A person in normal health with good medical history who voluntarily gives blood or plasma for therapeutic use.
Donor, first time	Someone who has never donated either blood or plasma.
Donor, paid or professional	Donor who willingly donates blood against payment (money or kind)
Donor, prospective	Someone who presents him/her self ar a blood or plasma collection establishment and states his/her wish to give blood or plasma.
Donor, regular	Someone who routinely donates their blood or plasma (i.e. within the last two years), in accordance with minimum time intervals, in the same donation centre.
Donor, repeat	Someone who has donated before but not within the last two years in the same donation centre.
Donor, replacement or family	Donor recruited by a patient to endorse then to undergo therapy which requires blood transfusion. The recruited donor could be family or unrelated.
Dual sourcing	Using only a few suppliers for a single component.
Durability	A dimension of quality that refers to a product's ability to withstand stress or trauma.
E –	
Effectiveness	Measure of the extent to which planned activities are realized and planned results achieved - ISO 9000
Efficiency	Relationship between the result achieved and the resources used - ISO 9000
Employee involvement	Regular participation of employees in decision-making and suggestions. The driving forces behind increasing the involvement of employees are the conviction that more brains are better, that people in the process know it best, and that involved employees will be more motivated to do what is best for the organization.
Electronic data interchange (EDI)	Using computers to share data between customers and suppliers.
Empathy	A dimension of service quality that refers to the amount of caring and individualized attention exhibited by the service firm.
Empowerment	A management initiative designed to move decision making to the lowest level in the organization. Usually refers to giving employees decision-making and problem-solving authority within their jobs.
End user	The ultimate user of a product or service.
Engineering analysis	The process of applying engineering concepts to the design of a product, including tests such as heat transfer analysis, stress analysis, or analysis of the dynamic behavior of the system being designed.
Enterprise capabilities	Capabilities that make firms unique and attractive to customers.
Enterprise resource planning (ERP)	A system that integrates financial, planning, and control systems into a single architecture. Examples include the SAP R/3 system and Oracle.
EQAS	External quality assessment scheme

E –	
Error	A mistake possibly resulting in non-compliance or non-conformance; a deviation from accuracy or correctness.
Evaluation	Determination of the amount, value or significance by careful appraisal and study. Assessment of how relevant resources and capabilities are to generic strategies in generic internal assessment.
Event	An occurrence
Expert	Individual with appropriate qualifications and experience to provide technical advice to a Competent Authority inspector
Experimental training techniques	Training that is hands-on and provides the recipients of training the opporunity to experience in some manner the concepts that are being taught.
Exporter	A firm that sells its product in another country.
External customer	A person or organization outside your organization who receives the output of a process. Of all external customers, the end-user should be the most important.
External evaluation or audit or assessment	An audit, inspection, evaluation, investigation, assessment or survey performed by an outside party for the purposes of licensing, accreditation or certification (e.g. ISO, Health Inspectorate or Competent Authority)
External evaluator or auditor	One who performs an evaluation but is not an employee of the organization being evaluated.
External events	A term used in fault tree analysis. An external event is an event that is normally expected to occur and thus is not considered a fault when it occurs by itself.
External failure costs	These are monetary losses associated with product failure after the customer has possession of the product. These may include warranty or field repair costs.
External quality assessment	The external assessment of a laboratory's performance using samples of known but undisclosed content, and including comparison against other laboratories
External services	Service that are provided by companies other than yours.
External validation	Using benchmarking as a way to ensure that a firm's current practices are comparable to those being used by benchmark firms.
F –	
Facilities	Hospitals, clinics, manufacturers, and biomedical research institutions to which blood or blood components may be delivered.
Facilitation	Helping a team or individual achieve a goal. Often used in meeting or with teams to help the teams achieve their objectives.
Facilitator	Person who helps a team with issues of teamwork, communication, and problem-solving. A facilitator should not contribute to the actual content of the team's project, focusing instead as an observer of the team's functioning as a group.
Familiarization visit	An activity, that includes a visit to a blood establishment in order for a candidate inspector to become familiar with its overall processes, functions and operations.

Quality Terminology. (Continued)

F –	
Failure costs	Two sets of costs — internal failure costs and external failure costs. Internal failure costs include those costs that are associated with failure during production, whereas external failure costs are associated with product failure after the production process.
Failure Mode Effects Analysis (FMEA)	A technique that systematically analyzes the types of failures which will be expected as a product is used, and what the effects of each "failure mode" will be.
Failure Mode Effects and Criticality Analysis (FMECA)	FMECA is an extensive but simple method for identifying ways in which an engineered system could fail. The primary goal of FMECA is to develop priorities for corrective action based on estimated risk.
Fault tree analysis	An analytical tool that graphically renders the combination of faults that lead to the failure of a system.
Features	A dimension of quality that refers to those attributes of a product
Final product definition	The process of articulating the final drawings and specifications for a product.
Financial benchmarking	Numerical ratios of firm performance such as return on equity, return on assets, and earnings per share.
Financial ratios	Numerical ratios of firm performance such as return on equity, return on assets, and earnings per share.
Fishbone or Ishikawa diagram	Another name for a Cause and Effect diagram, derived from the original shape of the diagram as used by its creator, Kaoru Ishikawa.
Fitness for purpose	Suitability of a product for the purpose for which it is intended
Five Ss	A process for inducing discipline in an organization.
5w2h	Who, what, when, where, why, how, and how much.
Flow chart	A graphical representation of a given process delineating each step. It is used to diagram how the process actually functions and where waste, error, and frustration enter the process.
Focus group	A group of people who are brought together and are asked to share their opinions about a particular product or service.
Force Field Analysis	A tool, developed by social psychologist Kurt Lewin, which is used to analyze the opposing forces involved in causing/resisting any change. It is shown in balance sheet format with forces that will help (driving forces) listed on the left and forces that hinder (restraining forces) listed on the right.
Forming	The first stage of team development, where the team is formed and the objectives for the team are set.
Frequency distribution	An organization of data, usually in a chart, which depicts how often an different events occur. A histogram is one common type of frequency distribution, and a frequency polygon is another.
Functional benchmarking	A type of benchmarking that involves the sharing of information among firms that are interested in the same functional issues.

G –	
Gantt chart	A bar chart that shows planned work and finished work in relation to time. Each task in a list has a bar corresponding to it. The length of the bar is used to indicate the expected or actual duration of the task.
Gap	The difference between desired levels of performance and actual levels of performance
Gap analysis	A term associated with the SERVQUAL survey instrument, gap analysis is a technique designed to assess the gap that can exist between a service that is offered and customer expectations.
Geometric modeling	A technique used to develop a computer-based mathematical description of a part.
GCP	Good Clinical Practice
Globalization	An approach to international markets that requires a firm to make fundamental changes in the nature of its business by establishing production and marketing facilities in foreign markets.
GLP	Good Laboratory Practice
GMP	Good Manufacturing Practice
Good manufacturing practice	That part of quality assurance which ensures that products are consistently produced and controlled to the quality standards appropriate for their intended use and legal requirements. All elements in the established practice that will collectively lead to final products or services that consistently meet appropriate specifications and compliance with national and international regulations.
Good practice	All elements in established practice that collectively will lead to final blood or blood components that consistently meet predefined specifications and compliance with defined regulations, or is being prescribed and used appropriately – safe and efficacious. There is good laboratory practice (GLP), good manufacturing practice (GMP) and good clinical practice (GCP).
Grade	Category or rank given to different quality requirements for products, processes or system having the same functional use
Green manufacturing	A method for manufacturing that minimizes waste and pollution. These goals are often achieved through product and process design.
Group decision support system	A computer system that allows users to anonymously input comments in a focus group type of setting.
Group technology	A component of CAD that allows for the cataloguing and standardization of parts and components for complex products.
Guideline	Document stating recommendations or suggestions - ISO 9000
H –	
Hard data	Measurements data such as height, weight, volume, or speed that can be measured on a continuous scale.
Hardware mock-ups	Physical representations of hardware that show designers, managers, and users how an eventual system will work
Haemovigilance	A set of organized surveillance procedures relating to serious adverse or unexpected events or reactions in donors or recipients, and the epidemiological follow-up of donors.

Quality Terminology. (Continued)

H –	
Heterogeneous	A characteristic of services that means that for many companies, no two services are exactly the same. For example, an advertising company would not develop the same advertising campaign for two different clients.
Hidden factory	A term introduced by Wickham Skinner that refers to firm activities that have no effect on the customer.
Histogram	A specialized bar chart showing the distribution of measurement data. It will pictorially reveal the amount and type of variation within a process
Horizontal deployment	A term that denotes that all of the departments of a firm are involved in the firm's quality efforts.
Hoshin planning	A method of strategic planning for quality. It helps executives integrate quality improvement into the organization's long-range plan. According to the GOAL/QPC Health Care Application Research Committee, "Hoshin Planning is a method used to ensure that the mission, vision, goals, and annual objectives of an organization are communicated to and implemented by everyone, from the executive level to the 'front line' level."
Hospital blood bank	A hospital unit which stores and distributes and may perform compatibility tests on blood and blood components exclusively for use within hospital facilities, including hospital based transfusion activities.
House of quality	Another name for quality function deployment
Human Resource Management (HRM)	The management of all aspects related to the human resource.
Human resource measures	Ratios that are used to measure the effectiveness of a firm's human resource practices.
I –	
Ideal quality	A reference point identified by Taguchi for determining the quality level of a product or service.
Imputability	The likelihood that a serious adverse reaction in a recipient can be attributed to the blood or blood component transfused, or that a serious adverse reaction in a donor can be attributed to the donation process.
Incident	Occurrence of importance that can lead to serious consequences.
Indicator	Quantitative measure of performance. Indicators are usually ratios comparing the number of occurrences a certain phenomenon and the number of times the phenomenon could have occurred.
Individual needs assessment	A method for determining training needs at the worker level prior to developing and implementing training programs. Often associated with company literacy programs.
Induction	An approach to theory development based on observation and description. Although the process of induction is useful, it is subject to observer bias and misperception.
Information	Meaningful data

I –	
Infrastructure	System of permanent facilities and equipment of an organization - ISO 9000
In-process inspection	The practice of inspecting work, by the workers themselves, at each stage of the production process.
Inspection	Conformity evaluation by observation and judgment accompanied as appropriate by measurement, testing or gauging - ISO 9000
Inspection schedule	A schedule prepared by the competent authority for an specific inspection. The schedule comprises the inspection content (based on the scope) and the time frame
Inspection team	A team comprising several individuals that perform an inspection. Very often an inspection team consists of two inspectors. One inspector will inspect the quality system and in the case of 'peer' inspections a technical specialist inspector may also be available
Inspection, external (regulatory)	An inspection carried out by the Health Inspectorate or Competent Authority or accreditation body. Formal and objective control according to adopted standards to assess compliance with the blood legislation and other relevant legislation and to identify problems. (This definition expands on the definitions given by the Directive 2002/98/EC and the CoE Guide).
Inspection, peer	A 'peer' inspection is carried out by inspectors from different facilities within the same blood establishment. The 'peer' inspection will require a multicentre structure of the same blood establishment that provides experts with equivalent skills and knowledge based at different locations. Alternatively, 'peer' inspections can be organised through the cooperation between national or regional blood services.
Inspection, self-	An inspection conducted by trained and competent representatives of the organisation but managerially independent of the department concerned. Note: There are several equivalent definitions for this term. The word self-inspection is very often used inter-alia with the terms 'audit' or 'internal-audit'
Inspector, lead	The lead inspector is responsible for coordinating the activity of the inspection 'team' and presenting the findings and outcomes of the self-inspection. In smaller blood establishment very often the inspections are carried out by a single inspector.
Inspectorate training programme	An inspectorate training programme covers general topics essential for the inspector, including principles of inspection techniques as well as specific and on-going training.
Installation qualifications	The verification that equipment and support systems are correctly installed and capable of consistently operating within the limits established by6 their design and required by a process.
Intangible	A characteristic of services that means that services (unlike manufactured goods) cannot be inventoried or carried in stock over a long period of time.
Interested party	Person or group having an interest in the performance or success of an organization - ISO 9000

Quality Terminology. (Continued)

I –	
Interference checking	A feasibility test for product designs to make sure that wires, cabling, and tubing in products such as airplanes don't conflict with each other.
Internal auditor or evaluator	One who works within the facility and performs an audit or evaluation, but is not responsible for the operations of the area being audited or evaluated.
Internal customer	Someone within your organization, further downstream in a process, who receives the output of your work.
Internal failure costs	Losses that occur while the product is in possession of the producer. These include rework and scrap costs.
Internal quality assessment or evaluation	The assessment of an institution's overall quality system by 'splitting' a sample into two and processing one normally and the other through the normal system but as a 'blind' sample and comparing the results with the normally identified sample.
Internal services	Services that are provided by internal company personnel. For example, data processing personnel are often considered providers of internal services.
Internal validation	Method of studying the quality system to find gaps in quality deployment.
Interrelationship digraph	A tool designed to help identify the causal relationships between the issues affecting a particular problem.
Investigation	Ability to find sources of competitive advantage in generic internal assessment.
Involuntary services	A classification for services that are not sought by customers. These include hospitals, prisons, and the Internal Revenue Service.
ISO	International Organization for Standardization. The organization that support the ISO Quality Standards Series.
ISO 9000 series	A set of voluntary worldwide quality standards applicable to organizations, the purpose of which is to provide guidance for suppliers in quality management and to provide generic requirements against which a customer can evaluate the adequacy of a supplier's quality system.
J –	
Job analysis	The process of collecting detailed information about a particular job. This information includes tasks, skills, abilities, and knowledge requirements that relate to certain jobs.
Just-in-time (JIT)	(1) A method for optimizing processes that involves continual reduction of waste; (2) The Toyota Motor Company production system; (3) An umbrella term that encompasses several Japanese management techniques.
Just-in-time (JIT) instruction	Training given as needed for immediate application, without lag time and the usual loss of retention.
Just-in-time (JIT) purchasing	An approach to purchasing that requires long-term agreements with few suppliers

K –	
Kaizen	A Japanese word meaning continuous improvement through constant striving to reach higher standards.
Key business factors (KBF)	Those measures or indicators that are significantly related to the business success of a particular firm.
KJ method	Another name for the affinity diagram, after its inventor, Kawakita Jiro.
Knowledge growth system	A compensation system that increases an employee's pay as he or she establishes competencies at different levels relating to job knowledge in a single job classification.
Knowledge work	Jobs that consist primarily of working with information.
L –	
Label control	A process that assures that labels, as controlled documents, are used according to specified protocols in the production process
Law of diminishing marginal returns	A law that stipulates that there is a point at which investment in quality improvement will become uneconomical.
Leader behaviour	A view of leadership stating that leadership potential is related to the behaviors an individual exhibits.
Leadership	The process by which a leader influences a group to move toward the attainment of a group of super-ordinate goals.
Leader skills	A view of leadership stating that leadership potential is related to the skills possessed by an individual.
Leading	The power relationship between two or more individuals where the power is distributed unevenly.
Learning curve effect	A theoretical concept that suggests that the more you do something, the better you become at doing it.
Licensing	A method of reaching international markets that does not require the establishment of international supply chains or marketing arms.
Life testing	A facet of reliability engineering that concerns itself with determining whether a product will fail under controlled conditions during a specified life.
Line-stop authority	The approval authority to stop a production line whenever a problem is detected.
Loss to society	According to Taguchi, this occurs every time a dimension in a product varies from its target dimension. This is associated with Taguchi's "ideal quality."
Lot tolerance percent defective (LTPD)	The maximum level of percent defective acceptable in production lots.
M –	
Maintenance, preventive maintenance	Such activities as cleaning, adjusting, modifying, overhauling, repairing a piece of equipment to assure its performance is in accordance with quality requirements. Maintenance of a software system includes correcting software errors, adapting software to a new environment or making enhancement to software
Malpractice	The result of mistakes made by a professional service provider.
Management	Coordinated activities to direct and control an organization - ISO 9000
Management by fact	A core value that focuses on data-based decision making.

Quality Terminology. (Continued)

Management system	System to establish policy and objectives and to achieve those objectives - ISO 9000
Manufacture	All steps in propagation or manufacture and/or preparation of products including but not limited to, filling, testing, labeling, packaging, and storage by the manufacturer.
Manufacturer	Any legal person or entity engaged in the manufacture of a product that is subject to license under Law.
Manufacturing-based	Dimensions of quality that are production related.
Manufacturing system design	The process of designing a manufacturing system.
Market share data	A comparative measure that determines relative positions of firms in the marketplace.
Matrix diagram	A brainstorming tool that can be used in a group to show the relationships between ideas or issues.
Mean	The average of a group of measurement values. Mean is determined by dividing the sum of the values by the number of values in the group.
Measurement	Set of operations having the object of determining the value of a quantity - ISO 9000
Measurement management system	Set of interrelated and interacting elements necessary to achieve metrological confirmation and continual control of measurement processes – ISO 9000
Measurement process	Set of interrelated resources, activities, and influences related to a measurement - ISO 9000
Measuring equipment	Measuring instrument, software, measurement standard, reference material or auxiliary apparatus or combination thereof to realize a measurement process – ISO 9000
Median	The middle of a group of measurement values when arranged in numerical order. For example, in the group (32, 45, 78, 79, 101), 78 is the median. If the group contains an even number of values, the median is the average of the two middle values.
Meeting management	A term that refers to the effective management of meeting in an organization.
Metacraftmanship	Metacraftsmanship is a term used to tie together the many ideas shared by quality improvement, reengineering, management, leadership, and customer-driven production. Although these theories have much in common, they are often treated as separate and disparate approaches to improving a business. Metacraftsmanship focuses on overcoming the losses to society which are engendered by specialization, and suggests ways of getting complex organizations to work the way a single craftsman would.
Metrological characteristics	Distinguishing feature which can influence the results of measurement – ISO 9000
Metrological confirmation	Set of operations required to ensure that measuring equipment (3.10.4) conforms the requirements for its intended use – ISO 9000

M –	
Metrological function	Function with administrative and technical responsibility for defining and implementing the measurement management system – ISO 9000
Mission statement	A written declaration of the purpose of an organization or project team. Organizational mission or vision statements often include an organizational vision for the future, goals, and values.
Mode	The most frequently occurring value in a group of measurements
Moment of truth	In a service context, the phrase "moment of truth" refers to the point in a service experience at which the customer expects something to happen.
Monitoring	Control of an operation (performance) for a special purpose and over a period of time
Mourning	The final stage of the team life cycle, where team members regret the ending of the project and the breaking up of the team.
MR chart	A chart for plotting variables when samples are not possible.
Multilevel approach	Term used to depict state quality award programs that include two levels: a top level based on the full-Baldrige criteria and a second level based on the Baldrige-lite approach.
Multiple skills systems	A method for developing employees so that they can perform more than a single task.
Multi-user-CAD system	Computer aided design systems that are networked so that multiple designers can work on a single design simultaneously.
N –	
Natural work groups	A term used to describe teams that are organized according to a common product, customer, or service.
New seven (7) tools	Managerial tools that are used in quality improvement
Noise	In the context of quality management, noise is essentially variability. For example, if you are making ketchup, noise in the process comes from variations in the quality of incoming tomatoes, in changes in ambient temperature and humidity, in variations in machinery performance, in variations in the quality of human factors, etc.
Nominal group technique	Technique used to encourage creative thinking and new ideas, but is more controlled than brainstorming. Each member of a group writes down his or her ideas and then contributes one to the group pool. All contributed ideas are then discussed and prioritized.
Non-compliance	Not meeting required standards
Non-compliance, critical	Any non-compliance in a process or a written procedure which directly affects the safety of the donor or patient.
Non-compliance, major	A serious non-compliance in a process or a written procedure but does not on its own affect the safety of the donor or patient.
Non-compliance, other significant	A non-compliance in a system or process or there is insufficient information to classify it as a major or critical. Note: There could be a combination of several "other" significant non-compliances, none of which on their own may be major or critical, but may together represent a major or critical non-compliance. These should be clearly explained and reported as such.

Quality Terminology. (Continued)

N –	
Nonconformity, non-conformance	Non-fulfilment of a requirement - ISO 9000
Norming	The third stage of team development, where the team becomes a cohesive unit, and interdependence, trust, and cooperation are built.
Non-random variation	Controllable variation
Np chart	A control chart indicating the number of defective units in a given sample.
O –	
Objective evidence	Data supporting the existence or verity of something - ISO 9000
Observation	An inadequacy in a system or process that is not a failure to comply with a standard. Observations obtained during an inspection or audit, are 'non-compliances' where action to be taken by the blood establishment is suggested.
Occurrence	An event or outcome contrary to the expected. The word 'occurrence' is often used to describe such events before they are further classified as errors, accidents, complaints, deviations, and the like.
Off-line experimentations	A method for determining the best configurations of processes. Usually uses a design of experiments (DOE) format such as the Taguchi method or Plackett-Burman experiments.
On-the-job training	Training that an employee receives at work during the normal work day.
Operating characteristic (OC) curve	An assessment of the probability of accepting a shipment, given the existing level of quality of the shipment.
Operating results	Measures that are important to monitoring and tracking the effectiveness of a company's operations.
Operating qualification	The demonstration that the system, using worst-case variables, will effectively and reproducibly result in products that meet performance specifications.
Operational auditing	Modern auditing practices that focus on operational efficiencies.
Operational system	A collection of related processes within the path of workflow.
Ordinal data	Ranked information
Organization	Group of people and facilities with an orderly arrangement of responsibilities, authorities and relationships - ISO 9000
Organizational design	The process of defining the best structure to meet company objectives.
Organizational learning	The sum of the changes in knowledge among the employees of a firm.
Organizational structure	Orderly arrangement of responsibilities, authorities and relationships between people - ISO 9000
Orthogonal arrays	Experimental design tools that ensure independence between iterations of an experiment.
Over-the-wall syndrome	Difficulties that arise when different types of engineers work in totally different departments in the same firm.

P –	
p chart or percent chart	A chart used to monitor proportion defective. A control chart that determines the stability of a process by finding what percentage of total units in a sample are defective.
Paper prototypes	A series of drawings that are developed by the designer on CAD systems and are reviewed by decision makers prior to acceptance.
Paradigm	A way of thinking about a given subject that defines how one views events, relationships, ideas, etc. within the boundaries of that subject.
Parallel processing in focused teams	Performing work simultaneously rather than sequentially.
Parameter design	Designing control factors such as product specifications and measurements for optimal product function.
Pareto analysis	An economic concept identified by Joseph Juran that argues that the majority of quality problems are caused by relatively few causes. This economic concept is called Pareto's law or the 80/20 rule. Juran dichotomized the population of causes of quality problems as the vital few and the trivial many.
Pareto chart	Chart used to identify and prioritize problems to be solved.
Pareto's Law (the 80/20 rule)	80 percent of the problems are a result of 20 percent of the causes.
Pareto principle	The idea that a few root problems are responsible for the large majority of consequences. The Pareto principle is derived from the work of Vilfredo Pareto, a turn-of-the-century Italian economist who studied the distributions of wealth in different countries. He concluded that a fairly consistent minority, about 20% of people, controlled the large majority, about 80% of a society's wealth. This same distribution has been observed in other areas and has been termed the Pareto principle. It is defined by J.M. Juran as the idea that 80% of all effects are produced by only 20% of the possible causes.
Partnering	An approach to selling in foreign markets that involves the collaborative effort of two organizations.
Passive data gathering	This occurs when the customer initiates the data gathering for a firm such as filling out a customer complaint card or sending an e-mail. The firm provides the mechanism for feedback, the customer must initiate the use of the mechanism.
Passively solicited customer feedback	A method of soliciting customer feedback that is left to the customer to initiate, such as filling out a restaurant complaint card or calling a toll-free complaint line.
Pay-for-learning programmes	Programmess that involve compensating employees for their knowledge and skills rather than singularly for the specific jobs they – perform
Perceived quality	A dimension of quality identified by David Garvin that refers to a subjective assessment of a product's quality based on criteria defined by the observer.
Performance	A dimension of quality that refers to the efficiency in which a product performs its intended purpose.

Quality Terminology. (Continued)

P –	
Performance benchmarking	A type of benchmarking that allows initiator firms to compare themselves against benchmark firms on performance issues such as cost structures, various types of productivity performance, speed of concept to market, and quality measures.
Performing	The fourth stage of team development, where a mutually supportive, steady state is achieved.
Physical environment	The geographic area that is in the proximity of an organization.
Pie chart	A chart that compares groups of data to the whole data set by showing each group as a "slice" of the entire "pie." Pie charts are particularly useful for investigating what percentage each group represents.
Plan-Do-Check-Act (PDCA) cycle	A process for improvement pioneered by W. E. Deming.
Policy	A definite action that is adopted for a purpose.
Policy deployment	Another name for hoshin planning.
Population	Total set of items from which a sample set is taken.
Precision	Reproducibility of the quantifiable outcomes of processes and procedures
Prevention costs	Costs associated with preventing defects and imperfections from occurring.
Preventive action	Action taken to prevent the recurrence of potential non-conformity, defect or other cause of error Action taken to eliminate the cause of a potential nonconformity or other potentially undesirable situation - ISO 9000
Preventive maintenance	Maintaining scheduled up-keep and improvement to equipment so equipment can actually improve with age.
Prioritization grid	A tool used to make decisions based on multiple criteria.
Procedure	Specific activity that forms the basic unit of a process Specified way to carry out an activity or a process - ISO 9000
Process	A series of steps or actions that lead to a desired result or output System of activities which uses resources to transform inputs into outputs - ISO 9000
Process benchmarking	A type of benchmarking that focuses on the observation of business processes including process flows, operating systems, process technologies, and the operation of target firms or departments
Process capability	1. A statistical measure indicating the inherent variation for a given event in a stable process, usually defined as the process width divided by 6 sigma. 2. Competence of the process, based on tested performance, to achieve certain results.
Process capability index	Measurement indicating the ability of a process to produce specified results. Cp and Cpk are two process capability indices.
Process charts	Tools for monitoring process stability.
Process control	Acrivities, measurements, techniques, etc., to keep operating processes in control to meet process goals

P –	
Process decision programme chart	A tool that is used to help brainstorm possible contingencies or problems associated with the implementation of some program or improvement.
Process description	A written document that describes how a particular process (e.g., a quality system essential) functions in a given facility.
Process improvement	The continuous challenge of a process using the results of internal/external assessments, patient/customer feedback and occurrence reports to improve performance.
Process improvement team	Teams that are involved in identifying opportunities for improving select processes in a firm.
Process performance qualification	Establishing confidence that equipment, reagents, and ancillary systems are capable of consistently operating within established limits and tolerances to establish that the process is effective and reproducible.
Producer's risk	The risk associated with rejecting a lot of material that has acceptable quality.
Product	Result or outcome of a process - ISO 9000 A tangible good that is produced for a customer.
Product-based	The context of Garvin's quality dimensions.
Product benchmarking	A type of benchmarking that firms employ when designing new products or upgrades to current products.
Product data management	A method for gathering and evaluating product-related data
Product design and evaluation	Activities that include the definition of the product architecture and the design, production, and testing of a system (including its subassemblies) for production.
Product design engineering	A form of engineering that involves activities associated with concept development, needs specification, final specification, and final design of a product.
Product idea generation	The process of generating product ideas from external and internal sources.
Product liability	The risk a manufacturer assumes when there is a chance that a consumer could be injured by the manufacturer's product.
Product marketing and distribution preparation	The process of developing the marketing-related activities associated with a product or service.
Product manufacture, delivery and use	Stages of the supply chain.
Product performance qualification	The comprehensive testing of performance attributes of product(s) resulting from a validation study.
Product traceability	The ability to trace a component part of a product back to its original manufacturer.
Productivity ratios	Ratios that are used in measuring the extent to which a firm effectively uses its resources.
Proficiency testing	Overall assessment of a laboratory's ability to perform certain processes, including equipment, personnel, reagents, etc.

Quality Terminology. (Continued)

P –	
Profound organizational learning	Quality-based learning that occurs as people discover the causes of errors, defects, and poor customer service in a firm.
Project	Unique process consisting of a set of coordinated and controlled activities with start and finish dates undertaken to achieve an objective conforming to specific requirements including the constraints of time, cost and resources - ISO 9000
Project charter	A document showing the purposes, participants, goals, and authorizations for a project.
Prototyping	An iterative approach to design in which a series of mock-ups or models are developed until the customer and the designer come to agreement as to the final design.
Pugh matrix	A method of concept selection used to identify conflicting requirements and to prioritize design tradeoff.
Purpose	A statement at the beginning of a procedure (SOP) that describes why the procedure exists.
Q –	
QAS	Quality assessment scheme
Qualification	Combination of personal attributes, minimum education, training, work and audit experience, and competencies possessed by an auditor - ISO 9000
Qualification process	Process to demonstrate the ability to fulfill specified requirements
Quality	Totality of characteristics of an entity that bear on its ability to satisfy stated and implied needs Ability of a set of inherent characteristics of a product, system or process to fulfill requirements of customers and other interested parties - ISO 9000
Quality assurance (QA)	The overall range of activities and systems that provide confidence within the organization and authorities that all quality requirements are met. Part of quality management focused on providing confidence that quality requirements are fulfilled - ISO 9000
Quality at the source	A method of process control whereby each worker is responsible for his or her own work and performs needed inspections at each stage of the process.
Quality audit	A systematic and independent examination to determine whether quality activities and related results comply with planned arrangement and whether these arrangement are implemented effectively and are suitable to achieve objectives.
Quality characteristic	Inherent characteristic of a product, process or system derived from requirement - ISO 9000
Quality circles	Brainstorming sessions involving employees of a firm whose goal is improving processes and process capability.

Q –	
Quality control (QC)	Checks put in place to ensure that processes, procedures and products meet the quality requirements Part of quality management focused on fulfilling quality requirements - ISO 9000
Quality Control/Assurance (QC/QA) Unit	One or more individuals designated by, and reporting directly to, management with defined authority and responsibility to assure that all quality assurance policies are carried out in the organization.
Quality Department	The identified and authorized department within an organization responsible for the overall development, organization and management of quality and quality systems
Quality dimensions	Aspects of quality that help to better define what quality is. These include perceived quality, conformance, reliability, durability, and so on.
Quality evaluation	Systematic examination of the extent to which an entity is capable of fulfilling specified requirements Progression in the principles of a quality system from inspection, quality control, quality assurance, total quality management
Quality function deployment (QFD)	QFD involves developing a matrix that includes customer preferences and product attributes. A QFD matrix allows a firm to quantitatively analyze the relationship between customer needs and design attributes.
Quality improvement	Part of quality management focused on increasing effectiveness and efficiency - ISO 9000
Quality improvement system	The result of the interactions between the various components that defines the quality policy in a firm.
Quality improvement team	A group of employees that take on a project to improve a given process or design a new process within an organization.
Quality function deployment (QFD)	A technique used to translate customer requirements into appropriate goals for each stage of product or service development and output. The two approaches to quality function deployment are known as the House of Quality and the Matrix of Matrices.
Quality loop or quality spiral	Conceptual model of interacting activities that influence quality at the various stages from identification of the needs to the assessment of satisfaction
Quality loss function (QLF)	An algebraic function that determines economic penalties that the customer incurs as a result of purchasing a nonconforming product.
Quality management	Coordinated activities to direct and control an organization with regard to quality - ISO 9000
Quality management analysis (QMA)	A study in which a firm's level of maturity relating to quality practices is assessed.
Quality management system	System to establish a quality policy and quality objectives and to achieve those objectives - ISO 9000
Quality Manager	The appointed, responsible and authorized individual within an organization with the responsibility for developing and managing the quality system
Quality Manual	Document specifying the quality management system of an organization - ISO 9000

Quality Terminology. (Continued)

Q –	
Quality measures	Ratios that are used to measure a firm's performance in the area of quality management.
Quality objective	Something sought, or aimed for, related to quality - ISO 9000
Quality Officer	An individual who works within the quality department of an organization and who is primarily concerned with the day-to-day operation and running of the quality system
Quality plan	Document specifying the quality management system elements and the resources to be applied in a specific case - ISO 9000
Quality planning	Part of quality management focused on setting quality objectives and specifying necessary operational processes and related resources to fulfill the quality objectives - ISO 9000
Quality policy	Overall intentions and direction of an organization related to quality as expressed by top management - ISO 9000
Quality programme	The combination of quality systems and the design to accomplish the overall quality objectives in an organization.
Quality requirement	Requirement for inherent characteristics of a product, process or system - ISO 9000
Quality system	Organizational structure, procedures, processes, and resources needed to implement quality requirements
Quality system essentials (QSE)	Processes within a quality system that are necessary ro ensure the quality of the finished products/services.
Quarantine	Non-authorization to proceed to next stage of a process until specified standards / conditions are met
R –	
R chart or range chart	A variables chart that monitors the dispersion of a process.
Random variation	Variation that is uncontrollable
Reactive customer-driven quality (RCDQ)	A state that is characterized by a supplier "reacting" to the quality expectations of a customer rather than proactively anticipating customer needs and expectations
Readiness	Used in a leadership context, the term refers to the extent to which a follower has the ability and willingness to accomplish a specific task.
Ready-fire-aim	A method that focuses on getting new technology to market and then determining how to sell the products.
Recall procedures	Steps for taking defective products from market.
Record	Document stating results achieved or providing evidence of activities performed - ISO 9000
Redundancy	A technique for avoiding failure by putting backup systems in place that can take over if a primary system fails. For example, many redundant systems are used on the space shuttle to protect the crew if a primary system fails.
Re-engineering	(1) A method for making rapid, radical changes to a company's organization and processes; (2) Taking apart a competitor's products to see how they are designed and then designing similar products.

R –	
Registration	A formal process by which any facility that prepares components from whole blood (other than red cells by centrifugation or separation) or modifies blood components (by washing, irradiation, leukocyte reduction by methods other than bedside filtration) receives a facility registration number that is different from the licensing number. Registered and licensed establishments are inspected by a competent authority (e.g., Health or Pharmaceutical Inspectorate)
Re-grade	Alteration of the grade of a nonconforming product in order to make it conform to requirements.- ISO 9000
Regression analysis	A statistical technique used to determine the best mathematical expression to describe the relationship between a response and independent variables.
Relationship management	A method for developing long-term associations with customers.
Release	Authorization to proceed to next stage of a process - ISO 9000
Reliability	Propensity for failure of a product or component
Repair	Action taken on a non-conforming product to make it conform to the requirements
Replications	Number of runs of an experiment
Requirement	Expression of need as defined quantitative or qualitative requirements Need or expectation that is stated, customarily implied or obligatory - ISO 9000
Responsible person	An individual formally designated as being responsible for the quality of defined operations or outcomes within an organization
Responsiveness	A dimension of service quality that refers to the willingness of the service provider to be helpful and prompt in providing service.
Retrospective validation	Validation for a product already in distribution based upon accumulated production, testing and control data.
Revalidation	Validation that is required when there are 1) changes in packaging, formulation, supplies, equipment, or processes that could impaxt on product effectiveness or characteristics; or 2) change in product characteristics. The extend of the revalidation will depend upon the nature of the changes and how they affect different aspects of production that they have previously been validated for.
Reverse engineering	The process of dismantling a competitor's products to understand the strengths and weaknesses of the designs
Review	Activity undertaken to ensure the suitability, adequacy, effectiveness and efficiency of the subject matter to achieve established objectives - ISO 9000
Rework	Action on a nonconforming product to make it conform to the requirement.
Risk assessment	Method to assess and characterise the critical parameters in the functionality of an equipment, system or process
Robust	The ability of a product or service to function appropriately regardless of external conditions and other uncontrollable factors.

Quality Terminology. (Continued)

R –	
Robust design	Designing such that an increase in variability will not result in defective products.
Run chart	Also known as a line chart, or line graph. A chart that plots data over time, allowing you to identify trends and anomalies.
S –	
Sample	A part representing a whole.
Sample standard deviation chart (s chart)	Control chart in which the standard deviation of the subgroup is tracked to determine the variation within a process over time. Sample standard deviation charts are usually paired with average charts for complete analysis.
Sampling plan	A determination of how data are to be gathered and evaluated.
Scatter diagram or plot	A scatter plot used to examine the relationships between variables.
Scope	A statement of all areas to which a policy, process or procedure is applicable
Scrap	Action on a nonconforming product to preclude its originally intended use – ISO 9000
Selection	The process of evaluating and choosing the best qualified candidate for a particular job
Self-assessment	The ongoing evaluation of process and quality indicator data within an organization to determine if processes are in control.
Self-directed work team	Work teams that have a considerable degree of autonomy.
Self-direction	A term that refers to providing autonomy to employees (or other recipients of training) in terms of facilitating their own training needs.
Sequential or departmental approach to design	An approach to design that requires product designers, marketers, process designers, and production managers to work through organizational lines of authority to perform work.
Serious adverse event	Any untoward occurrence associated with the collection, testing, processing, storage and distribution, of blood and blood components that might lead to death or life-threatening, disabling or incapacitating conditions for patients or which results in, or prolongs, hospitalisation or morbidity.
Serious adverse reaction	An unintended response in donor or in patient associated with the collection or transfusion of blood or blood components that is fatal, life threatening, disabling, incapacitating, or which results in, or prolongs, hospitalisation or morbidity.
Service	Intangible product that is the result of at least one activity performed at the interface between the supplier and customer - ISO 9000
Services blueprinting	A chart that depicts service processes and potential fail points in a process.
Service reliability	A dimension of service quality that refers to the ability of the service provider to perform the promised service dependably and accurately.
Serviceability	A dimension of quality that refers to a product's ease of repair

S –	
SERVQUAL	A survey instrument designed to assess service quality along five specific dimensions consisting of tangibles, reliability, responsiveness, assurance, and empathy.
Seven tools of quality	Quality improvement tools that include the histogram, Pareto chart, check sheet, control chart, cause-and-effect diagram, flowchart, and scatter diagram.
Shewhart cycle	Another name for the Plan-Do-Check-Act cycle. It is also sometimes called the Deming cycle.
Shitsuku	A term that refers to the discipline required to maintain the changes that have been made in a workplace.
Signal factors	Factors in a Taguchi experiment that are not under control of the operator. Examples include small variations in ambient temperature and variability in material dimensions.
Situational leadership model	A model of leadership proposed by Hersey and Blanchard that clarifies the interrelation between employee preparedness and effectiveness in leadership.
Societal environment	The portion of a firm's environment pertaining to cultural factors such as language, business customs, customer preferences, and patterns of communication.
Soft data	Data that cannot be measured or specifically quantified, such as survey data that asks respondents to provide their "opinion" about something.
Software	Intellectual product consisting of information on a support medium - ISO 9000
Sole-source filters	External validation measures of quality programs such as the Baldrige criteria and ISO 9000.
Sole sourcing	Using only one supplier for a single component.
SOP	Standard operating procedure
Special causes	Causes of variation in a process that are not inherent in the process itself but originate from circumstances that are out of the ordinary. Special causes are indicated by points that fall outside the limits of a control chart.
Specification	Document stating requirements - ISO 9000
Specification limit	An engineering or design requirement that must be met in order to produce a satisfactory product.
Stability	The likelihood a process will be random
Standard	Minimum level required
Standard operating procedure	Written instructions for the performance of a specific procedure
Statistical Process Control (SPC)	A technique that is concerned with monitoring process capability and process stability.
Statistical Quality Control (SQC)	Analysis and control of quality through the use of statistical techniques, essentially the same as SPC.
Statistical thinking	Deming's concept relating to data-based decision making.
Storming	The second stage of team development, in which the team begins to get to know each other but agreements have not been made to facilitate smooth interaction among team members.

Quality Terminology. (Continued)

S –	
Strategic benchmarking	A type of benchmarking that involves observing how others compete. This type of benchmarking typically involves target firms that have been identified as "world class."
Strategic partnership	An association between two firms by which they agree to work together to achieve a strategic goal. This is often associated with long-term supplier-customer relationships.
Strategy	(1) The art of planning military operations; (2) What a firm does; (3) A firm's long-term plan for attaining objectives.
Stretch target	A challenging goal or objective requiring significant effort to achieve.
Structural measures	Measures that include objectives, policies, and procedures that are followed by a firm.
Structural variation	Variation caused by recurring system-wide changes such as seasonal changes or long-term trends.
Superordinate goals	Goals that transcend individual needs to reflect group objectives.
Supplier	Organization or person that provides a product - ISO 9000
Supplier audit	The auditing portion of supplier development programmes.
Supplier certification or qualification programmes	Programmes designed to certify suppliers as acceptable for a particular customer.
Supplier development programmes	Training and development programmes provided by firms to their suppliers.
Supplier evaluation	A tool used by many firms to differentiate and discriminate among suppliers. Supplier evaluations often involve report cards where potential suppliers are rated based on different criteria such as quality, technical capability, or ability to meet schedule demands.
Supplier partnering	A term used to characterized the relationship between suppliers and customers when a high degree of linkages and interdependencies exist.
Supplier qualification	Acrivities designed to assure that materials or services obtained from a supplier peform as expected in a given process.
Supply chain	A network of facilities that procures raw materials, transforms them into intermediate subassemblies and final products, and then delivers the products to customers through a distribution system.
Surveying	Generating a list of strengths and weaknesses in a firm in generic internal assessment.
System	Set of interrelated or interacting elements - ISO 9000
System checks	Quality indicators used to determine if operational activities are in control.
System reliability	The probability that components in a system will perform their intended function over a specified period of time.
Systems review	A management viewpoint that focuses on the interactions between the various components (i.e., people, policies, machines, processes, and products) that combine to produce a product or service. The systems view focuses management on the system as the cause of quality problems.

T –	
Tampering	Dr. Deming cautions against tampering with systems that are "in control." It is very common for management to react to variation which is in fact normal, thereby starting wild goose chases after sources of problems which don't exist. Tampering with stable processes actually increases variation.
Tangibles	A dimension of service quality that refers to the physical appearance of the service facility, the equipment, the personnel, and the communications material.
Target firm or organization	The firm that is being studied or benchmarked against.
Task environment	The portion of a firm's environment pertaining to structural issues such as the skill levels of employees, remuneration policies, technology, and the nature of government agencies.
Task needs assessment	The process of assessing the skills that are needed within a firm.
Team	A group of individuals working to achieve a goal with activities requiring close coordination.
Team building	A term that describes the process of identifying roles for team members and helping the team members succeed in their roles.
Teamware	Computer software that is used in making group decisions
Technical expert	Person who provides specific knowledge or expertise with respect to a particular subject field to be audited - ISO 9000:2000
Technology feasibility statement	A feasibility statement used in the design process to assess a variety of issues such as necessary parameters for performance, manufacturing imperatives, limitations in the physics of materials, and conditions for quality testing the product.
Technology selection for product development	The process of selecting materials and technologies that provide the best performance for the customer at an acceptable cost.
Test	Technical operation that consists of the determination of one or more characteristic of a given product, process or service according to a specified procedure - ISO 9000
Third party/subcontractor	Any organisation that provides a service to a procurement organisation or a Blood Establishment on the basis of a contract or written agreement. Includes donor or blood testing laboratories, contract sterilisers and user hospitals which store blood components pending human application.
360-degree evaluation	A method for evaluating performance with input from supervisors, peers, and employees.
Three spheres of quality	Quality management, assurance, and control
Three T's	The task, treatment, and tangibles in service design.
Tiger teams	Teams with a specific defined goal and a short time frame to attain the goal.

Quality Terminology. (Continued)

T –	
Time keeper	Team member who keeps track of time spent on each agenda item during team meetings. This job can easily be rotated among team members.
Tolerance design	The act of determining the amount of allowable variability around parameters.
Top management	Person or group of people who direct and control an organization at the highest level - ISO 9000
Total Quality Human Resource Management (TQHRM)	An approach to human resources management that involves many of the concepts of quality management. The primary purpose of this approach is to provide employees a supportive and empowered work environment.
Total Quality Management	Management approach of an organization centered on quality based on the participation of all its members and aiming at long term success through customers satisfaction, and benefits to all members of the organization and to society
Traceability	Ability to trace the history, application or location of that which is under consideration - ISO 9000
Trace-back	Process of investigating a report of a suspected transfusion-associated adverse reaction in a recipient in order to identify a potentially implicated donor.
Training needs analysis	The process of identifying organizational needs in terms of capabilities, task needs assessment in terms of skill sets that are needed within the firm, and individual needs analysis to determine how employee skills fit with company needs.
Training needs assessment	A process for gathering organizational data relative to finding areas where training is most needed.
Training programme design	A term that describes the process of tailoring a course or set of courses to meet the needs of a company.
Trait dimension	A view of leadership that states that leadership potential is related to the "traits" of an individual, such as height.
Transcendent	A definition of quality that states that quality is something we all recognize but we cannot verbally define.
Tree diagram	A chart used to break any task, goal, or category into increasingly detailed levels of information. Family trees are the classic example of a tree diagram. In PathMaker, the structure of the tree diagram is identical to that of the cause & effect diagram.
Trend	A movement or process output data in a specific direction, the general movement over a period of time of some statistical progressive change.
Type I error	Rejecting something that is acceptable. Also known as an alpha error.
Type II error	Accepting something that should have been rejected. Also known as beta error.
U –	
u chart	A chart used to monitor the number of defects in sequential production lots.

U –	
Underdeveloped events	A term used in fault tree analysis. Undeveloped events are faults that do not have a significant consequence or are not expanded because there is not sufficient information available.
User-based	A definition of service or product quality that is customer centered.
V –	
Validation	Confirmation and provision of objective evidence that the requirements for a specific intended use or application have been fulfilled - ISO 9000:2000
Validation protocol	A written plan stating how validation will be conducted, including test parameters, product characteristics, production equipment, and decision points on what constitutes acceptable results.
Value added	Each time work is done to inputs to transform them into something of greater usefulness as an end product.
Value-based	A definition of quality relating to the social benefit from a product or service.
Value chain	A tool, developed by Michael Porter, that decomposes a firm into its core activities.
Value chain activities	Porter's chain of activities, including inbound logistics, production, and outbound logistics.
Value system	A network of value chains.
Variable	A measurement.
Variables data	Data that is measured on a continuous and infinite scale such as temperature, distance, and pressure rather than in discreet units or yes/no options. Variables data is used to create histograms, some control charts, and sometimes run charts.
Variance	A measure of deviation from the mean in a sample or population.
Variety	The range of product and service choices offered to customers
Variation	Change in the output or result of a process. Variation can be caused by common causes, special causes, tampering, or structural variation.
Verification	Confirmation and provision of objective evidence that specified requirements have been fulfilled - ISO 9000:2000
Vertical deployment	A term denoting that all of the levels of the management of a firm are involved in the firm's quality efforts.
Virtual teams	Teams that do not physically meet but are linked together through intranets and the Internet.
Vision	Often incorporated into an organizational mission (or vision) statement to clarify what the organization hopes to be doing at some point in the future. The vision should act as a guide in choosing courses of action for the organization.
Voice of the customer	A term that refers to the wants, opinions, perceptions, and desires of the customer.
W –	
Whack-a-mole	A novel term that describes the process of solving a problem only to have another problem surface.
Work environment	Set of conditions under which a person operates - ISO 9000
Working prototype	A functioning mock-up or model of a product.

Quality Terminology. (Continued)

W –	
Worse case	A set of conditions encompassing upper and lower processing limits and circumstances, including those within standard operating procedures, which poise the greatest chance of process and product failure when compared to ideal conditions. Such conditions do not necessarily induce process or product failure. Note: This definition applies to conditions needing to be evaluated, as applicable, in process validation.
X –	
X chart	A chart used to monitor the mean of a process for population values
$\bar{\bar{x}}$ chart	A chart that monitors the mean of a process for variables
Y –	
Z –	
Zero defects	Philip Crosby's recommended performance standard that leaves no doubt regarding the goal of total quality. Crosby's theory holds that people can continually move closer to this goal by committing themselves to their work and the improvement process.

Annex 4 – Human Development Index (HDI) Ranking

HDI ranking (http://hdr.undp.org/en/media/HDR_2011_EN_Tables.pdf).

Index

B

C

D

E

F

Q

R